# Global Perspectives on Reproductive Rights and Policies

Maja Pucelj
*EMUNI University, Slovenia*

Magdalena Matusiak-Frączczak
*University of Łódź, Poland*

IGI Global
Scientific Publishing
Publishing Tomorrow's Research Today

Published in the United States of America by
IGI Global
701 E. Chocolate Avenue
Hershey PA, USA 17033
Tel: 717-533-8845
Fax: 717-533-8661
E-mail: cust@igi-global.com
Web site: https://www.igi-global.com



Library of Congress Cataloging-in-Publication Data

CIP Pending
ISBN: 979-8-3693-7837-3
EISBN: 9798-3-693-7839-7

Vice President of Editorial: Melissa Wagner
Managing Editor of Acquisitions: Mikaela Felty
Managing Editor of Book Development: Jocelynn Hessler
Production Manager: Mike Brehm
Cover Design: Phillip Shickler

British Cataloguing in Publication Data
A Cataloguing in Publication record for this book is available from the British Library.

# Table of Contents

# Detailed Table of Contents



Following the landmark Supreme Court decision to overturn Roe v. Wade in the Dobbs v. Jackson Women's Health Organization case of 2022, the United States has witnessed a surge in state-level abortion bans. This paper employs Carol Bacchi’s “What’s the problem represented to be?” approach to policy analysis to scrutinize and compare problem representations in the context of these abortion bans and the broader realm of human rights. Through a critical lens, we explore the contrasting problem representations: “violations of the rights of unborn children” in abortion bans versus “violations of women’s equal rights” in human rights discourse. Although these representations appear contradictory, feminist theory reveals nuanced inequalities perpetuated by both. This paper emphasizes that the current frameworks surrounding abortion do not provide women with equal access to their rights. Thus, it calls for a more comprehensive and equitable approach to address the complexities of reproductive autonomy post-Roe v. Wade.

There has been a long-running debate between the fetal rights and reproductive rights of women surrounding the topic of abortion. The world is divided into the groups of pro-life and pro-choice. Amid this debate, India, despite having an issue of female infanticide due to its social history and structure, has proactively taken a stand through legislation and adjudication for the 'reproductive rights of women.' The commendable efforts in Indian jurisdiction through the 2021 Amendment to the 'Medical Termination Act, 1971' along with its few limitations and the recent developments by the Supreme Court of India, have been examined in this chapter.



Discussion on reproductive health became prominent in the second half of the 20th century. The Declaration of the universality of human rights energized a right-based approach to reproductive health. Many women realized that without reproductive rights the questions on their dignity, equality, liberty, and life would become meaningless. This right-based approach got momentum in USA and extended to other countries, including India. But both these countries did not consider right to abortion as an absolute right. In India, the enactment of Medical Termination of Pregnancy Act, 1971 considered it as a limited right. The US judiciary in its Roe judgment in 1973 considered it under right to privacy in the ambit of right to liberty but only as a limited right. However, this judgment was overruled by the Dobbs judgment in 2022. In this context, this chapter attempts to compare the perspectives of both USA and India on reproductive health.

This chapter provides a comprehensive analysis of the legal frameworks governing reproductive rights and policies, covering their historical evolution, international and regional contexts and national implementations. It examines key international treaties including CEDAW, ICESCR and the Sustainable Development Goals, and their influence on global reproductive health policies. It also explores regional legal frameworks in Europe, Africa and the Americas, and their impact on national laws. A comparative analysis of national approaches highlights variations in legal traditions and effectiveness in safeguarding reproductive rights. The chapter also addresses key issues in reproductive health like contraception, maternal health, abortion laws and assisted reproductive technologies (ART), assessing legal status, barriers and successful interventions. The chapter underscores the critical role of legal frameworks in ensuring access to reproductive health services and protecting individual rights.



"The more law the less justice."- Marcus Tullius Cicero The reproductive challenges are very common now a days in a modern world particularly in the urban inhabitants of an Indian society and almost in every western cultures globally and due to stereotype society adult humans aren't aware of their reproductive rights and duties and they have to knock the doors of the courts despite of numerous legislations and reproductive case precedents of abortion, Assisted Reproductive technology, Surrogacy challenges in their respective legislations. The reproductive challenges are mainly due to infertility issues, unsafe abortion, lack of awareness in STD's (sexually transmitted diseases), HIV, forced pregnancies etc. The authors in this chapter will explore about surrogacy and abortion laws as a solution to the reproductive challenges and proposes an effective remedy for the dispute's settlement mechanism.

The critics argue that commercial surrogacy would result in commodification of pregnancy, exploitation of economically vulnerable women in the lower social strata and ultimately leads to depersonalised reproduction process. However, the advocates of commercial surrogacy contend that commercial surrogacy provides financial stability to the surrogate mother and is a boon for those infertile parents who want to safeguard their privacy and are reluctant to involve their family members or relatives as surrogate mothers. This research study aims to explore and analyse compensation models in commercial surrogacy arrangements across different jurisdictions in the context of ensuring equitable treatment and protection of human rights of surrogate mothers. In meticulous detail, this study examines the ethical, legal, cultural and economic dimensions, particularly regarding the compensation offered to surrogate mothers for their labour.



Reproductive health and rights encompass a broad range of issues, including family planning, maternal health, sexual health education, and access to safe and legal abortion. While these areas are often viewed through a lens that primarily considers women's roles and responsibilities, the involvement of men is equally crucial. Lack of male engagement in reproductive health perpetuates gender inequality. By reinforcing the notion that reproductive health is solely a woman's domain, societal norms continue to marginalize women and restrict their autonomy. This not only affects women's health and well-being but also impedes progress towards achieving gender equality and empowering women in India.

# Preface

Today's society is striving to intensify the debate on reproductive rights in connection with their restriction. With the aim to critically assess that debate, we prepared a monograph, titled *Global Perspectives on Reproductive Rights and Policies*. This edited volume aims to act as a crucial resource for understanding and addressing the crucial challenges, which evolve around reproductive rights in today's complex social and political landscapes.

If we want to engage in the discussion about such intensive interventions in human rights, we need to research and debate and ensure that we bring together knowledge from different disciplines — including law, medicine, politics and ethics. With the aforementioned act, we aim to equip our readers with the comprehensive insights they need to tackle pressing issues such as abortion legislation, in vitro fertilization policy and the influence of non-state actors. The evidence presented in this book goes beyond mere academic engagement; it is an indispensable tool for advocacy and informed decision-making. By examining legal frameworks and ethical dilemmas in different cultural contexts, we provide a deeper understanding of how reproductive rights are shaped and contested around the world. This research is critical for professionals, researchers, students and policy makers who want to engage in meaningful dialogue and bring about change.

This volume is particularly concerned with the urgent need for informed debate on contentious issues such as abortion and reproductive technologies. The research included here illuminates the ethical considerations and social consequences of these issues and offers practical guidance for resolving conflicts between competing rights. By presenting case studies and comparative analysis, we aim to promote understanding of the different perspectives that influence reproductive rights and enable readers to engage effectively in their own contexts.

We encourage reader to consider the critical role of research and adequate discussion in promoting reproductive rights and shaping policies that respect and uphold human dignity. We believe that through in-depth research, we can address the challenges of current debates on reproductive rights and pave the way for a more equitable future. This discussion should surpass discussion without considering the impact of such invasion on women's rights.

We are grateful to the authors whose expertise and insights have shaped this work, and we invite our readers to join us in this important conversation. Together, through informed research and advocacy, we can champion reproductive rights as a fundamental aspect of human rights.

To begin this exploration of Global Perspectives on Reproductive Rights and Policies, we present a detailed overview of each chapter, which together illuminate pressing reproductive rights challenges and opportunities in a variety of contexts.

Chapter 1, "Whose Rights Prevail? Exploring Problem Representations in Post-Roe v. Wade Abortion Policies," examines the post-Roe v. Wade landscape in the United States, specifically the rise of state-level abortion bans following the Supreme Court's 2022 decision. Utilizing Carol Bacchi's analytical framework, this chapter critically compares the opposing representations of rights—those of unborn children versus women's equal rights—highlighting the nuances of feminist theory. The authors call for a more equitable approach to reproductive autonomy that transcends the current divisive narratives.

Chapter 2, "Polish Abortion Ruling (2020) From the Perspective of International Law: Some Critical Remarks on Methodology and Reasoning," critiques the controversial ruling by the Polish Constitutional Tribunal, questioning its legal validity and methodological integrity. The analysis reveals significant flaws in judicial reasoning and the use of international law, shedding light on the broader implications for the relationship between legislative bodies and constitutional courts. This chapter serves as a cautionary tale about the importance of sound legal practices in safeguarding reproductive rights.

Chapter 3, "Revisiting the Paradigm of Abortion-Related Reproductive Health Laws in the European Union," offers a comprehensive examination of abortion laws across EU member states, juxtaposing liberal frameworks with more restrictive approaches. By analyzing historical developments and socio-economic factors influencing access to abortion, this chapter emphasizes the complexities inherent in reproductive health laws and the vital role of judicial interventions.

Chapter 4, "Reproductive Rights as a Human Rights Challenge With Special Focus on Abortion: Insights From Poland and Slovenia," focuses on the contested nature of women's right to abortion in light of recent judicial decisions in Poland and Slovenia. The chapter explores the resulting social movements and legal frameworks, assessing the current status of women's reproductive rights and their implications for global human rights discourse.

Chapter 5, "Abortion and Women: Intersects of Religion, Law, and Society – A Perspective From Muslim Majority Countries," delves into the intricate dynamics surrounding abortion in Muslim-majority countries. This chapter explores the historical evolution, legal landscapes, and ethical perspectives that shape societal attitudes towards abortion, ultimately examining their impact on women's rights and health.

Chapter 6, "Contours of Choice: Interpreting the Medical Termination of Pregnancy Act 1971 in the Context of Women's Rights," analyzes India's *Medical Termination of Pregnancy Act, 1971*, highlighting the ongoing debate between fetal rights and women's reproductive rights. The chapter discusses legislative amendments and recent Supreme Court rulings, showcasing India's proactive stance on reproductive rights amid its complex social realities.

Chapter 7, "Right-Based Approach to Reproductive Autonomy: A Comparative Study Between Indian and US Judiciaries," presents a comparative study of reproductive health perspectives in the United States and India. By examining how each country addresses reproductive rights, particularly abortion, this chapter highlights the limitations of current legal frameworks while advocating for a more expansive understanding of reproductive autonomy.

Chapter 8, "Legal Frameworks Governing Reproductive Rights and Policies," provides a thorough analysis of the historical and contemporary legal frameworks affecting reproductive rights globally. The chapter discusses key international treaties and regional approaches, emphasizing the critical role of law in ensuring access to reproductive health services.

Chapter 9, "Reproductive Challenges and Rights of Surrogates: A Mixed Methods Study From Indian Urban Inhabitants," explores the multifaceted reproductive challenges faced by urban Indian populations, particularly concerning surrogacy and abortion laws. The authors advocate for increased awareness of reproductive rights and propose effective dispute resolution mechanisms to address ongoing challenges.

Chapter 10, "Navigating Human Rights and Ethical Challenges in Compensation Models of Commercial Surrogacy: Comparative Analysis," critically examines compensation models in commercial surrogacy arrangements, considering the ethical and legal implications of these practices. The chapter seeks to balance the interests of surrogate mothers with the need for equitable treatment, underscoring the complexities of commodification in reproductive health.

Chapter 11, "Men's Role in Reproductive Health and Rights: Understanding the Involvement and Impact of Men in the Reproductive Health Decisions of Women in India," emphasizes the importance of male involvement in reproductive health decisions. By addressing societal norms that marginalize men's roles, this chapter advocates for a more inclusive approach that promotes gender equality and empowers women.

Chapter 12, "Complexities of Assisted Reproductive Technology: Exploring Legal Framework, Ethical Debate, and Religious Beliefs," investigates the legal, ethical, and religious debates surrounding Assisted Reproductive Technologies (ART).

This chapter highlights the advancements and controversies within ART, calling for ongoing dialogue to navigate the challenges posed by rapid technological changes.

Chapter 13, "Human Genome and Embryo Editing: Featuring Global Standards for Ethical, Legal, and Social Issues," explores the ethical and legal dimensions of genome and embryo editing technologies. This chapter stresses the need for global standards that prioritize reproductive justice and equity, addressing the potential for these technologies to deepen existing inequalities.

Together, these chapters contribute to a richer understanding of reproductive rights and policies worldwide. As we delve into these critical issues, we invite our readers to engage deeply with the complexities of reproductive autonomy and the imperative for informed advocacy.

As we conclude this preface to *Global Perspectives on Reproductive Rights and Policies*, we are reminded of the vital importance of the discussions presented within these pages. The challenges surrounding reproductive rights are not just legal or political; they are profoundly human, affecting individuals and communities in deeply personal ways. Each chapter serves as a testament to the complex interplay of law, ethics, and social values that shape reproductive policies worldwide.

Our collective commitment to informed research and advocacy is more crucial than ever. The insights offered here provide not only a thorough analysis of existing frameworks and practices but also illuminate paths toward equitable solutions. By understanding the nuances of reproductive rights across different cultural contexts, we empower ourselves and our readers to engage in meaningful dialogue and drive positive change.

This book stands as a resource for legal professionals, policymakers, scholars, and advocates alike, offering evidence-based insights and practical guidance. We hope it inspires a renewed commitment to the principles of justice and equity in reproductive health. Together, through collaboration and rigorous inquiry, we can champion reproductive rights as an essential facet of human rights, fostering a future where all individuals can exercise their autonomy and make informed choices about their reproductive lives.

We extend our heartfelt gratitude to the contributors for their invaluable work and to our readers for their engagement with these critical issues. May this volume inspire action, reflection, and ongoing dialogue about the importance of preserving women's rights as we collectively navigate the complexities of reproductive rights in our diverse global landscape.

**Maja Pucelj**
*EMUNI University, Slovenia*

**Magdalena Matusiak-Fracczak**

*University of Lódz, Poland*

# Chapter 1
# Whose Rights Prevail?
## Exploring Problem Representations in Post-Roe v. Wade Abortion Policies

**Akash Bag**
https://orcid.org/0000-0001-8820-171X
*Adamas University, Kolkata, India*

**Anwesha Ghosh**
https://orcid.org/0000-0003-4167-2121
*Amity Law School, Amity University, Kolkata, India*

**Tejaswini Tripathy**
https://orcid.org/0009-0000-5672-2377
*National Law University, Odisha, India*

## ABSTRACT

*Following the landmark Supreme Court decision to overturn Roe v. Wade in the Dobbs v. Jackson Women's Health Organization case of 2022, the United States has witnessed a surge in state-level abortion bans. This paper employs Carol Bacchi's "What's the problem represented to be?" approach to policy analysis to scrutinize and compare problem representations in the context of these abortion bans and the broader realm of human rights. Through a critical lens, we explore the contrasting problem representations: "violations of the rights of unborn children" in abortion bans versus "violations of women's equal rights" in human rights discourse. Although these representations appear contradictory, feminist theory reveals nuanced inequalities perpetuated by both. This paper emphasizes that the current frameworks surrounding abortion do not provide women with equal access to their rights. Thus, it calls for a more comprehensive and equitable approach to address*

DOI: 10.4018/979-8-3693-7837-3.ch001

*the complexities of reproductive autonomy post-Roe v. Wade.*

## INTRODUCTION

The controversial topic of abortion, which falls under the category of sexual and reproductive health and rights, is still hotly debated worldwide. Concerning figures highlight how serious this discussion is: 41% of women globally struggle with various restrictive abortion laws, while 28% of women live in nations where abortion is either completely outlawed or only allowed in extreme cases ("*The world's abortion laws*" 2023). According to the World Health Organization (WHO), 23,000 women lose their lives each year as a result of unsafe abortion procedures, and a startling 700 million women of reproductive age do not have access to safe and legal abortion services ("*The world's abortion laws*" 2023). Numerous international organizations and courts have firmly acknowledged the relevance of access to safe abortion as a fundamental human right (Jain, 2023). In this sense, the right to abortion is inextricably linked to the rights to autonomy and privacy, liberty and security of person, equality and non-discrimination, equal protection under the law, health, and life, and freedom from torture and other cruel treatment, as well as the right to reap the rewards of scientific advancement. The Committee on the Elimination of Discrimination Against Women (CEDAW) and the Human Rights Committee have solidified this complex viewpoint of abortion's place within the framework of human rights (Erdman, 2017; Rebouché, 2016; Pizzarossa & Skuster, 2021).

Notably, two crucial international instruments explicitly recognize abortion as a right, namely the CEDAW which is included in Article 12, and the ICCPR is illustrated in the general comment no. 36 (2018) of Article 6. These legal grounds emphasize the significance of abortion in the context of human rights, which does not conform to the boundaries of countries and cultures, necessitating reflection and analysis. A review of the abortion law: the right to an abortion under certain circumstances is also a way of protecting women's rights. Interestingly, this includes the right to an abortion in rape or incest cases. This particular feature has been safeguarded by court rulings, including those made by the Committee on the Elimination of Discrimination Against Women in the *L.C. v. Peru* (Ngwena, 2013) and the Human Rights Committee in the *V.D.A. case*, where it represented *LMR v. Argentina* (Fine et al., 2017). Now that we are back in the United States, abortion is the main topic of this investigation. It has led to an extensive and complex discussion that has fluctuated over time. But in 1973, a turning point was reached when the Supreme Court rendered a historic ruling in *Roe v. Wade*, which essentially made abortion a constitutionally protected right across the country (Kaufman et al., 2022). When we fast-forward to 2022, we experience the effects of change. By rejecting the *Roe v. Wade* precedent, the Supreme Court's decision in the *Dobbs v. Jackson Women's Health Organization* case heralded a seismic shift. This historic ruling made it possible for states to prohibit abortion, allowing for limitations on a right that had previously been acknowledged.

Examining the country more closely shows that 44 of the 50 states that make up the United States have some abortion prohibition in place. Of them, thirteen states have outlawed abortion completely, and thirteen more have only allowed it up until the moment of fetal viability. Given the complexity and diversity of the abortion issue in the United States, it is critical to acknowledge the various points of view that are engaged. In the interest of clarity and analytical rigor, this paper will refer to these viewpoints as the "*pro-life movement*" and the "*pro-choice movement*." An estimated 25 million unsafe abortions are performed each year, and these dangerous procedures are thought to be responsible for 7.9% of maternal deaths ("Information series: Sexual and Reproductive Health and Rights", 2020). It is important to remember that the most vulnerable populations impacted by this problem are people with low incomes and members of marginalized and disadvantaged communities. A startling fact becomes apparent: almost all deaths caused by unsafe abortions occur in nations where access to abortion services is restricted by law or practice (Ganatra et al., 2017; Starrs et al., 2018). A startling 287,000 women died either during or after pregnancy and childbirth in 2020 (Yamin, 2023). This alarming figure highlights the enormous risks connected to pregnancy and unsafe abortions. As a result, it becomes clear that women's access to abortions is a fundamental human right that must be protected. This right is intrinsically linked to other human rights, especially the rights to health and life (Fine et al., 2017). When the U.S. Supreme Court ruled against the long-standing protection of abortion rights established by the *Roe v. Wade* decision in the case of *Dobbs v. Jackson Women's Health Organization* in June 2022, the landscape of abortion rights in the United States underwent a seismic shift. Several states nationwide passed numerous restrictive legislation due to this historic time (Chen et al., 2023).

States, including Alabama, Texas, Arkansas, Louisiana, and Tennessee, passed some of the strictest laws (Sherman et al., 2024). Except for rape or incest instances, these states outlawed abortions outright from the moment of conception, albeit they did make an exemption for circumstances in which a woman's life was in danger. The impact of these strict prohibitions on women's rights, particularly their sexual and reproductive rights—which are recognized as essential elements of human rights—has provoked heated discussions and divisive disagreements ("*Human rights crisis*", 2023). However, as Berer (2023) stated, CEDAW has urged the United States to guarantee women's rights to safe and legal abortion and align them with the Women's Rights Convention. The influence of the current state of abortion rights can be seen to be very crucial in the present global dimensions, which are much more than the American borders (Kaufman et al., 2022). Some of the questions that have been raised include whether abortion prohibitions are a violation of the rights of individuals or not that has been raised in some of the discussions. That is why it is possible to point out that making strict antiabortion legislation does not necessarily lead to the reduction of abortions. In contrast, several works suggest that such limitations contribute to raising the rates of unsafe abortions, which is rather dangerous for women. Also, prior research has provided unto an understanding on the nature of politics on the advancement of the abortion issue. Our study centers on this complex relationship between the judiciary and politics (Luna, 2020; Ziegler, 2020). Here, our objective is to understand and analyze the history of current restrictions on abortion and their potential consequences from a gender perspective. Analyzing the nature of these abortion prohibitions effectively requires the application of critical policy analysis techniques. Therefore, for this paper, we adopted Carol Bacchi's critical policy analysis framework known as "*What's the problem represented to be?*" or W. P. R. (Bacchi, 2009). In this way, one may understand the legislation policies, comprehend how governance is executed, and evaluate the impacts on the people who are subjected to those policies. In the following section, we apply this lens and utilize a back-end synthesis of the five analyzed abortion prohibition statutes in the United States to explicate the cumulative mechanisms behind the distribution of legal structure and its repercussions. This paper pays particular attention to five U.S. abortion prohibition statutes in an attempt to analyze how they portray the problem as faced by international human rights policies. The state statutes from the United States under analysis are the ones from Texas, Alabama, Louisiana, Tennessee, and Arkansas. However, we shall also briefly examine the positions of these nations about abortion laws by analyzing General Comment 31 of ICCPR and treaty body monitoring on CEDAW. As we know, prior research has established that comprehensive bans on abortion are a violation of human rights. Therefore, instead of reiterating the issue at hand, this section must analyze the nuances of the problem representation and unfold the outcomes that stem from it. Three main questions guide our analysis:

a) Firstly, our main focus is to establish the kind of problem representation that the recent U.S. abortion prohibitions present and how this differs from the problem representation in the ICCPR and CEDAW using Carol Bacchi's What's the problem represented to be? (Bacchi, 2009) technique.
b) We will attempt to describe how the concept of rights is articulated and construed in the context of the problem representation in the material under analysis.
c) We will also consider the problem representation in more detail from the gender perspective and discuss possible gender aspects and impact.

## LITERATURE REVIEW

Women's Sexual and Reproductive Health and Rights (SRHR) share links with so many human rights as shown below. As per the international human rights norms, it consists of such rights as the right to life, the ban on torture, the right to health, the right to private life, the right to education, and non-discrimination (Carpenter, 2020). The Committee on Economic, Social, and Cultural Rights (CESCR) and the Committee on the Elimination of Discrimination against Women (CEDAW) have agreed that sexual and reproductive health is a women's right. However, this claim has been controversial. This right is complex. Hence, the body of information and research on it is vast. We understand this subject domain more deeply by papering past research and material. In this quest, we try to find patterns that may explain elements' complex interactions and identify gaps in the literature that require more research.

### Global Abortion Rights

Global abortion rights are investigated from several angles and themes. However, certain essential tenets and findings repeat in this complex landscape. A basic premise in abortion research is that strict abortion regulations do not eliminate abortions but rather increase unsafe abortions (Ganatra et al., 2017). A Guttmacher-Lancet Commission report estimates 25 million unsafe abortions per year, proving this (Starrs et al., 2018). Another widely accepted conclusion is that restrictive or criminalized abortion laws violate international human rights law, especially when a pregnant woman's life is in danger, or the pregnancy is caused by rape, incest, or severe fetal abnormalities ("Information series: Sexual and Reproductive Health and Rights", 2020). Distinguished scholars like Johanna B. Fine, Katherine Mayall, and Lilian Sepúlveda have addressed the subject in their paper, "*The Role of International Human Rights Norms in the Liberalization of Abortion Laws Globally*" (Fine et al., 2017). Restrictive abortion regulations violate women's rights to health, privacy, and, in some cases, freedom from harsh, inhumane, and humiliating treatment. (Fine et al., 2017). This violation of women's autonomy and dignity violates international justice and human rights. Abortion perception is also heavily influenced by race, financial status, religion, and history. This contextual relativity emphasizes the need for nuanced abortion research. Keertana Kannabiran Tella's "*Abortion Rights, Reproductive Justice, and the State: International Perspectives*." emphasizes this issue's importance in the U.S. Tella correctly points out that the American political atmosphere and the probable reversal of *Roe v. Wade* affect reproductive rights worldwide (Tella, 2024).

## The U.S. Abortion Right Before Dobbs v. Jackson Women's Health Organization

Many scholars have studied abortion in the U.S. due to its controversial debate. The recent judicial case of Dobbs v. Jackson Women's Health Organization has sparked several opinions and focal points in this discourse. The American abortion issue often centers on politics. Numerous studies have examined the relationship between politics and abortion discourse, arguing that political currents shape it. This research agrees that political power drives the abortion issue. Pro-life and pro-choice movements change with the political climate. In their book "*The End of Roe v. Wade: Inside the Right's Plan to Destroy Legal Abortion*," Robin Marty and Jessica Mason Pieklo delve into the ways the conservative right-wing has targeted the abstraction of abortion rights through legal actions (Marty & Pieklo, 2019). The explanation that follows demonstrates the influence of political ideologies on the discourse surrounding abortion. Mary Ziegler's magnum opus, "*Abortion and the Law in America: Roe v. Wade to the Present*," explains the complex relationship between politics and abortion through a systematic review of abortion policy in the United States since *Roe v. Wade*. provides an evaluation of the state of abortion access in the United States before and after *Roe v. Wade*. By critically analyzing the details of the case, Ziegler's comprehensive examination enlightens the reader on how political processes impact abortion-related judicial milestones. Similarly, she warns against fixating on the potential reversal of *Roe v. Wade*, stating that it could exacerbate the site beyond the politicization of abortion, scholarly discussions also take into account the experiences of low-income individuals, women of color, and native women in particular. It is noteworthy to emphasize that the focus should remain on the targeted populations, who experience systemic inequality amplified in terms of sexual and reproductive health care because abortion policy impacts different population groups differently. Zakiya Luna's "*Reproductive Rights as Human Rights: Women of Color and the Fight for Reproductive Justice*" (Luna, 2020). supports this inclusive and equitable appeal. Luna effectively emphasizes the need to address these underprivileged populations' distinct issues in the abortion debate. Religion and abortion debate are also common themes in research. This complex debate includes how religious beliefs and institutions shape abortion views. Religious issues remain essential to U.S. abortion debates.

## The U.S. Abortion Right After Dobbs v. Jackson Women's Health Organization

The landmark Supreme Court decision in *Dobbs v. Jackson Women's Health Organization* and the subsequent wave of abortion bans across the U.S. in 2022 have sparked a large body of research on its effects. This substantial paper corpus emphasizes a negative outlook on the ruling and its far-reaching effects. Researchers have studied the complex effects, particularly on women and society, and how they affect human rights. Ziegler argues that *Roe v. Wade* did not simply determine the abortion debate. It claims that the abortion controversy has escalated since this precedent was overturned. Yvonne Lindgren's insightful "*Dobbs v. Jackson Women's Health and the Post-Roe Landscape*" (Lindgren, 2022) supports this pre-court claim. Lindgren's paper shows that Roe v. Wade is not the key problem. This analysis also highlights the conflict between the verdict, the accompanying bans, and international human rights norms. The U.S. fails to defend these rights, it is argued (Kaufman et al., 2022). The Universal Declaration of Human Rights (UDHR) Article 12 protects the right to privacy, health, and healthcare, which such stringent laws violate (Kapoor, 2023). They are also accused of violating the right to equality and non-discrimination, which Article 26 of the International Covenant on Civil and Political Rights (ICCPR) (Xing et al., 2023) and Article 16. e of CEDAW upholds (Xing et al., 2023).

Articles 6 and 12 of the ICCPR charge further violations of the right to life and health. These laws are said to violate the U.N. treaty against torture and harsh, inhuman, or humiliating treatment, raising the threat of inhumanity and degradation. Finally, Article 17 of the ICCPR's right to privacy is said to be violated. Ramanpreet Kaur Chhabra and Dr. Varinder Kaur's "*Comparative Analysis of Abortion Laws Through the Lens of Human Rights*" (Chhabra & Kaur, 2022) and Amanda Misasi's "*Abortion Is a Right: Pursuing International Remedies for U.S. Human Rights Law Violations*" (Miasi, 2022) explore these claims from a human rights perspective. The Human Rights Watch briefing document highlights the international conventions the U.S. abortion bans violate (Chen et al., 2023). The U.S. has ratified the ICCPR, ICERD, and C.A.T. The document also refers to the CRPD, C.R.C., and ICESCR. The Committee on the Elimination of Discrimination against Women (CEDAW) has condemned the new U.S. legislation for violating human rights (Berer, 2023).

## THEORETICAL UNDERPINNINGS

This discussion revolves around Carol Bacchi's question, "*What's the problem represented to be*?" (W.R.P.) method, which thoroughly analyzes laws and policies (Bacchi, 2009). Bacchi's method thoroughly examines the policy idea beyond its surface level. However, it is crucial to understand that the W.R.P. approach is based on a revolutionary way of understanding "*problems*" beyond simple methodology and analytical instruments. The first step in using the W.P.R. technique effectively is understanding the fundamental philosophical framework underpinning it. This viewpoint deviates from the traditional "*problem-solving*" approach and emphasizes understanding problem representation and problematization. The fundamental idea is that "*problems*" are dynamic, malleable entities tied to social dynamics and governance. Since the definition of a "*problem*" depends on the observer's viewpoint, this analysis—which looks at how different viewpoints on abortion are viewed—is fascinating. Bacchi uses the theoretical idea of problematization as a crucial instrument for policy analysis within the framework of the W.R.P. method. The term "*problematicization*" by Bacchi (2009) has become popular in modern social theory, frequently used to emphasize the necessity of rigorously challenging accepted "*truths*." With inspiration from thought leaders like Paulo Freire, problematization is "*a pedagogical practice that disrupts taken-for-granted 'truths'*" and "*as a 'strategy for developing a critical consciousness.'*" (Bacchi, 2012). In contrast, Michel Foucault presents two perspectives on problematization: first, like Freire, it entails questioning prevailing "*truths*," and second, "*a way into thinking behind particular forms of rule*" (Bacchi, 2009). Notably, Bacchi cites the relevance of Foucault's exact definition of problematization within the framework of her methodology. This convergence of theoretical foundations highlights the significant consequences of Bacchi's W.P.R. approach in revealing the complex character of policy issues—like the divisive topic of abortion—by analyzing the perspective from which they are viewed.

Critical discourse analysis uses "*problematization*" to mean more than just representing an object or creating one through words. Instead, it involves a complex interaction of discursive and non-discursive processes that give something the capacity to be true or untrue, making it a contemplatable object for moral reflection, scientific research, or political analysis (Bacchi, 2009).

"*What's the problem represented to be?*" by Carol Bacchi, three main ideas underpin the W.P.R. approach:

a) Individuals and civilizations are governed by problematization.
b) Problematization and its representations should be studied before isolated "problems."

c) The necessity to question the problematizations' premises and implications (Bacchi, 2009).

Bacchi's W.P.R. technique uses problematization in two ways based on these concepts. First, propositions A and B focus on how issues are understood as '*problems*,' revealing cognitive processes that shape governance (Bacchi, 2009). Second, as mentioned in statement c, the phrase is used to question problematizations critically. The W.P.R. approach emphasizes "*problem representation*," or understanding the hidden 'issue' in-laws and regulations. Unlike the 'real,' representation in the W.P.R. approach establishes a policy 'issue' (Bacchi, 2009). Discourse is key to the W.P.R. approach since it defines what can be thought, written, or spoken about a social object or practice. Discourse shapes our worldview. W.P.R. uses leading questions to analyze policies and laws (Bacchi, 2009). The methods chapter will address these problematization-related problems. Policy and laws are not just about "*problem-solving*"; they also portray problems and how that representation impacts policy. Feminist legal theory is used to analyze the selected statutes. Our technique lets us assess how well these laws address feminist objections and concerns. We focus on specific feminist critiques that shed light on the law's treatment of the female perspective and women's societal roles rather than exploring feminist philosophy in general. The current study cannot cover the large and complex body of feminist theory studies. Instead, we'll focus on feminist critiques, including the lack of women, male privilege, the public/private contradiction, and intersectionality. Two key ideas underpin all feminist perspectives, "*the first is an observation – the world has been shaped by men, particularly white men, who for this reason possess larger shares of power and privilege; the second is an aspiration – all feminists believe that women and men should have political, social, and economic equality.*" (Edwards, 2010). Feminists aim to correct historical inequalities caused by a world constructed by and for men and achieve a condition of equality.

Feminists share the aim of gender equality, but their views on how to achieve it vary. Feminist theory's diversity of thinking produces diverse perspectives to help us analyze the chosen laws. We will begin with a feminist critique of the lack of women in law and human rights. Feminist researchers argue that this system's long-standing exclusion of women from decision-making neglects women's rights, interests, concerns, wants, and wishes. This exclusion is especially obvious when judicial questions are interpreted by men or women who have internalized and followed masculine elite norms and interests. Thus, men's perspectives dominate women's legal experiences (Edwards, 2010). The second criticism is that human rights law favors men. The legal system favors and prioritizes men's experiences and reality while ignoring or marginalizing women's. Feminist theorists claim that men's experiences have affected international human rights rules from creation to interpretation and application (Charlesworth & Chinkin, 2022). We have failed to address harms that primarily or severely affect women (Charlesworth & Chinkin, 2022). Cultural feminism holds that, like conventional psychology theories, the legal system favors a male-centric worldview and marginalizes women. The legal institution's hierarchical structure, adversarial format, and objective of abstractly balancing competing rights make it patriarchal. The final critique is that men dominate the public domain and women the private (Edwards, 2010). Critics say the rule emphasizes the public arena, ignoring women's private concerns. The public/private dichotomy is blamed for women's legal exclusion, especially when it overlaps with official accountability for human rights abuses. Additionally, this hierarchical attitude that prioritizes the male-conceived public domain over the domestic sphere perpetuates tyranny. Men worry about government oppression, whereas women worry about men's private persecution. This paradox also explains why women's rights violations are often ignored (Edwards, 2010).

Radical feminism believes the public/private duality conceals and legitimizes men's dominance over women. Catherine MacKinnon, a radical feminist, claims that males dominate and women submit in social relations (MacKinnon & Jaggar, 1994). She believes a gender- and sex-based hierarchical society keeps women down (Fisher & Tallant, 2016). The crucial question from this perspective is whether policies or legislation perpetuate gender- or sex-based subordination. An alternative legal interpretation proposes that the law should prioritize freedom from systemic sex subordination over gender-blindness. This feminist critique follows liberal feminism. As an ideology, liberal feminism seeks gender equality in all public spaces (Charlesworth & Chinkin, 2022). This includes equal political representation, paid work, education, and market services for women. Liberal feminists aim to alter the legal system by removing legislative barriers that prevent women from equal treatment in public. Liberal feminism has been criticized, nevertheless. One criticism suggests that pursuing "*sameness*" with men may force women to adapt to a male-dominated culture. Thus, this method may give women access to a society shaped by men's values and objectives. Liberal feminism strives to remove gender-based inequities, but critics wonder whether it frees women from a male-dominated worldview.

Our third critique examines how the judicial system essentializes women, reinforcing a communal female identity. Traditional roles like mothers and wives, which depend on men, shape this group identity. This essentialism is flawed because women are generally limited to a binary perspective of sex distinction in the legal system, such as "*the strong man*" and "*the weak woman*," or "*the male subject*" and "*the female object*" (Edwards, 2010). The legal context also makes essentialism problematic since it homogenizes women's experiences, believing they all have the same experience. Due to their identities and backgrounds, women experience life differently. This is where intersectionality matters. Intersectionality is the interaction of multiple identities and how they can create privilege and disadvantage. Feminist scholars believe an intersectional approach is necessary to understand and address marginalized women's complex and unique experiences with numerous intersecting identities. These ideas also question traditional views about how women should behave and handle crises like assault. Advocates and decision-makers must be alert to avoid replacing gender-based stereotypes with new victim categories like sex/race, class, or sexuality. Intersectional feminism emphasizes how identities interact and affect people's experiences and vulnerabilities (Edwards, 2010). These feminist criticisms will be used to analyze the problem representations in selected U.S. abortion restrictions and human rights abortion policies. We will examine how these critiques—including the legal exclusion of women, the primacy of the male perspective, and the public/private dichotomy—can be used to evaluate these laws and these representations. We will also use multiple discrimination and intersectionality to understand how these problem representations may disadvantage different groups of women with multiple intersecting identities.

## ANALYSIS

### Policies

#### U.S. Abortion Ban Policies

Following the Supreme Court's decision to reverse *Roe v. Wade*, a landmark ruling in American legal history—as demonstrated by the *Dobbs v. Jackson Women's Health Organization* case (Sherman et al., 2024)—many states have taken the initiative to outlaw abortion. This divisive topic has sparked significant legal and ethical discussion. One of the main points of contention in this discussion is the question of whether a fetus is considered a child. It is generally agreed upon among these state laws that life begins at conception. The legislative documents unambiguously communicate this fundamental principle. For example, the law in Louisiana states unequivocally that "*every unborn child is a human being from the moment of conception*," and the definition in Tennessee defines an "*unborn child*" as "*an individual living member of the species, homo sapiens, throughout the entire embryonic and fetal stages of the unborn child from fertilization until birth*" (Jaffe, 2020). Additionally, certain laws go even further. This definitional clarity is the cornerstone of the entire legal system about the prohibition of abortion. The specific purpose for which these restrictions were put in place was to protect human life. However, it is important to remember, that the argument over the rights of the unborn child and the point at which life genuinely begins is a long-running and intricate one. Arguments supporting the equal rights of the unborn child to those of born humans—that is, adults and children—have been discussed for a long time. Legislative efforts to give rights to underprivileged groups who had not previously been granted legal safeguards have historically resulted in profound societal changes. Examples of such revolutionary legislative initiatives include the abolition of slavery and the provision of legal safeguards to native communities. The House Bill from Alabama bases its reasoning on this supposition.

Natural law is famously upheld in the U.S. Declaration of Independence, which states that "*all men are created equal.*" Based on natural law, this fundamental concept asserts that all people are equal from their formation. Numerous historical movements, such as the American civil rights movement, the women's suffrage movement, the Nuremberg war crimes trials, and the anti-slavery campaign, have relied heavily on this idea. These movements' capacity to draw attention to the universal fact of human equality was crucial to their success. The justification presented in the legislation of Alabama and Arkansas is strong. They make a comparison between historically underprivileged communities that have experienced various forms of injustice and unborn children. They argue that unborn infants should have the same rights and protections as these disadvantaged populations. Both states use particular analogies that highlight past injustices experienced by the African American population to emphasize this argument.

Arkansas and Alabama draw attention to a pivotal moment in history: the upholding of segregation by the Supreme Court in the *Plessy v. Ferguson* case. They claim that because this ruling grossly violated the rights of Black people, it amounted to a grave crime against humanity. Employing an analogy, they contend that the legalization of abortion under *Roe v. Wade* should likewise be seen as a crime against humanity since it is believed to deprive the unborn child of their rights. It is interesting to observe that the legislation of the other three states does not specifically mention this comparison, even though Arkansas and Alabama specifically promote it. However, this legal viewpoint highlights how crucial it is to recognize the rights and safeguards of unborn children in the larger framework of past battles for justice and equality. A common theme throughout the chosen laws under examination is their emphasis on the rights of unborn infants. Notably, while Tennessee, Texas, Alabama, and Louisiana refer to their bans as the "*Human Life Protection Act,*" Arkansas gives its act a more specific name, calling it the "*Arkansas Unborn Child Protection Act.*" This terminology communicates the main goal of these regulations, which is further supported by the language and content used in them.

The reference in Alabama's law to the November 6, 2018, constitutional amendment, which proclaimed the state's public policy as one that acknowledges and respects the sanctity of unborn life and the rights of unborn children, highlights this commitment. A similar goal is stated in Arkansas, where the state's legislation expressly aims to protect unborn children's lives and outlaw abortion. This rhetorical emphasis highlights a significant viewpoint in the abortion debate, which is that the problem is not just about a woman's right to choose as the pro-choice movement advocates but also about the rights of the unborn child at its core. The necessity to "*recognize and support the sanctity of unborn life and the rights of unborn children*" is echoed in the legislation language. It is significant to notice that the legal rules about exceptions demonstrate this focus on the rights of the unborn child. These exclusions usually apply to circumstances where the woman's life or health is seriously jeopardized. The laws always expressly permit medical procedures that are required to keep a pregnant woman from dying or being in significant danger of dying from a physical ailment or to keep a pregnant woman's life-sustaining organ from being severely or permanently impaired in Louisiana.

Furthermore, when looking at the financial elements of these measures, the focus is mostly on restricting public funding for abortions. For example, Amendment 68 of the Arkansas Constitution states that public monies may not be used for abortions unless the mother's life is in danger. It also outlines the state's commitment to preserve the life of every unborn child from conception until birth. It's important to note that Louisiana, Alabama, and Arkansas laws all expressly mention financial constraints; the laws of the other two states do not. This emphasizes both the states' statutory commitment to limiting public funding for abortions and their general emphasis on the rights and sanctity of unborn children.

## Human Rights Abortion Policies

In the context of the human rights debate, the complex nuances surrounding abortion laws require serious thought. It has been the focus of intense discussion and interpretation by numerous committees, even if it may not be expressly recognized as a stand-alone right in any international human rights treaty. The argument that the right to an abortion falls under the category of several different human rights for women is the result of these discussions (Cook & Dickens, 2003). To clarify, abortion is addressed as a right under the Convention on the Elimination of All Forms of Discrimination Against Women (CEDAW), which approaches the issue from the standpoint of family planning and protecting women from unsafe abortions. According to CEDAW's Article 16(e), women have the equal rights to choose how many children to have and how far apart to have them. Moreover, it gives people the necessary knowledge, instruction, and resources to execute their rights.

This clause has been widely interpreted to include the right to an abortion as well as other rights related to sexual and reproductive health. *L.C. v. Peru* is a noteworthy legal precedent that is worth looking into. In this instance, it was vehemently argued and later upheld that the victim's rights were violated by the denial of access to abortion under many articles of the CEDAW, including 1, 2, 3, 5, 12, and 16 (e) in addition to General Recommendation No. 24. The decision confirmed the claim that several human rights tools and ideas could be used to justify the right to an abortion. In the context of the human rights debate, the complex nuances surrounding abortion laws require serious thought. It has been the focus of intense discussion and interpretation by numerous committees, even if it may not be expressly recognized as a stand-alone right in any international human rights treaty. The argument that the right to an abortion falls under the category of several different human rights for women is the result of these discussions (Sutton & Borland, 2019).

Maternal mortality rates and the right to an abortion are discussed in detail in CEDAW General Recommendation No. 24, which relates to Article 12 of the Convention. It highlights how important it is to give priority to preventing unintended pregnancies through two important channels: sex education and comprehensive family planning. The guideline also emphasizes how crucial it is to lower maternal death rates by offering prenatal care and safe parenting services. In addition, General Recommendation No. 24 urges that laws that prohibit abortion be reexamined. It calls on legislators to change these kinds of regulations so that severe penalties for women who seek abortions are removed (Todd-Gher & Shah, 2020). This viewpoint is consistent with a more comprehensive human rights framework that aims to protect women's autonomy and well-being concerning reproductive health. Regarding the International Covenant on Civil and Political Rights, a significant advancement happened in 2019 when General Comment No. 36 on Article 6, which deals with the right to life, specifically mentioned abortion. This statement makes it clear that although states are allowed to implement laws to control voluntary pregnancy termination, these laws cannot contradict any other Covenant-guaranteed rights or the right to life of expectant mothers or girls (Alston, 1990).

Practically speaking, this means that any limitations on a woman or girl's right to an abortion shouldn't do any of the following: risk their life, cause them to suffer physical or mental suffering that violates Article 7 of the Covenant, discriminate against them, or trespass into their private without permission. This interpretation emphasizes how crucial it is to make sure that any laws about abortion uphold and defend the fundamental rights that women and girls have under international law. Within the debate on human rights, the affirmation of the right to an abortion, along with other specific rights, comes before this principle is formally stated in a general comment. This claim is supported by the Human Rights Committee's earlier jurisprudential history, evident in instances decided before 2019. These instances demonstrate the Committee's changing position as they consider the right to an abortion concerning several other rights. A key component of this discussion is Article 2 of the International Covenant on Civil and Political Rights, which deals with protection against discrimination. Article 3, which emphasizes the idea of equal rights for men and women, complements it. Furthermore, four current instances have referred to Article 7, which deals with protection against torture and cruel, inhuman, or degrading treatment or punishment, as well as Article 17, which outlines the right to privacy. These instances include, among others, *Mellet v. Ireland* (2016), *Whelan v. Ireland* (2017), *V.D.A. v. Argentina* (2011)· and *K.L. v. Peru* (2005). It is important to note that Article 6, which guarantees the right to life, plays a central role in this discussion and is discussed concerning the *K.L. v. Peru* case. The intersection of the right to abortion and these fundamental rights, as explained by historical legal decisions, creates a complex and nuanced discourse that merits rigorous analysis in this intricate web of human rights jurisprudence. The interaction of these clauses highlights the development of human rights law and encourages a more thorough analysis of the ramifications for the larger legal system.

## What's The Problem Represented to Be?

The policies and terminology ingrained in them indicate the transition of the abortion debate in the United States toward a different direction. One noteworthy finding is the noticeable shift in focus from the rights of women to the rights and welfare of unborn infants. The names "Human Life Protection Act" and "*Arkansas Unborn Child Protection Act*," which highlights the changed emphasis, are two clear examples of the language used to characterize these measures. The language used in these statutes is instructive in that it indicates that abortion has moved from being a woman's problem to one that is primarily focused on the health of the unborn. The wording employed in this legislation, which continuously promotes the defense of the rights and lives of unborn children, further clarifies this change in emphasis. These policies' notable tactic is to contrast unborn children with historically marginalized and oppressed populations, which serves to emphasize further how important it is to protect unborn children. Furthermore, it is instructive that these statutes make no mention of pregnant women at all. It supports the claim made by the pro-choice movement that women and their rights are no longer the main focus of these programs. Rather, they take a completely different tack, emphasizing how the rights of unborn children are allegedly violated. The lawmakers argue that because abortion ends pregnancies, it ends the lives of unborn children, and for this reason, it is problematic. According to this definition, abortion is defined as the taking of a child's life because it holds that life begins at conception. Feminist criticisms of this problem representation are welcome, mainly because women are noticeably absent from the legal discourse. Women's rights are only mentioned in extraordinary circumstances, like when a woman's life is in danger or she is seriously hurt. In the end, the legal system disregards women's rights, wants, and desires when their voices are not included in the framework. Furthermore, the masculine perspective's preference is the subject of another important feminist criticism. Due to their inattention to the actual realities of women impacted by the problem representation, these rules unintentionally support the masculine perspective. These laws prioritize protecting unborn children over the particular difficulties associated with abortion and childbirth that affect women exclusively, even though abortion is a matter that predominantly impacts women.

A different way to look at the problem representation is to look closely at how the money is distributed, especially where it is going or not going. Regarding these almost complete prohibitions on abortion, the law only deals with money considerations concerning limiting access to government insurance, indicating that public funds will not be used or made available for these treatments. While the laws do not state clearly where this money is to be allocated, it is possible to deduce where they are to be allocated by looking at the location of the withdrawals. Analyzing the abortion question through the lens of international human rights legislation produces a clear picture of the dilemma. Different representations of the issue depend on which articles or comments are being examined. Investigating the underlying presuppositions and assumptions is crucial when analyzing the issue of representation found in U.S. laws, which revolves around the violation of the rights of unborn children and suggests outlawing abortion as a remedy. Our goal is to identify the implicit prior information that underlies this problem depiction. It is important to make clear that these presumptions provide insights into cultural values and the subconscious of society, not always legislators' opinions (Bacchi, 2009). The fundamental aspect of these programs is their preference for the rights of unborn children over those of women, which creates a difficult comparative analysis between the two. This begs the question of which group these policies value and see as more significant. One could contend that these laws subtly support the rights of unborn children over those of women, reflecting the pervasive notion that women are less valuable than men in society. Women have endured a long history of persecution, discrimination, and limited rights. To demonstrate this point, let us consider that the U.S. did not enact legislation prohibiting wage discrimination based on a person's sex for individuals performing the same job until 1963. This was followed by the outlawing of sex-based discrimination in education in 1972 and the achievement of women's credit card ownership rights in 1974. These legal firsts show how far we've come and emphasize how long women have been oppressed. Moreover, differences continue even in the presence of laws protecting equal rights. According to the Pew Research Center, women's earnings as of 2022 were only 82% of men's, highlighting the persistent gender disparities in society (Kochhar, 2023). The differences in women's rights and opportunities reflect ingrained cultural presumptions. To thoroughly analyze the assumptions underlying problem representation, we can follow Bacchi's advice and look at the policy framework's categories, important concepts, and binaries.

A binary with the separate components of woman and kid emerges. The distinguishing feature of binaries is that one side is frequently excluded or marginalized concerning the other. Furthermore, a hierarchy is implied by binaries by nature, with one side being given greater privileges and valued more highly than the other (Bacchi, 2009). The central binary in the context of these policies is woman/child. The policies depend on how these two groups' rights are valued and assessed. After a thorough analysis, it is clear that the child's viewpoint is seen as more significant and valuable than the other. One of the main ways that these policies pose problems is by giving the rights of unborn infants precedence over those of mothers. The policies being discussed involve basic ideas that are somewhat ambiguous, allowing for various interpretations based on varying ideological viewpoints (Bacchi, 2009). Two key ideas are particularly relevant. The first is the controversial concept of life and its origin, which was previously discussed concerning these policies.

These bills depict unborn children as a vulnerable population that is prone to serious injustices and rights violations. This is supported by a juxtaposition that compares historical horrors like the Holocaust and racial segregation to the act of abortion. On the other hand, those who seek or carry out abortions are almost always portrayed as possible violators of the unborn child's rights, except in the very rare situation in which there is a risk to the life of the individual. Notable is the glaring absence of women as unique, independent beings; instead, they are primarily shown as simply wombs of unborn children. Examining the fundamental assumptions and presuppositions that these abortion prohibition laws are based on makes it impossible to ignore how similar they are to feminist criticisms, especially radical feminism's core principles. According to these criticisms, the purpose of these laws is to maintain women's place as inferiors (Edwards, 2010). From a radical feminist standpoint, these statutes are viewed as the primary source of gender inequality in the legal system.

Examining the presumptions and assumptions in international accords like the International Covenant on Civil and Political Rights (ICCPR) and the Convention on the Elimination of All Forms of Discrimination Against Women (CEDAW) reveals a different interpretation. In this particular context, it might be argued that the provisions and clauses about abortion rights are predicated on the notion that women and girls are not entitled to the same rights as males and so require further protection. This viewpoint implies that racism and discrimination against women continue to be widely held beliefs despite the existence of treaty articles intended to prevent such practices. An underlying belief that women are fundamentally inferior persists on both the national and international levels but with a particular emphasis on the latter, where this belief is based on the idea that women are weak creatures in need of safeguards. Notably, international instruments that emphasize women's rights, including the right to an abortion, as essential components of broader women's rights include the International Covenant on Civil and Political Rights (ICCPR) and the Convention on the Elimination of All Forms of Discrimination Against Women (CEDAW). The study also emphasizes how women's rights are not given enough consideration in debates around abortion restrictions, which primarily center on the rights of unborn children. Some laws may recognize a woman's right to life as an exception, but her other rights—such as her choice and bodily autonomy—are frequently disregarded. When comparing how abortion regulations are portrayed in the United States, where the emphasis is still predominantly on women's rights, the disregard is made more apparent. Proactive steps are being taken in New York to support abortion rights and protect those who provide abortion care. Governor Hochul has moved to guarantee state support for reproductive health services through expanding the Family Planning Grant Program in 2023 (McNamara et al., 2023). This includes addressing racial inequities in maternal mortality as well as lowering rates of maternal death (McNamara et al., 2023). There is a stark difference between the women's rights-focused strategy of New York and the abortion-banning approaches of other states. This disparity highlights a significant omission from the restrictions on feminist criticism, as already mentioned. It draws attention to how noticeably absent the viewpoint of women is from the creation of these laws. Women's rights beyond the right to life would probably be given more thorough consideration if their voices were included in the legislative process.

The frequency of unsafe abortions is another issue that the prohibitions fail to address sufficiently. In the past, women have sought abortions even when they were forbidden, and this is still the case in nations where abortion is still outlawed. The main issue in many nations where abortion is illegal is the large number of unsafe abortions, which put women's health at grave risk. A WHO and Guttmacher Institute analysis found that between 2010 and 2014, almost 45% of all abortions were considered unsafe (Ganatra et al., 2017). Despite this, previous studies have claimed that the prohibitions fail to acknowledge this issue. The prohibitions also fail to consider the feminist critique of intersectionality, highlighting how the bans may specifically impact women with various identities. This element remains unexplored because these rules fail to address the diverse experiences and obstacles women who identify as several genders encounter. A contrasting viewpoint can be found by consulting international human rights agreements like the International Covenant on Civil and Political Rights (ICCPR) and the Convention on the Elimination of All Forms of Discrimination Against Women (CEDAW).

The statement highlights a perceived oversight in the consideration of the rights of the unborn child or fetus in international laws such as CEDAW and ICCPR, which primarily focus on women's rights in abortion debates. While these laws affirm a woman's right to choose an abortion, they do not explicitly address or impose restrictions on this right. International human rights legislation typically grants rights only from the point of birth, leading to the conclusion that unborn children have no recognized rights, including the right to life. This omission creates room for interpretation and debate. Even in countries where abortion is legal, restrictions often revolve around the fetus's potential viability outside the mother's womb. The right to abortion, being a complex concept intertwined with other rights, lacks precise definitions and restrictions, allowing for ongoing discussions and debates. The study questions the lack of formal acknowledgment of abortion as a fundamental human right and explores the implications of its absence. It argues that the marginalization of abortion rights to other rights is rooted in the failure to establish them as distinct rights. A feminist analysis suggests that the omission stems from viewing abortion as a matter confined to women's private lives, diminishing its importance compared to issues affecting men in the public domain. The critique extends to intersectionality, highlighting the oversight of various groups of women with unique needs and challenges in policy discussions.

Furthermore, the study criticizes how the lack of explicit recognition reduces women to a collective identity, sidelining their diverse perspectives and experiences. The focus on unborn child rights in abortion discourse sidelines women's concerns and the challenges they face in unintended pregnancies. The study also highlights how policy representations can perpetuate stigma against women seeking abortions, framing them as responsible for the perceived violation of the unborn child's rights. This stigma may lead to social alienation and exclusion of women and girls seeking abortion services. The study relates this perspective to feminist criticism, arguing that it reflects essentialism by portraying women as wrongdoers needing government intervention rather than individuals with inherent rights. Furthermore, these policies have significant long-term implications. Abortions have always occurred and will continue to do so even if they are outlawed, as was previously mentioned. But they will turn illegal and dangerous, increasing the risk and mortality rates for mothers and increasing the complexities and hazards associated with unsafe abortions. Furthermore, these regulations would limit access to safe abortion services, which will mostly impact low-income women who cannot afford to fly to neighboring jurisdictions for the procedure. Examining intersectionality becomes possible since different groups of women will suffer from various disadvantages. Abortion access will be restricted for some due to state laws prohibiting the procedure, therefore making it a class issue. The poor will be forced to either accept unintended pregnancies or undergo dangerous home abortions; only the wealthy will be able to afford healthcare. According to data from the Guttmacher Institute in 2014, women who made less than 25% of the federal poverty line performed 49% of abortions, while low-income women performed 26% of the procedures, and middle-class or upper-class women performed 25% (Jerman et al., 2023). This data shows how women with low incomes will be disproportionately impacted by laws prohibiting abortion, even if they may not have the means to seek care elsewhere.

Additionally, because the majority of those with the lowest incomes are people of color, notably Black and Hispanic people, this class issue also becomes entwined with racial inequality. For example, in 2019–2020, the median annual income of non-Hispanic black women aged 20–29 was only $19,200, while that of Hispanic women was $20,600 ("*Statistics at a Glance,*" 2023). In comparison, the median income of white women was $25,500, and Asian women was $31,900. Remarkably, 60% of abortions in 2014 occurred in the age range of 20–29 (Jerman et al., 2023). Given their greater propensity to seek abortions and their low financial resources, these figures indicate that women of color, especially black and Hispanic women in the 20–29 age range, will be the group most negatively impacted by abortion laws. Abortion laws can be analyzed from a variety of angles and can have a substantial impact on a variety of populations.

First of all, these policies might put more women with impairments at a disadvantage. There are hazards associated with pregnancy by nature, but these risks are compounded for women who have underlying health conditions or disabilities, such as an 11-fold increased chance of maternal death ("*NIH Study Suggests,*" 2021). Furthermore, if abortion becomes the sole option available in their state, these women might not be able to move elsewhere due to physical or mental limitations. They are more likely to become pregnant unintentionally as a result of this circumstance, which could have serious repercussions for both them and their unborn children. From the standpoint of international human rights, several implications exist. Women's viewpoints may be suppressed in terms of rhetoric, even in treaties such as the ICCPR and CEDAW, because abortion is not explicitly recognized as a separate right but rather is included in the package of rights. This could lessen the focus on abortion as a unique issue.

However, these tools support gender equality by advancing the idea that women have equal rights. This, too, is debatable because some contend that women are presented as helpless victims who depend on men for protection. The practical ramifications are as follows: women's rights can be enhanced and given greater possibilities and choices if abortion laws are upheld. Safe and legal abortions can lower the dangers and consequences that come with risky practices. Furthermore, rates of maternal mortality and morbidity could drop dramatically if access to and affordability of reproductive healthcare were ensured. On the other hand, people who hold moral or religious views that life begins at conception can argue that abortion violates the rights of unborn children. Arguments based on religion and morality are frequently used in the abortion debate, especially in areas of the United States known as the "*bible belt*" that are heavily influenced by conservative Christianity. Religion and morality are not specifically stated in the legislation themselves, but they are utilized to support the problematic portrayal of abortion prohibitions (Abadi & Gal, 2018). However, these debate-relevant characteristics are frequently discussed in social media and public conversation.

It's crucial to remember that arguments in favor of abortion rights and religious freedom from nonreligious or other religions can balance out arguments in favor of religion. It is possible to argue against the problem depiction of violations of the unborn child's rights, particularly in light of the absence of a generally agreed-upon definition of the beginning of life. While some claim it starts at conception, others say that it does not begin until birth or viability ("*State Bans on Abortion,*" 2024). A case can be made for women's human rights to be equally protected from a human rights standpoint. Proponents contend that women should have equal rights in all spheres, including those that do not directly affect men but are within their rights. However, similar justifications for abortion prohibitions, such as moral objections and religious convictions, can be used to refute this viewpoint. This subject may also be impacted by the ongoing controversy regarding the exact moment life begins, with some arguing that it may not occur at birth.

## CONCLUSION

The study discusses findings related to recent abortion restrictions in the United States and the broader context of abortion rights as human rights. It highlights the fundamental opposition between the issue representations used in the U.S. abortion restrictions and the human rights paradigm. The U.S. restrictions emphasize the sanctity of life from conception, prioritizing the rights of unborn infants over women's right to abortion. In contrast, the human rights approach prioritizes and defends women's equal rights, emphasizing potential violations resulting from restrictive abortion laws. The stark disparities in these representations underscore the contention in the abortion debate, particularly regarding the relative importance of rights and differing views on the beginning of life. The study notes that these opposing representations may contribute to inconsistency with and potential violations of basic human rights. A feminist analysis raises concerns about the marginalization of women in U.S. abortion legislation and the potential essentialization of women as helpless victims in human rights-based abortion laws. Both representations invite feminist critiques, highlighting the need for changes that accurately reflect women's perspectives and promote gender equality within the legal system. The research anticipates potential outcomes and sheds light on the motivations behind the legislation. However, it emphasizes the need for future studies to fully understand the implications of recent abortion restrictions, considering factors such as maternal mortality rates, morbidity rates, and the prevalence of unsafe abortions.

The study concludes by emphasizing the importance of comprehensive investigation and evaluation to determine whether prioritizing unborn children's rights over women's rights is appropriate.

## REFERENCES


Abadi, M., & Gal, S. (2018, May 2). *The rust belt, the corn belt, and every other "belt" in the USA: Business insider india*. Business Insider. https://www.businessinsider.in/the-rust-belt-the-corn-belt-and-every-other-belt-in-the-usa/articleshow/64002711.cms

Alston, P. (1990). The Unborn Child and Abortion under the Draft Convention on the Rights of the Child. *Human Rights Quarterly*, 12(1), 156–178. DOI: 10.2307/762174 PMID: 11655994

Bacchi, C. (2012). Why Study Problematizations? Making Politics Visible. *Open Journal of Political Science*, 02(01), 1–8. DOI: 10.4236/ojps.2012.21001

Bacchi, C. L. (2009). *Analysing policy: What's the problem represented to be?* Pearson.

Berer, M. (2023). Challenging the US Supreme Court's Majority Ruling on Roe v. Wade at the International Human Rights Level. *Health and Human Rights*, 25(1), 195–206. PMID: 37397425

Carpenter, M. (2020). The OHCHR background note on Human Rights Violations Against Intersex People. *Sexual and Reproductive Health Matters*, 28(1), 1731298. Advance online publication. DOI: 10.1080/26410397.2020.1731298 PMID: 32204689

Charlesworth, H., & Chinkin, C. (2022). *The Boundaries of International Law: A Feminist Analysis*. Manchester University Press. DOI: 10.7765/9781526163592

Chen, R., Gordon, M., Chervenak, F., & Coverdale, J. (2023). Addressing Moral Distress after Dobbs v. Jackson Women's Health Organization: A Professional Virtues-Based Approach. *Academic Medicine*, 99(1), 12–15. DOI: 10.1097/ACM.0000000000005476 PMID: 37816216

Chhabra, R. K., & Kaur, V. (2022). Comparative Analysis of Abortion Laws through the lens of Human Rights Laws. *International Journal of Law Management and Humanities*, 5(3), 47–66.

Cook, R. J., & Dickens, B. M. (2003). Human Rights Dynamics of Abortion Law Reform. *Human Rights Quarterly*, 25(1), 1–59. DOI: 10.1353/hrq.2003.0003 PMID: 15719517

Edwards, A. (2010). *Violence Against Women Under International Human Rights Law*. Cambridge University Press. DOI: 10.1017/CBO9780511779671

Erdman, J. N. (2017). Theorizing Time in Abortion Law and Human Rights. *Health and Human Rights*, 19(1), 29–40. PMID: 28630539

Fine, J. B., Mayall, K., & Sepúlveda, L. (2017). The Role of International Human Rights Norms in the Liberalization of Abortion Laws Globally. *Health and Human Rights*, 19(1), 69–80. PMID: 28630542

Fisher, A., & Tallant, J. (2016). Judith Jarvis Thomson on Abortion. In *How To Get Philosophy Students Talking: An Instructors Toolkit*. essay, Routledge.

Ganatra, B., Gerdts, C., Rossier, C., Johnson, B. R.Jr, Tunçalp, Ö., Assifi, A., Sedgh, G., Singh, S., Bankole, A., Popinchalk, A., Bearak, J., Kang, Z., & Alkema, L. (2017). Global, regional, and subregional classification of abortions by safety, 2010–14: Estimates from a bayesian hierarchical model. *Lancet*, 390(10110), 2372–2381. DOI: 10.1016/S0140-6736(17)31794-4 PMID: 28964589

*Human rights crisis: Abortion in the United States after Dobbs*. Human Rights Watch. (2023, April 18). https://www.hrw.org/news/2023/04/18/human-rights-crisis-abortion-united-states-after-dobbs

*Information series: Sexual and Reproductive Health and Rights*. UN Human Rights Office. (2020). https://www.ohchr.org/en/women/information-series-sexual-and-reproductive-health-and-rights

Jaffe, S. (2020). US Supreme Court upholds abortion rights, for now. *Lancet*, 396(10244), 85–86. DOI: 10.1016/S0140-6736(20)31518-X PMID: 32653060

Jain, D. (2023). Supreme Court of India judgement on abortion as a fundamental right: Breaking new ground. *Sexual and Reproductive Health Matters*, 31(1), 2225264. Advance online publication. DOI: 10.1080/26410397.2023.2225264 PMID: 37395544

Jerman, J., Jones, R. K., & Onda, T. (2023, August 11). *Characteristics of U.S. Abortion Patients in 2014 and Changes Since 2008*. Guttmacher Institute. https://www.guttmacher.org/report/characteristics-us-abortion-patients-2014

Kapoor, S. (2023, May 10). Abortion: Comparative Study between Indian Laws and US Laws. Retrieved August 18, 2024,.

Kaufman, R., Brown, R., Martínez Coral, C., Jacob, J., Onyango, M., & Thomasen, K. (2022). Global impacts of Dobbs v. Jackson Women's Health Organization and Abortion Regression in the United States. *Sexual and Reproductive Health Matters*, 30(1), 2135574. Advance online publication. DOI: 10.1080/26410397.2022.2135574 PMID: 36383177

Kochhar, R. (2023, March 1). *The Enduring Grip of the Gender Pay Gap*. Pew Research Center. https://www.pewresearch.org/social-trends/2023/03/01/the-enduring-grip-of-the-gender-pay-gap/

Lindgren, Y. (2022). Dobbs v. Jackson Women's Health and the Post-Roe Landscape. J. Am. Acad. Matrimonial Law., 35, 235.

Luna, Z. (2020). *Reproductive Rights as Human Rights: Women of Color and the fight for Reproductive Justice.* New York University Press. DOI: 10.18574/nyu/9781479894369.001.0001

MacKinnon, C. A. (1994). Toward Feminist Jurisprudence. In A. M. Jaggar (Ed.), *Living with Contradicitons* (1st ed.). essay, Routledge.

Marty, R., & Pieklo, J. M. (2019). *The End of Roe V. Wade: Inside the Right's Plan to Destroy Legal Abortion.* IG Publishing.

McNamara, K., Poverman, M., Nádas, M., Mallow, M., & Gerber, S. (2023). Privileging Midwives for Abortion Care. *Journal of Midwifery & Women's Health*, 68(6), 769–773. DOI: 10.1111/jmwh.13577 PMID: 37850529

Miasi, A. (2022, November 28). *Abortion is a right: Pursuing international remedies for U.S. human rights law violations.* Platform for Peace and Humanity. https://peacehumanity.org/2022/11/28/abortion-is-a-right-pursuing-international-remedies-for-u-s-human-rights-law-violations/

Ngwena, C. G. (2013). A Commentary on LC v Peru: The CEDAW Committee's First Decision on Abortion. *Journal of African Law*, 57(2), 310–324. DOI: 10.1017/S0021855313000107

*NIH Study Suggests Women with Disabilities have Higher Risk of Birth Complications and Death.* National Institutes of Health. (2021, December 15). https://www.nih.gov/news-events/news-releases/nih-study-suggests-women-disabilities-have-higher-risk-birth-complications-death

Pizzarossa, L. B., & Skuster, P. (2021). Toward Human Rights and Evidence-Based Legal Frameworks for (Self-Managed) Abortion: A Review of the Last Decade of Legal Reform. *Health and Human Rights*, 23(1), 199–212. PMID: 34194213

Rebouché, R. (2016). Abortion rights as human rights. *Social &amp. Social & Legal Studies*, 25(6), 765–782. DOI: 10.1177/0964663916668391

Sherman, C., Witherspoon, A., Glenza, J., & Noor, P. (2024, July 29). Tracking abortion laws across the united states. *The Guardian.* Retrieved from https://www.theguardian.com/us-news/ng-interactive/2024/jul/29/abortion-laws-bans-by-state

Starrs, A. M., Ezeh, A. C., Barker, G., Basu, A., Bertrand, J. T., Blum, R., Coll-Seck, A. M., Grover, A., Laski, L., Roa, M., Sathar, Z. A., Say, L., Serour, G. I., Singh, S., Stenberg, K., Temmerman, M., Biddlecom, A., Popinchalk, A., Summers, C., & Ashford, L. S. (2018). Accelerate progress—sexual and reproductive health and rights for all: Report of the guttmacher– lancet commission. *Lancet*, 391(10140), 2642–2692. DOI: 10.1016/S0140-6736(18)30293-9 PMID: 29753597

*State Bans on Abortion Throughout Pregnancy*. Guttmacher Institute. (2024, July 25). https://www.guttmacher.org/state-policy/explore/state-policies-abortion-bans

*Statistics at a Glance: Earnings of Women Aged 20–59, by Age Group and Race/Ethnicity*. Social Security Administration. (2023). https://www.ssa.gov/policy/docs/factsheets/at-a-glance/earnings-women-age-race-ethnicity.html

Sutton, B., & Borland, E. (2019). Abortion and Human Rights for Women in Argentina. *Frontiers*, 40(2), 27–61. DOI: 10.1353/fro.2019.a730152

Tella, K. K. (2024). *Abortion Rights, Reproductive Justice and the State: International Perspectives*. Routledge India.

*The world's abortion laws*. Center for Reproductive Rights. (2023). https://reproductiverights.org/maps/worlds-abortion-laws/

Todd-Gher, J., & Shah, P. K. (2020). Abortion in the Context of COVID-19: A Human Rights Imperative. *Sexual and Reproductive Health Matters*, 28(1), 1758394. DOI: 10.1080/26410397.2020.1758394 PMID: 32308156

Xing, E., Owda, R., Loder, C., & Collins, K. (2023). Abortion rights are Health Care Rights. *JCI Insight*, 8(11), e171798. Advance online publication. DOI: 10.1172/jci.insight.171798 PMID: 37288659

Yamin, A. E. (2023). Five Lessons for Advancing Maternal Health Rights in an Age of Neoliberal Globalization and Conservative Backlash. *Health and Human Rights*, 25(1), 185–194. PMID: 37397427

Ziegler, M. (2020). *Abortion and the Law in America: Roe v. Wade to the present*. Cambridge University Press.

## ADDITIONAL READING


Aiken, A. R. A., Digol, I., Trussell, J., & Gomperts, R. (2017). Self-reported outcomes and adverse events after medical abortion through online telemedicine: Population-based study in the Republic of Ireland and Northern Ireland. *BMJ (Clinical Research Ed.)*, 357, j2011. DOI: 10.1136/bmj.j2011 PMID: 28512085

Baum, S. E., Ramirez, A. M., Larrea, S., Filippa, S., Egwuatu, I., Wydrzynska, J., Piasecka, M., Nmezi, S., & Jelinska, K. (2020). It's not a seven-headed beast: Abortion experience among women that received support from helplines for medication abortion in restrictive settings. *Health Care for Women International*, 41(10), 1128–1146. DOI: 10.1080/07399332.2020.1823981 PMID: 33156737

Beynon-Jones, S. M., & Sheldon, S. (2023). Repercussions of overturning Roe v. Wade for women across systems and beyond borders. *Reproductive Health*, 20(1), 123. https://reproductive-health-journal.biomedcentral.com/articles/10.1186/s12978-022-01457-0 PMID: 37612745

Ferguson, L., & Gill, A. (2023). The fall of Roe v. Wade: The fight for abortion rights is universal. *BMJ*. https://www.bmj.com/content/377/bmj.n1618

Lewandowska, M. (2022). Feminist theory drafting injustice: Overturning Roe v. Wade, spillover effects, and the disproportionate impact on women of color. *Gender & Society*, 36(5), 689–711. DOI: 10.1177/08912432221110344

McGovern, M., & Abdelmonem, A. (2022). Constitutionalizing reproductive rights (and justice). In Dixon, M. (Ed.), *Reproductive Rights and Justice: New Perspectives* (pp. 123–145). Oxford University Press., https://academic.oup.com/edited-volume/34710/chapter/296430744

Rao, R. (2023). From choice to reproductive justice: De-constitutionalizing abortion rights. *International Journal of Law and Politics*, 15(3), 345–367. https://academic.oup.com/edited-volume/34710/chapter/296430744

Thompson, L. (2023). From reproductive rights to reproductive justice: Abortion in the United States. *Journal of Feminist Studies*, 42(2), 101–119. https://academic.oup.com/edited-volume/34710/chapter/337816966

## KEY TERMS AND DEFINITIONS

**Abortion Policies:** These are legal measures that have been enacted and put in place by governments as means of regulating the performance, prohibition, or restriction of abortions. There are differences between countries and states and that is because each has its own culture, religion, and political system.

**Abortion Bans:** Abortion bans are legal actions that make abortions legal either in no circumstances or after a certain number of weeks with a few conditions. The said bans are usually put forward from moral, religious, or political standpoints and are influential in deciding women's reproductive autonomy.

**Problem Representations:** In policy analysis, problem representations represent the way how the problem, such as abortion, is framed and defined in the view of policymakers and media, which affects the subsequent population perception and policy solutions. The framing can focus on some aspects and ignore or play down others when it comes to things such as abortion.

**Roe v. Wade:** It emerged in 1973 as a U. S Supreme Court case that liberalized abortion across the country: it gave a woman a right to an abortion before the fetus is capable of surviving outside the womb. It was widely applauded and has set a precedent for women's reproductive rights but this decision has also received legal challenges and criticism over time.

**Human Rights:** The rights libertied in the case of abortion refer to the rights allowing women to conduct safe, legal, and affordable abortions. Limitations to abortion have been considered as infringement of women's rights to privacy, autonomy and health.

**Feminist Theory:** Feminist analysis looks at abortion from a vantage point that seeks to uphold the equality of women where they have equal freedom to choose for their bodies. It opposes the power relations that attempt to control women and for that, it emphasizes the ability to have a safe abortion as part of the Gender Justice.

# Chapter 2
# Polish Abortion Ruling (2020) From the Perspective of International Law:
## Some Critical Remarks on Methodology and Reasoning

**Marcin Gorski**
*Faculty of Law and Administration, University of Lodz, Poland*

## ABSTRACT

*The 2020 "judgment" of the Polish Constitutional Tribunal on abortion raises many doubts. The primary problem concerns its status. But this dictum is affected by other dysfunctions pertaining to the methodological technique, the method of constructing judicial reasoning, the application of international law and the references to the rulings of international courts, as well as the consequences of the "judgment" for the perception of the relationship between the legislature and the constitutional court. The aim of this chapter is to analyse critically the extreme methodological poverty of the Constitutional Tribunal's argumentation and the obvious, actually even "schoolboy", errors affecting judicial reasoning. So, let us tell a story about manifest errors, intellectual shamelessness and argumentative abuses and manipulations.*

DOI: 10.4018/979-8-3693-7837-3.ch002

## INTRODUCTION

The 2020 "judgment" ("Judgment" of the Constitutional Tribunal, Poland, October 22, 2020, K 1/20) of the adjudicating panel on abortion is the Poland's second constitutional review of the Polish Act of 7th January 1993 on family planning, protection of the human foetus and the conditions for the admissibility of termination of pregnancy. One should explain that in this chapter the references to the aforementioned "ruling" or "judgment" shall be put in brackets in order to highlight the lack of its constitutional legitimacy, and we shall as well endeavour to avoid referring to „Constitutional Court" as its invalid composition results in the duty to avoid treating this body as the Constitutional Court as provided for in the Constitution of the Republic of Poland. Instead, we shall attempt to employ, as far as possible, terms like "adjudicating panel" etc.

In 1997 the Constitutional Court held that a provision allowing for termination of pregnancy in the event of difficult living conditions or a difficult personal situation of the pregnant woman violated the constitutional principle of the rule of law (Ruling of the Constitutional Tribunal, Poland, May 28, 1997, K 26/96). Already in that ruling the Constitutional Court addressed the context of international law by holding that:

> *"[t]he position that human health should be subject to legal protection also in the prenatal phase is directly confirmed by the Convention on the Rights of the Child. Article 24, paragraph 1 of the Convention reads that States Parties recognize the right of the child to the enjoyment of the best possible state of health (...). The second paragraph of this article reads that States Parties shall strive to ensure the full realization of this right and in particular shall take appropriate measures to: (...) d) provide mothers with appropriate prenatal and postnatal care. Therefore, regardless of the wording of paragraph 10 of the preamble to the Convention, in the light of which the concept of a child employed in the Convention should also include a child before birth, Article 24 contains a direct indication that the right to the enjoyment of the best possible state of health also includes a conceived child. Only in this way can the obligation resulting from paragraph 2 to provide mothers with prenatal care be explained. This obligation was not introduced with a view to the interests of the pregnant woman herself but, as is clearly stated in Article 24, paragraph 2 in principio, in order to ensure the full realization of this right (i.e. specified in par. 1). Clearly, this concerns guarantees for the conceived child to enjoy the best possible state of health" (K 26/96, op. cit., in chapter 3).*

Clearly, the discussed provision does not lead to the conclusions derived by the Constitutional Tribunal in 1997. On the contrary, an indispensable element of the right to health guaranteed by Article 24 CRC is the right to reproductive health. As rightly noted by John Tobin:

> *"Both the ESCR and CRC Committees have explained that the right to health includes not only entitlements to health care and related services but freedoms including 'the right to control one's health and body, including sexual and reproductive freedom and the right to be free from interference such as the right to be free from torture, non-consensual medical treatment and experimentation'" (Tobin, 2019, p. 909; see also pp. 914-915).*

The perspective of a woman's right to reproductive health and to make decisions on pregnancy was abandoned in this (infuriatingly patronizing) passage of the Constitutional Court's reasoning of its 1997 decision. Also, it is surprisingly superficial when it persuades that "clearly" the right of a woman to enjoy "appropriate pre-natal and post-natal health care" must lead to any kind of prohibition of abortion.

But, the 2020 "judgment" of the Polish Constitutional Tribunal regarding abortion raises doubts on so many more levels. Of course, the primary ambiguity concerns the status of the "judgment" itself, i.e. whether it constitutes, in formal terms, a judgment or is it just the view of a group of people with a partially undetermined constitutional status on what they believe stems from the Polish Constitution and other acts randomly quoted and abused in their so-called "argumentation". But this dictum is affected by yet another kind of dysfunction. In the present chapter, we shall analyse the abortion "judgment" of the Polish Constitutional Tribunal from the perspective of the methodological technique, the method of constructing judicial reasoning, the application of international law and the references to the rulings of international courts, as well as the consequences of the "judgment" for the perception of the relationship between the legislature and the constitutional court. Therefore, the aim of this chapter is to appraise critically the extreme methodological impoverishment of the Constitutional Tribunal's argumentation and the obvious, actually even "schoolboy", errors affecting judicial reasoning. So, let us tell a story about manifest errors, intellectual shamelessness and argumentative abuses and manipulations.

The issue of the legal status of the adjudicating panel's "ruling" of 22nd October 2020 in case K 1/20 shall not be elaborated in-depth here. The author of this chapter generally shares the position expressed in the legal expert opinion on the legal nature of this "ruling", developed by the Team of Advisors for the Control of the Constitutionality of Law at the Speaker of the Senate of the 10th term (Chmaj et al., 2020), as well as he fully endorses the analysis of the Poland's constitutional breakdown presented broadly by Wojciech Sadurski who pointed out at the process of gradual "switching-off" of democratic guarantees of the rule of law: the "remaking" of the Constitutional Tribunal (i.e. subjecting it, through the violation of the Constitution and politically-driven judicial nominations, to *voluntas politica*), further dismantling of checks and balances through disactivating the public prosecution service (in its role of the guarantor of the rule of law) and imposing the system of repressions on political triggers on the judiciary, and finally assaulting individuals' rights (Sadurski, 2019, pp. 58-161).

However, this broader political context in which the "ruling" was delivered is, obviously, important for understanding properly its significance. Basically, the adjudicating panel pretending to be a properly functioning constitutional court demonstrated its actual motivation and function, namely, that it no longer plays the role of a constitutional adjudicator, being the protector of the constitutional regime of the state and fundamental rights and freedoms of individuals, but rather, to implement a political agenda of a particular political force standing behind the panel.

Therefore, the "reasoning" of the "judgment" did not intend to achieve the goals normally determining the reasoning of any constitutional court, being – among others – to persuade the general public that particular constitutional values are actually protected in the legal system and result in that a particular norm of statutory legislation must be declared null and void – that is, in the Kelsen's words, "to secure the legality of the state's functions" (Kelsen, 2015, p. 22; also Kelsen, 2007, p. 149 and subsequent). The adjudicating panel, instead, simply endeavoured to implement a particular political agenda. The fact that the Constitution of Poland is silent about the moment when the constitutional protection of human life begins and that it left for the ordinary legislator to decide on the legal determinants of termination of pregnancy was therefore no impediment for the adjudicating panel because its decision and argumentation was subject, so to speak, to other criteria and paradigms than those applicable to constitutional adjudication. But, again, even though these more general issues need to be seen as the general background of the "ruling" discussed in this chapter, neverthelees they not the core business of this paper as we are focusing here on deficient and abusive interpretation of international law.

Therefore, leaving aside the formal reservations, which had already been discussed in more detail in the aforementioned legal expert opinion, and later also defined to some extent in the judgment of the ECtHR in *XERO FLOR v. Poland* (ECtHR, 7 May 2021, *XERO FLOR w Polsce sp. z o.o. v. Poland*, appl. no. 4907/18) and ultimately in *M. L. v. Poland* (ECtHR, *M.L. v. Poland,* 14 December 2023, appl. no. 40119/21, at 160-176), directly in the context of the "ruling" discussed in this paper, it is necessary to present briefly the reasoning of the adjudicating panel in this case, if it even is perceptible at all, and to make a critical analysis of it. Let us briefly note, though, that when it comes to the problem of constitutional legitimacy of the persons in the adjudicating panel, the ECtHR held in *XERO FLOR v. Poland* (in §§ 290-291) that:

*"the Court has established that the fundamental rule applicable to the election of Constitutional Court judges was breached, particularly by the eighth-term Sejm and the President of the Republic (see paragraphs 275 and 277-278 above). The eighth-term Sejm proceeded to elect three Constitutional Court judges, including [Mariusz Muszyński], on 2 December 2015, even though the respective seats had already been filled by the three judges elected by the previous Sejm. The President of the Republic refused to swear in the three judges elected by the previous Sejm, and received the oath of office from the three judges elected on 2 December 2015. In the light of the foregoing, and having regard to the three-step test set out above (see paragraphs 248-251 above), the Court considers that the applicant company was denied its right to a "tribunal established by law" on account of the participation in the proceedings before the Constitutional Court of Judge [Mariusz Muszyński], whose election was vitiated by grave irregularities that impaired the very essence of the right at issue".*

In *M. L. v. Poland* the Strasbourg Court added that (§ 173):

*"Judges J. Piskorski and J. Wyrembak, who likewise sat on the bench, were elected in 2017 and 2018 respectively in order to replace two other judges who had been elected together with Judge M. Muszyński by the eighth-term Sejm in a procedure which the Court has already found to be in breach of Article 6".*

As we explained, the latter case concerned the composition of the panel directly in K 1/20.

## LACK OF JUDICIAL DIALOGUE AND CONSTITUTIONAL BENCHMARKING

Any constitutional court in Europe caring about the persuasive power of its argumentation and the chances for a general reception and acceptance of its stances seeks for precedents in other jurisdictions in the European constitutional space, thus entering into judicial dialogue and trying to create the impression that its reasoning and understanding of constitutional principles is not an isolated one (one can call it "argumentative mainstreaming"). The "ruling" discussed here infamously lacks any such attempts. It is all the more traceable when one realises that difference between this "ruling" and its analogues in other European states in approaching the interpretation of international law.

For instance, the Spanish Constitutional Court in its 2023 ruling (Tribunal Constitucional de España, Sentencia 44/2023, 23 May 2023, available at https://hj.tribunalconstitucional.es/es/Resolucion/Show/29434, Retrieved on October 10, 2024) included methodologically accurate references to the European Convention and case-law of the ECtHR or the extensive presentation of international non-binding documents. It noted, among others, that (see chapters II.22.B and II.2.C in fine):

*"The European Court of Human Rights (ECtHR) [...] adopts a dynamic and evolving approach as a way of interpreting the Convention to ensure that its rights are practical and effective. According to it, the Court must have regard to the changing conditions within the respondent State and within Contracting States generally and respond, for example, to any evolving convergence as to the standards to be achieved (ECtHR judgments of 11 July 2002, Goodwin v. United Kingdom, § 74, and of 28 May 2002, Stafford v. United Kingdom, §§ 68-69). It has projected the specific context of voluntary termination of pregnancy (ECtHR of 16 December 2010, A. B. and C. v. Ireland, § 234). Consensus has therefore been invoked to justify a dynamic interpretation of the Convention".*

The adjudicating panel (in K 1/20) also failed to draw any inspiration (even if critically) from the constitutional courts outside Europe, e.g. the Supreme Court of the United States (SCOTUS: *Griswold v. Connecticut*, 381 U.S. 479 (1965), 7 June 1965, on the right to use of contraceptives as an element of the right of marital privacy being within the penumbra of specific guarantees of the Bill of Rights; *Roe v. Wade*, 410 U.S. 113 (1973), 22 January 1973, a long-controlling case holding that the Due Process Clause protecting the right to privacy against state action, including a woman's right to terminate her pregnancy; *Planned Parenthood of Southeastern Pa. v. Casey*, 505 U.S. 833 (1992), 29 June 1992, another long-controlling case holding that an undue burden exists, and therefore a provision of law is invalid, if its purpose or effect is to place substantial obstacles in the path of a woman seeking an abortion before the foetus attains viability; *Stenberg v. Carhart*, 530 U.S. 914 (2000), 28 June 2000, upholding *Roe v. Wade* and holding that under the Fourteenth Amendment, a state cannot pass an anti-abortion law that does not include an exception for the health of the mother. It also cannot pass a law that criminalizes partial-birth abortions unless it is thoroughly clear that it does not extend to other forms of abortion), or international bodies competent in respect of human rights questions pertaining to abortion (Committee on the Elimination of Discrimination against Women, *L.C. v. Peru*, CEDAW/C/50/D/22/2009, 4 November 2011, at 7.12–7.14, finding, among others, that "the lack of legislative and administrative measures regulating access to therapeutic abortion condemns women to legal insecurity in so far as protection of their rights is completely at the mercy of gender prejudices and stereotypes" – see 7.12). Neither did the adjudicating panel invoke the extensive case-law of the ECtHR on termination of pregnancy viewed from the perspective of Article 2 (See e.g. ECtHR (GC), *Vo v. France,* 8 July 2004, appl. no. 53924/00, *Mehmet Şentürk and Bekir Şentürk v. Turkey,* 9 April 2013, appl. no. 13423/09, or (GC) *Evans v. the United Kingdom*, 10 April 2007, appl. no. 6339/05 (at 54), all insisting generally on the "absence of any European consensus on the scientific and legal definition of the beginning of life"), Article 3 (See e.g. ECtHR, *R. R. v. Poland,* 26 May 2011, appl. no. 27617/04) or Article 8 (See e.g. ECtHR, *P. and S. v. Poland,* 30 October 2012, appl. no. 57375/08, *Tysiąc v. Poland,* 20 March 2007, appl. no. 5410/03, or (GC) *A, B and C v. Ireland,* 16 December 2010, appl. no. 25579/05) of the Convention, i.e. from the different angles that one might possibly see the competing interests at stake in such cases. Finally, no attention was paid in the "ruling" discussed here to voluminous statements, analysis and positions adopted by international human rights bodies such as the Human Rights Committee, the Committee on the Elimination of Discrimination against Women, the Committee against Torture (CAT Committee), the Committee on Economic, Social and Cultural Rights or the Committee on the Rights of the Child (Shah, Jacob, 2023, pp. 343-344).

The intellectual impoverishment of the "ruling" discussed in this chapter manifests, among many other features of its "reasoning", in that unlike so many (unmentioned therein) positions of international authorities or constitutional (judicial) courts' decisions mentioned above, it adopts an extremely biased and thus completely flawed viewpoint on the whole complexity of problems pertaining to fundamental rights and involved in the questions of legality of termination of pregnancy. The "reasoning" of the "ruling" is limited to the "foetal perspective", while missing the issue of the fundamental rights of a pregnant woman. The question whether, and to what extent, women should be allowed to terminate pregnancies is answered by referring strictly and exclusively to the (alleged) guarantee of pre-natal phase of life of an "unborn child", whereas women's rights such as dignity, privacy, or freedom from tortures and inhuman or degrading treatment were left unaddressed.

It is indeed disappointing that comparative or international references were not included in the "ruling" discussed here, and, as we shall see, instead the adjudicating panel chose to decorate its "argumentation" with random and inaccurate passages invoking that what it had seemingly believed to have been the state of international law.

## The "Judgment"

The ruling commented in this chapter was issued following the consideration of the motion by a group of Members of the Parliament requesting the Constitutional Tribunal to examine the compliance of Article 4a sec. 1 item 2 and Article 4a sec. 2, first sentence, of the Act of 7th January 1993 on family planning, protection of the human foetus and the conditions for the admissibility of termination of pregnancy, with Article 30 (this provision reads that „The inherent and inalienable dignity of a human shall be the source of freedom and human and civil rights. It is inviolable, and the respect of and the protection thereof shall be the duty of public authorities") of the Constitution of the Republic of Poland in that the former provisions legalize "eugenic practices" (one should clarify that the allegedly "eugenic practices" are understood in the "ruling" as the termination of pregnancy where "prenatal tests or other medical indications indicate a high probability of severe and irreversible impairment of the foetus or an incurable disease that threatens its life").in relation to an unborn child, thus denying it respect for and protection of human dignity, and possibly – in the event if the former provisions were found compatible with Article 30 of the Constitution – to examine the compliance of the same provisions of the Act on Family Planning with Article 38 in conjunction with Article 30 and Article 31 sec. 3 (this provision reads that „Restrictions on the exercise of constitutional freedoms and rights shall only be established by a statute and only when necessary in a democratic state for the protection of its security or public order, or for the protection of the environment, health or public morals, or the freedoms and rights of other persons") and with Article 38 (This provision reads that „The Republic of Poland shall ensure legal protection of life to every human being") in conjunction with Article 32 sec. 1 and 2 (these provisions read, respectively, that "Everyone is equal before the law. Everyone has the right to equal treatment by public authorities" and that "No one may be discriminated against in political, social or economic life for any reason") of the Constitution of the Republic of Poland by legalizing "eugenic practices" pertaining to the right to life of an unborn child and making the protection of the right to life of an unborn child dependent on its health condition, which constitutes prohibited direct discrimination. Furthermore, the applicants also requested a ruling on the compliance of the same provisions of the Family Planning Act with Article 38 in connection with Article 31 sec. 3 and in connection with Article 2 (this provision reads that "The Republic of Poland is a democratic state based on the rule of law implementing the principles of social justice") and Article 42 (this article provides that: „Only those who have committed an act prohibited under penalty by the law in force at the time of its commission are subject to criminal liability. This principle does not prevent punishment for an act that at the time of its commission constituted an offence under international law. Anyone against whom criminal proceedings are conducted has the right to defence at all stages of the proceedings. In particular, they may choose a defence attorney or, under the principles specified in the law, use a public defender. Everyone is presumed innocent until their guilt is established by a final court judgment") of the Constitution of the Republic of Poland by legalizing the termination of pregnancy without sufficient justification by the need to protect another constitutional value, right or freedom and by using unspecified criteria for this legalization, thus violating the constitutional guarantees for human life.

The adjudicating panel, by a majority vote (separate opinions, with different directions of argumentation, were submitted by L. Kieres, P. Pszczółkowski, Z. Jędrzejewski, M. Muszyński and J. Wyrembak) held that "Article 4a sec. 1 item 2 of the Act of 7 January 1993 on family planning, protection of the human foetus and the conditions for the admissibility of termination of pregnancy (…) is inconsistent with Article 38 in conjunction with Article 30 in conjunction with Article 31 sec. 3 of the Constitution of the Republic of Poland". Out of the chronicler's duty, and also to reflect the spirit of the times in which the "decision" was made and for the benefit of future generations, let us only add that in the issuance of the "ruling", apparently with a sense of joyful freedom from the principle of *nemo iudex in causa sua*, participated two former members of the Sejm (chamber of the Parliament) of the Republic of Poland, who had taken part in the (as noted by the dissenting judge L. Kieres) "voting on all draft amendments to the contested act, processed in the years 2012-2019", and "one of them was a signatory to the motion of the group of members of parliament initiating the proceedings in this case" (both quotations come from the dissenting opinion of Judge L. Kieres in case K 1/20). In other words, one of the judges assigned to this case has been simultaneously a petitioner of this very case. The other one „only" shaped the disputed law while deliberating and voting on it as a member of the Parliament. The "judge"-rapporteur of this case was Mr. Justyn Piskorski whose nomination to the Constitutional Court violated the Constitution and Article 6 ECHR (the right to a tribunal established by law).

Of course, the commented "ruling" uses, even more strongly than the Constitutional Tribunal's ruling in case K 26/96 (Ruling of the Constitutional Tribunal, Poland, May 28, 1997, K 26/96), terminology with a strong predominance of ideological over juridical provenance (e.g. "child in the prenatal period", "child in the prenatal phase of life", "eugenic nature [of the questioned legalizing premise] within the meaning of liberal eugenics", etc.). The narrative of the "judgment" reminds of a political manifesto rather than an ideologically restrained judicial reasoning.

## The Central Element of the "reasoning"

In a rather troublesome and exhausting attempt to establish the fundamental idea underlying the position of the adjudicating panel in case K 1/20, it seems that one can point to chapter III.3.3.3. of the reasoning *in fine*. The adjudicating panel, having reported on the discussion devoted to the provision concerning the protection of life as part of the work of the Constitutional Committee of the National Assembly (it was a body established in the early 1990' responsible for drafting the Constitution), came to the conclusion that "the intention of the legislator was – in the absence of *expressis verbis* indication in the Constitution of the temporal limits of human life and its legal protection or the exclusion of the Tribunal's jurisdiction in this respect – to leave to the Constitutional Tribunal the issue pertaining to the binding determination of the meaning of the concept of a human being on the basis of Article 38 of the Constitution". This is, let us note, probably the most original approach to the role of the constitutional court known not only to Polish but also to the universal practice of constitutional review. Let us rephrase that in the opinion of the adjudicating panel, it has become a "positive legislator" (a constitutional law-maker), filling, while explicitly performing the role of a substitute for the ordinary legislator, the decision-making spaces intentionally left (as expressly confirmed by the adjudicating panel) by the legislator. This thought could, let us add somewhat maliciously, be developed only a little in order to assume that in the face of such a dictum, freed by the bench adjudicating in case K 1/20 from the burden of doubts potentially arising from Article 10 sec. 2 of the Constitution (the principle of the separation of powers – Article 10 sec. 2 of the Constitution reads that "Legislative power is exercised by the Sejm and the Senate, executive power by the President of the Republic of Poland and the Council of Ministers, and judicial power by the courts and tribunals"), the ordinary legislator became an unnecessary element of the landscape of constitutional bodies of the state, abdicating – in the rather exotic opinion of the adjudicating bench – in favour of the constitutional court. Quite amusingly, this stance of the adjudicating panel could be easily criticized for exactly identical reasons as those advanced by the Reagan's Republican critics against *Roe v. Wade*, i.e. abusive judicial activism replacing the rule of the people with the judicial interpretative tyranny (Ziegler, 2018, p. 204).

This construction of the principle of democracy does not seem to be challengeable from the perspective of e.g. the ECHR, even though the said principle, or the democratic system as its "product", is "guaranteed by Article 3 of Protocol No. 1" (Costa, 2008, p. 5), because "the text of the Convention does not provide any significant clues as to the definition of the concept of *political democracy*, and the ECtHR has, through its case law, contributed to the clarification of this notion only in an indirect and oblique way, unsurprisingly dealing more with what can be called the "individual" dimension of democracy than addressing the obvious political implications" (Ninatti, Arcari, 2015, p. 182). In other words, the ECHR protects certain individual guarantees which amalgamate in a mechanism contributing towards the protection of the principle of democracy, but it does not, at least in the present state of interpretation of the Convention, protect democracy against the usurpation of the legislative power by judicial bodies. Nevertheless, the open and clear assumption of the power to decide on the content of the law by the constitutional court seems uncommon from the point of view of the axiological foundations of the Convention, an indispensable element of which is the respect for the principle of democracy.

## Abusive and Superficial Interpretations of International Law

The further reasoning of the adjudicating panel in case K 1/20 was devoted to determining the meaning of the term "human being" employed in Article 38 of the Constitution (protection of life to every human being). This part of the "reasoning" is characterised – let us put it clear – by intellectual poverty and ostentatiously shameless manipulations of the instruments quoted and some randomly chosen comments scarcely invoked.

In his essay on the procedural dimension of the rule of law, Jeremy Waldron pointed out that legal philosophers "tend to emphasize formal elements of the rule of law", one of them being to "rule by clear and determinate legal norms, norms whose meaning is not so obscure or contestable as to leave those who are subject to them at the mercy of official discretion" (Waldron, 2023, p. 160). Having made this remark at the outset, Waldron summarised what he called a "laundry list" of characteristics necessary for the rule of law and added "a list of procedural characteristics which are equally indispensable", naming as one of them "a right to hear reasons from the tribunal when it reaches its decision, which are responsive to the evidence and arguments" and remarked that "these requirements are often associated with terms such as *natural justice* and as such they are important parts of the rule of law" (Waldron, 2023, pp. 161-162). And when discussing the significance of the legal argumentation and predictable interpretation for the rule of law, he concluded that:

> *"[c]ourts, hearings and arguments – those aspects of law are not optional extras; they are integral parts of how law works; and they are indispensable to the package of law's respect for human agency. To say that we should value aspects of governance that promote the clarity and determinacy of rules for the sake of individual freedom, but not the opportunities for argumentation that a free and self-possessed individual is likely to demand, is to sell short what the rule of law rests upon: respect for the freedom and dignity of each person as an active intelligence" (Waldron, 2023, p. 176).*

Indeed, one cannot imagine the rule of law without a proper judicial argumentation: a methodologically accurate judicial interpretation allowing for precise, predictable and convincing determination of applicable rules. It is all the more important in case of constitutional courts deciding on the constitutionality of legislative provisions, where their findings have impact on the society as a whole and not "just" on the parties to a particular individual dispute. Instead of meticulously and carefully, with the utmost precision, fine-tuning the interpretation of the provisions of the Constitution, in the "ruling" analysed in this chapter the adjudicating panel attempted to make the impression that Poland is actually internationally bound to prohibit abortion and opened this "argumentation" by holding *ex cathedra* (without any relevant substantiation) that "firstly, the legal obligation to protect human life in the prenatal phase is based on the acts of international law by which the Republic of Poland is bound". Let us analyse in some greater details which international instruments were cruelly abused and how.

## Article 6 ICCPR (Or Rather, What the Panel Thought it Meant)

For this purpose, a reference was made to Article 6 ICCPR. Let us recall that Article 6(1) ICCPR reads that (italics added)„Every human being has the inherent right to life. This right shall be protected by law. No one shall be arbitrarily deprived of his life" (in French: "Le droit à la vie est inhérent à la personne humaine. Ce droit doit être protégé par la loi. Nul ne peut être arbitrairement privé de la vie", in Spanish: "El derecho a la vida es inherente a la persona humana. Este derecho estará protegido por la ley. Nadie podrá ser privado de la vida arbitrariamente", in Russian: "Право на жизнь есть неотъемлемое право каждого человека. Это право охраняется законом. Никто не может быть произвольно лишен жизни"). The adjudicating panel held in that context that "although unambiguous statements on the subjective scope of this right are avoided", yet the fact that the term "human being" was only employed (apart from the preamble) in Article 6 ICCPR, is sufficient to conclude that "under the ICCPR, a "human being" should be understood as a human being, both before and after birth".

Let us remarks on the outset of critical analysis of this fragment of the "reasoning" that the adjudicating panel failed to consider the general rule of interpretation of treaties, as codified in Article 31 VCLT ("A treaty shall be interpreted in good faith in accordance with the ordinary meaning to be given to the terms of the treaty in their context and in the light of its object and purpose"), but instead the "argumentation" was limited to a linguistic analysis of the ICCPR, for some unknown reason, in the Polish language which is not an authentic language of the Covenant (see Article 53, paragraph 1 of the ICCPR, reading that „The present Covenant, of which the Chinese, English, French, Russian and Spanish texts are equally authentic, shall be deposited in the archives of the United Nations"), failing in consequence to notice the significant discrepancy in the wording of Article 6, paragraph 1, ICCPR in the authentic languages of the Covenant: the term *human being* was employed in the English version of the provision, while in the French and Spanish versions it was phrased as "human person" (personne humaine, persona humana), but in the Russian version the term "man" („человек") was used and similar term was employed in the Arabic language ( .), while in the (simplified) Chinese version it was simply "everyone"( ).

and finally failing to draw any conclusions as required by Article 33(4) VCLT (or actually failing to notice the very "existence" of this norm of universal customary international law). Let us recall that Article 33(4) VCLT reads that „Except where a particular text prevails in accordance with paragraph 1, when a comparison of the authentic texts discloses a difference of meaning which the application of articles 31 and 32 does not remove, the meaning which best reconciles the texts, having regard to the object and purpose of the treaty, shall be adopted". The grammatic "analysis" of the text of a treaty in a language that is not an authentic language of that treaty brings about nothing relevant and constitutes a pointless effort since it clarifies literally nothing.

Also, the General Comment No. 36 of 2018 was not even noticed (Human Rights Committee, 2018) which is an important cognitive source in determining the meaning of the right to life in the context of termination of pregnancy, nor was any attention paid to the *travaux préparatoires* of the Covenant as supplementary means of interpretation, which – by the way – have been collected and interestingly commented on in the easily available literature (United Nations General Assembly 1955, pp. 82-85; also – *passim* – Joseph, Schultz, Castan, 2004), or the circumstances of the treaty's conclusion (see Article 32 VCLT; also Le Bouthillier, 2011, pp. 852-858). Finally, not a single piece of scholarly writing was noticed by the adjudicating panel, nor any international(e.g. Human Rights Committee, 2005; also Human Rights Committee, 2016, where it held that "The Committee notes the author's claim that the State party's criminalization of abortion subjected her to a gender-based stereotype of the reproductive role of women primarily as mothers, and that stereotyping her as a reproductive instrument subjected her to discrimination. The Committee considers that the differential treatment to which the author was subjected in relation to other similarly situated women failed to adequately take into account her medical needs and socioeconomic circumstances and did not meet the requirements of reasonableness, objectivity and legitimacy of purpose. Accordingly, the Committee concludes that the failure of the State party to provide the author with the services that she required constituted discrimination and violated her rights under article 26 of the Covenant" – at 7.11.) or domestic case-law.

These obvious and astonishing technical deficiencies make the comments of the adjudicating panel in case K 1/20, concerning the interpretation of the concept of "human being" as employed in Article 6 ICCPR, devoid of any relevant substantive value and erred at a rudimentary ("schoolboy") level. Let us clarify here that the error of the adjudicating panel cannot be justified by the fact that such, let's call it, oversimplifications also affected the views expressed at the scholarly level in Poland (Czech, 2011, in chapter 4, entitled, quite amusingly, „The Science of the Origin of Human Existence and the Judge's "Private" View", in Polish: *Nauka o początkach istnienia istoty ludzkiej a „prywatny" pogląd sędziego,* where the reader can learn, for example, that "the view that a human being exists from the moment of conception is also accepted in the case law", with the only "case law" cited by the author being the judgment of the Constitutional Tribunal in case K 26/96. Unfortunately, the author's considerations did not include either the achievements of the Human Rights Committee or the ECtHR, as one should assume probably because they do not constitute "case law" (which could be objectively defended, and even then without any hope of winning this fight, only in relation to the Human Rights Committee).

However, the author did not provide the reasons for such disqualification, which did not prevent him from *ex cathedra* criticizing the common court that issued the judgment he criticized, while holding that a judge should "know the provisions of the law and case law in relation to the problem of the beginnings of the existence of a human being". Probably the same remark should also be made to the author of such radical, and unfortunately poorly sourced, views). The adjudicating panel was bound to provide for methodologically proper interpretation of a treaty if it decided to invoke it. Instead, it expressed a few inapt and useless remarks with no meritorious significance whatsoever.

## Article 2 ECHR (Or Rather, Again, What the Panel Thought it Meant)

The same critical remarks apply to the comments pertaining to Article 2 ECHR (also sadly not spared by the adjudicating panel), where the "reasoning" of the adjudicating panel was limited to the following statement: "Similarly, Article 2, paragraph 1 of the Convention for the Protection of Human Rights and Fundamental Freedoms, signed in Rome on 4 November 1950, subsequently amended by Protocols No. 3, 5 and 8 and supplemented by Protocol No. 2 (…) provides that *Everyone's right to life shall be protected by law. No one shall be deprived of his life intentionally save in the execution of a sentence of a court following his conviction of a crime for which this penalty is provided by law*".

In this respect, perhaps the most glaring evidence of an abuse of interpretation is the failure of the adjudicating panel to note the judgment of the ECtHR which is of a paramount importance for the interpretation of the said provision of the Convention in the context discussed in the "ruling", namely *Vo v. France* (ECtHR, Grand Chamber, 8 July 2004, *Vo v. France,* appl. no. 53924/00), where the Grand Chamber clearly held that "Article 2 of the Convention is silent as to the temporal limitations of the right to life and, in particular, does not define "everyone" ("*toute personne*") whose "life" is protected by the Convention" (*Vo v. France,* at 75) and that "the issue of when the right to life begins comes within the margin of appreciation which the Court generally considers that States should enjoy in this sphere, notwithstanding an evolutive interpretation of the Convention" (*Vo v. France,* at 82). At the same time, the ECtHR held in *A., B., and C. v. Ireland* that "there is indeed a consensus amongst a substantial majority of the Contracting States of the Council of Europe towards allowing abortion on broader grounds than accorded under Irish law" (ECtHR [Grand Chamber], 16 December 2010, *A., B. and C. v. Ireland,* appl. no. 25579/05, at 235) and "given this consensus amongst a substantial majority of the Contracting States, it is not necessary to look further to international trends and views" (Ibidem), although it concluded (somewhat inconsequently) that "the

Court does not consider that this consensus decisively narrows the broad margin of appreciation of the State" (*A., B. and C. v. Ireland,* at 236). Judges Rozakis, Tulkens, Fura, Hirvelä, Malinverni and Poalelungi rightly noted in their dissent that:

*"According to the Convention case-law, in situations where the Court finds that a consensus exists among European States on a matter touching upon a human right, it usually concludes that that consensus decisively narrows the margin of appreciation which might otherwise exist if no such consensus were demonstrated. This approach is commensurate with the "harmonising" role of the Convention's case-law. Indeed, one of the paramount functions of the case-law is to gradually create a harmonious application of human rights protection, cutting across the national boundaries of the Contracting States and allowing the individuals within their jurisdiction to enjoy, without discrimination, equal protection regardless of their place of residence. The harmonising role, however, has limits. One of them is the following: in situations where it is clear that on a certain aspect of human rights protection, European States differ considerably in the way that they protect (or do not protect) individuals against conduct by the State, and the alleged violation of the Convention concerns a relative right which can be balanced – in accordance with the Convention – against other rights or interests also worthy of protection in a democratic society, the Court may consider that States, owing to the absence of a European consensus, have a (not unlimited) margin of appreciation to themselves balance the rights and interests at stake. Hence, in those circumstances the Court refrains from playing its harmonising role, preferring not to become the first European body to "legislate" on a matter still undecided at European level. Yet in the case before us a European consensus (and, indeed, a strong one) exists. We believe that this will be one of the rare times in the Court's case-law that Strasbourg considers that such consensus does not narrow the broad margin of appreciation of the State concerned" (A, B and C v. Ireland, dissent, at 5 and 6).*

Instead of drawing any conclusions from this highly controversial and vividly disputed judgment (and the minority's dissent), the adjudicating panel chose not to notice it at all.

## Article 2 of the EU Charter of Fundamental Rights (Or Rather, Again and Again, What the Panel Thought it Meant)

Further, the same strong criticism applies to the "comments" of the adjudicating panel on Article 2 of the Charter of Fundamental Rights of the European Union. The reference to the ChFR of the EU also can be quoted in "extenso" (as it is shockingly short): "Pursuant to Article 2(1) of the Charter of Fundamental Rights of the

European Union of 7 December 2000 (OJ EU C 202, 7.06.2016, p. 389; hereinafter referred to as: CFR), *[e]veryone has the right to life*".

In relation to the ChFR the adjudicating panel limited itself to selectively quoting the fundamental Polish commentary on the Charter, while holding that "the position according to which the right to life does not serve a human being who has not (yet) been born cannot be accepted, because it is clearly contrary to both the principle of human dignity, on which the right to life is based, and to the essence and function of the right guaranteed by Article 2 of the Charter" (Quotation comes from the reasoning in case K 1/20; see Kamiński, Wróbel. 2020, item 16 on Article 2), ignoring, however, other arguments of this commentary that did not fit the thesis adopted by the adjudicating panel, including the following: "This does not mean that the right to life applies to the period starting from conception" (In Polish: „Nie oznacza to jeszcze, że prawo do życia dotyczy okresu od zapłodnienia"). Of course, no conclusions at all were drawn from the explanations to the Charter (contrary to Article 6 TEU), which clarify that "[Article 2 ChFR and Articles 2 ECHR and Article 1 of Protocol No 6 to the ECHR] have the same meaning and the same scope, in accordance with Article 52(3) of the Charter", nor from the significance of the relationship between Article 2 ChFR and Article 2 ECHR, as required by Article 52(3) of the Charter (which, moreover, would have forced the adjudicating panel to reach for the "inconvenient" Strasbourg case-law).

## Some Randomly Chosen Other Provisions of International Law (Or Rather...)

In its hopeless and clumsy effort to outline the comparative legal context for the interpretation of Article 38 of the Constitution, the adjudicating panel did not miss the opportunity to refer to the Convention on the Rights of the Child (Article 1 and Article 6) and the Convention on the Rights of Persons with Disabilities (Article 10). Here, again, it (somewhat consequently, but still absolutely incorrectly at a rudimentary level) limited itself to insignificant linguistic observations, while referring, for unknown reasons, to the formulations used in the Polish (unauthentic) version of both of these conventions. Pursuant to Article 54 of the Convention on the Rights of the Child, "The original of the present Convention, of which the Arabic, Chinese, English, French, Russian and Spanish texts are equally authentic, shall be deposited with the Secretary-General of the United Nations. In witness thereof the undersigned plenipotentiaries, being duly authorized thereto by their respective Governments, have signed the present Convention".

As regards Article 1 CRC, the adjudicating panel's observations (supported additionally by the reference to Article 6 of the CRC and Recital 9 of the preamble to that Convention) that "significantly, for the purposes of that Convention, a *child* means any human being below the age of eighteen years, unless, in accordance with the law applicable to the child, the child reaches the age of majority earlier (Article 1)", were clearly erred, because this provision cannot, if correctly interpreted, serve to prove the thesis put forward in the justification about the alleged "prenatal" dimension of the definition of "child" expressed therein. In its superficial argumentation, the adjudicating panel did not take into account the interpretative achievements concerning the Convention on the Rights of the Child, the course of the *travaux preparatoires* and the importance that the parties to the Convention attached to the relationship between the reference to the Declaration of the Rights of the Child in Recital 9 of the preamble and the wordings of Article 1 and Article 6 of the CRC. Without going into lengthy arguments, let us just briefly point out that during the negotiations, proposals were made to include in Article 1 of the CRC the prenatal phase in the definition, as well as to include, directly in the definition, birth as the moment from which "childhood begins", but ultimately the compromise proposal of the Moroccan delegation was accepted, which gave the final shape to the wording of Article 1 of the CRC. As for the wording of Recital 9 of the Preamble, it was also the result of a compromise reached after stormy negotiations, and actually proposed by – funnily enough – the Polish delegation. As a result, when read together, Article 1 and Article 6 of the CRC and recital 9 of its Preamble leave the parties to this Convention free to determine in their national legislation the issue of including in the concept of "child" also the prenatal phase of human development (Detrick, 1999, pp. 51-57 and 133-136; also: Archard, Tobin, 2019, pp. 25-27). Therefore, these provisions are actually useless for demonstrating the thesis pushed intrusively by the adjudicating panel, that they were intended to constitute an argument in favour of the "prenatal" scope of the definition of "child" in the CRC and the protection of its right to life. But to know that and avoid these schoolboy errors, the adjudicating panel should have referred, as required by the general rule of interpretation of treaties, to the context, object and purpose of the CRC provisions which it instead chose to interpret in a violently deficient way, and established the genuine intention of the parties expressed in the text of this treaty.

## Some Other "Thoughts" of the Adjudicating Panel

The adjudicating panel, still desperately searching for the justification of its standing being nothing more than substituting the parliamentary decision with its own judgment, added that "the fact that the protection of human life is available in the prenatal phase is also reflected in ordinary legislation". Of course, the way of understanding the terms used in the Constitution, as given in ordinary legislation, is of no great importance for the interpretation of a provision of the Constitution. As the Constitutional Tribunal rightly pointed out:

*"When interpreting constitutional concepts, definitions formulated in lower-level acts cannot have a binding meaning that determines the manner of their interpretation. As has been repeatedly emphasized in the case law of the Tribunal, constitutional concepts are autonomous in nature with respect to the applicable legislation. This means that the meaning of individual terms adopted in statutes cannot determine the manner of interpreting constitutional provisions, because then the guarantees contained in them would lose any meaning. On the contrary, constitutional norms should impose the manner and direction of interpreting the provisions of other acts. The starting point for the interpretation of the constitution is the historically shaped and established in the legal doctrine understanding of the terms used in the text of this legal act" (judgment of the Constitutional Tribunal, Poland, April 27, 2005, P 1/05, and the case-law referred to therein; see also: Smolak, 2016, passim).*

This passage of the adjudicating panel's reasoning is therefore also incorrect.

The above "considerations" led the adjudicating panel to the strong conviction that "a child not yet born, as a man (Pol. "człowiek", which is the term describing a human being regardless of sex – add. MG) – a human being who is entitled to inherent and inalienable dignity, is a subject of the right to life, and the legal system – in accordance with Article 38 of the Constitution – must guarantee appropriate protection of this central value, without which this subjectivity would be erased". At the same time, however, the adjudicating panel countered this position with a slightly – as it should probably be described, if we were to follow the ideological terminology in which the "argumentation" was dressed – "liberal-eugenic" statement that "the constitutional and legal subjectivity of a child in the period before birth does not mean, however, that it is fully entitled to protection of all rights and freedoms guaranteed by the Constitution. They are related to a specific level of psychophysical and social maturity". If this remark of the panel were to also apply to the right to life, to which the preceding sentence refers, the impression would be created that the scope of protection granted by Article 38 of the Constitution would apparently be decided by "psychophysical and social maturity". Such an understanding of the position of the adjudicating panel would provoke conclusions, perhaps even dangerous for some members of the panel, that the degree of a person's "social maturity" would determine the scope of their right to life. Let us assume, however, that this fragment of the position of the adjudicating panel was just another lapse of judgment, from which the justification of the adjudicating panel's view was actually entirely built.

The further "considerations" of the adjudicating panel in the discussed case were a "natural consequence" of the adopted assumption about the adequacy of the application of the constitutional model in the form of Article 38 of the Constitution of the Republic of Poland to the assessment of the challenged regulation, referring to the embryopathological premise of the admissibility of the termination of pregnancy

(Article 4a sec. 1 item 2 of the Family Planning Act). In particular, the adjudicating panel found that the aforesaid provision of the Family Planning Act does not allow for the assumption that a high probability of severe and irreversible impairment of the foetus or an incurable disease threatening its life is to constitute a basis for an automatic presumption of violation of the well-being of a pregnant woman, while the mere indication of the potential burden of such defects on the child is of a "eugenic nature". The said provision lacks reference to measurable criteria for violating the mother's well-being justifying termination of pregnancy, i.e. a situation in which it would not be legally possible to require her to sacrifice a given legal value, and as a result, it held that "the limitation of the legal protection of life by means of [the reviewed provision] does not meet the requirements of usefulness, necessity and proportionality in the strict sense".

The judgment in question does not contain any reference, in the part covering the relationship between the good sacrificed (the good of protecting the fetus) and the good protected (the "good of the mother"), to define what the "good of the mother" is (let us note here that using the phrase "*mother's* good" in reference to the rights and freedoms of a woman who is pregnant but would like to terminate her pregnancy is another semantic and ideological abuse by the authors of the reasoning. Namely, a woman who is pregnant is not a "mother", but a pregnant woman. Since she desires to abort the foetus, she does not want and does not intend to become the mother of the future child. Semantically placing her at this stage and against her will in the role of "mother" is of course a deliberate move that serves to unjustifiably turn the hostility of the readers of the "ruling" (the general public) against such a woman. In our civilisation, parents of a child are – and rightly so – expected to make the most far-reaching sacrifices for the sake of their offspring. Therefore, describing a pregnant woman who seeks to terminate her pregnancy with the word "mother" is intended to shape the image of a parent who, contrary to our civilisational canon, not so much neglects their "parental" duties as wants to kill her own "child"). This is another structural and logical defect in the adjudicating panel's deliberations, which consists in conducting the proportionality test required by Article 31, Section 3 of the Constitution, without defining the legal values justifying interference with (according to the adjudicating panel) the "right to life" of the foetus as a "human being". Applying any proportionality test requires that the aim pursued must be first defined before the relation between that aim and the measures employed for its protection is measured. If one fails to do it, the „reasoning" turns into a useless prolixity.

Leaving aside the issue of the applicability of Article 38 of the Constitution as a model of constitutional review – which we deny – this element of the reasoning also makes the deliberations of the panel devoid of substantive value. But this does not, of course, prevent us from attempting to indicate the constitutional values that fill the concept of the "good of the mother" used by the adjudicating panel to – somehow and rather hopelessly – fill in the content of the "ruling". In this respect, one could indicate not only privacy (Article 47 of the Constitution) and reproductive autonomy (ibid.), but also, above all, dignity (Article 30 of the Constitution), as a principle that should be referred to when interpreting the meaning of other constitutional guarantees, including the guarantee of the right to privacy (dissenting opinion of Judge Marek Safjan annexed to the judgment of the Constitutional Tribunal, Poland, October 30, 2006, P 10/06). As indicated by the Constitutional Tribunal, "being the source of individual rights and freedoms, the concept of dignity determines the way in which the state understands and implements them. The prohibition of violating human dignity is absolute and applies to everyone. On the other hand, the obligation to respect and protect dignity has been imposed on the public authorities of the state. Consequently, all actions of public authorities should, on the one hand, take into account the existence of a certain sphere of autonomy, within which a person can fully realize themselves socially, and on the other hand, such actions cannot lead to the creation of legal or factual situations that deprive the individual of a sense of dignity" (Judgment of the Constitutional Tribunal, Poland, April 4, 2001, K 11/00). The possibility of a future assessment of the anti-abortion regulation in the context of these values, which are due to entities that have not been noticed so far in the analyses conducted by the Constitutional Tribunal in case K 26/96 (as rightly pointed out by Judge L. Garlicki in a dissenting opinion to this judgment) and by the adjudicating panel in the case discussed here – i.e. women – seems to be an open question.

## CONCLUSION

As we explained, the adjudicating panel who issued the "judgment" in the "abortion case" K 1/20, committed a series of grave "crimes" against interpretation of international law, let alone the Polish Constitution. To mention but a few, it failed to consider rules of customary international law, codified in the VCLT, concerning the interpretation of treaties, it operated on unauthentic texts of treaties which it chose to invoke (we intentionally abstain from employing the term "analysed"), or it failed to consider relevant international case law providing a useful point of reference in the interpretation of treaties. In the case of the ECHR, this basically means that the panel failed to "secure to everyone within [its] jurisdiction the rights and freedoms defined in Section I of this Convention" since it is precisely the ECtHR who is in charge of providing for authoritative interpretation of the Convention, because (as stipulated in Article 32 ECHR) "the jurisdiction of the Court shall extend to all matters concerning the interpretation and application of the Convention and the Protocols thereto" (Heri, 2024, p. 9).

It is also striking and saddening that the adjudicating panel decided to overlook some other instruments possibly shedding light on the issue at hand, such as the UN Convention on the Elimination of All Forms of Discrimination against Women, or international authorities such as *K.L. v. Peru* or *Mellet v. Ireland*, referred to above.

Instead of providing a meritorious and in-depth analysis of international law and practice, the adjudicating panel chose to decorate its erred (even when it comes to national Constitution) "reasoning" with random, defective and pointless references to what it entirely wrongly believed to have been international law and practice. This is what we call manipulation or abusive interpretation and this is because one cannot assume that the deficits of rudimentary knowledge of international law could so devastatingly impact law graduates claiming to be constitutional judges. It would actually shameful if it was not so amusingly helpless. Instead of strengthening the persuasive power of its findings, the adjudicating panel produced a teaching material for the course on "how not to interpret international law". It would be frightening too, indeed, should this "judgment" be an actual, lawful judgment, and not just some irrelevant, yet hilarious, piece of teaching material without normative significance.

## REFERENCES

Archard, D., & Tobin, J. (2019). The Definition of a Child. In J. Tobin (Ed.). *The UN Convention on the Rights of the Child.* Oxford: Oxford University Press.

CEDAW, *L.C. v. Peru*, CEDAW/C/50/D/22/2009, 4 November 2011.

Chmaj, M., . . .. (2020). Ekspertyza prawna w przedmiocie oceny prawnej orzeczenia TK z 22 października 2020 r. sygn. K 1/20, sporządzona w ramach Zespołu Doradców ds. kontroli konstytucyjności prawa przy Marszałku Senatu X kadencji. Retrieved October 9, 2024 from www.senat.gov.pl, pp. 1-43.

Costa, J.-P. (2008). *The links between democracy and human rights under the case-law of the European Court of Human Rights*. Paper presented in Helsinki on 5 June 2008. Retrieved September 12, 2024 from https://www.echr.coe.int/documents/d/echr/Speech_20080605_Costa_Helsinki_ENG, pp. 1-8.

Czech, B. (2011). Wykładnia prawa i niezawisłość sędziowska a zdrowy rozsądek (zagadnienia wybrane). In Gudowski, J., & Weitz, K. (Eds.), *Aurea praxis. Aurea theoria. Księga pamiątkowa ku czci Profesora Tadeusza Erecińskiego. Tom II.* LexisNexis.

Detrick, S. (1999). *A Commentary on the United Nations Convention on the Rights of the Child.* Martinus Nijhoff Publishers. DOI: 10.1163/9789004638693

Heri, C. (2024). Deference, Dignity and 'Theoretical Crisis': Justifying ECtHR Rights Between Prudence and Protection. *Human Rights Law Review*, 24, 1–19.

Human Rights Committee. (2005). K. L. v. Peru. 24 October 2005. CCPR/C/85/D/1153/2003.

Human Rights Committee (2018). General comment No. 36 (2018) on article 6 of the International Covenant on Civil and Political Rights, on the right to life, 30 October 2018. CCPR/C/GC/36,.

Human Rights Committee. (2016). Mellet v. Ireland. 31 March 2016. CCPR/C/116/D/2324/2013.

Joseph, S., Schultz, J., & Castan, M. (2024). *The International Covenant on Civil and Political Rights. Cases, Materials, and Commentary*. Oxford University Press.

Kamiński, I. C., & Wróbel, A. (2020). *Karta Praw Podstawowych Unii Europejskiej. Komentarz* (Wróbel, A., Ed.). C.H. Beck.

Kelsen, H. (2007). *General Theory of Law and State* (transl. by A. Wedberg). Clark: The Lawbook Exchange Ltd.

Kelsen, H. (2015). Wesen und Entwicklung der Staatsgerichtsbarkeit. In L. Vinx, *The Guardian of the Constitution : Hans Kelsen and Carl Schmitt on the Limits of Constitutional Law*. Cambridge: Cambridge University Press.

Le Bouthillier, Y. (2011). Article 32 Supplementary means of interpretation. In Corten, O., & Klein, P. (Eds.), *The Vienna Convention on the Law of Treaties: A Commentary*. Oxford University Press.

Ninatti, S., & Arcari, M. (2015). Patterns of Democracy In The Case Law of The EU Court of Justice And The European Court of Human Rights. *Polish Yearbook of International Law*, XXXV, 171–192.

Sadurski, W. (2019). *Poland's Constitutional Breakdown*. Oxford University Press. DOI: 10.1093/oso/9780198840503.001.0001

Shah, P. K., & Jacob, J. (2023). Beyond abortion decriminalization: human rights perspectives on the role of law in creating enabling environments for abortion access. In Ziegler, M. (Ed.), *The Research Handbook on International Abortion Law* (pp. 343–373). Edward Elgar Publishing Limited. DOI: 10.4337/9781839108150.00030

Smolak, M. (2016). *Wykładnia Konstytucji. Aktualne problemy i tendencje*. Wolter Kluwer.

Tobin, J. (2019). *The UN Convention on the Rights of the Child: A Commentary*. Oxford: Oxford University Press.

United Nations General Assembly (1955). *Draft International Covenants on Human Rights. Annotation prepared by the Secretary-General*, document of 1 July 1955, A/2929.

Waldron, J. (2023). *The Rule of Law and the Importance of Procedure* (in) *Thoughtfulness and the Rule of Law*, Cambridge-London: Harvard University Press.

Ziegler, M. (2018). *Beyond Abortion: Roe V. Wade and the Battle for Privacy*. Harvard University Press.

# Chapter 3
# Revisiting the Paradigm of Abortion-Related Reproductive Health Laws in the European Union

**Ravisha Sodha**
*Rajasthan High Court, Jodhpur, India*

**Hemendra Singh**
https://orcid.org/0000-0003-1160-8284
*O.P. Jindal Global University, Sonipat, India*

## ABSTRACT

*This chapter provides a detailed examination of abortion-related reproductive health laws within the European Union, focusing on their historical development, current legal frameworks, and the socio-economic factors that influence access to abortion services. It explores the diverse range of abortion laws across EU member states, highlighting the contrast between liberal approaches in countries such as Sweden and France and restrictive policies in nations like Poland and Hungary. The chapter also considers the impact of judicial interventions on shaping these laws and the broader implications for reproductive rights. Through this comprehensive analysis, the chapter aims to shed light on the complexities of abortion law within the EU and its relevance to women's reproductive health.*

DOI: 10.4018/979-8-3693-7837-3.ch003

## INTRODUCTION

The issue of abortion and reproductive health rights has long been a point of contention across European Union (EU) countries, with each nation reflecting a complex interplay of cultural, religious, legal, and political factors. In recent years, abortion laws across Europe have gained renewed attention due to evolving societal norms, increasing awareness of gender rights, and a growing emphasis on health as a fundamental human right. Countries within the EU demonstrate diverse approaches to abortion, from liberal frameworks that emphasize individual autonomy and freedom of choice, to more restrictive policies that focus on moral, religious, or cultural opposition to the practice. This spectrum of laws has ignited debates not only within national borders but also at the international level, where European policies on reproductive health are scrutinized for their impact on both women's rights and broader societal welfare (Mishtal, 2014).

Recent developments, such as the legalization of abortion in Ireland in 2018 and the tightening of abortion restrictions in Poland in 2020, have brought the issue of reproductive rights to the forefront of public discourse (Hogan, 2021). These contrasting approaches underscore the ongoing tension between progressive and conservative ideologies within the EU. On one hand, countries like France and Sweden continue to advance more liberal policies, providing broad access to abortion and reproductive healthcare services. On the other hand, countries such as Poland and Hungary have introduced more restrictive measures, placing greater limitations on abortion access and often aligning these policies with religious or traditional values (Hussein et al, 2018). These opposing trends reflect a broader societal struggle over the role of the state in regulating personal reproductive choices, and they raise important questions about the universality of reproductive rights within the EU.

A growing body of literature explores the impact of these divergent policies on women's health outcomes and broader social implications. Studies indicate that restrictive abortion laws are often linked to higher rates of unsafe abortions, which can result in severe health complications and increased maternal mortality rates (Berer, 2017). Conversely, more liberal policies that facilitate access to safe abortion services have been associated with improved reproductive health outcomes and greater gender equality (Sedghet al., 2016). The literature also highlights the intersectionality of reproductive rights, emphasizing how socio-economic status, geographic location, and ethnicity can influence access to reproductive healthcare. For instance, women from marginalized communities in countries with restrictive abortion laws face disproportionate barriers, compounding existing inequalities (Pheterson & Azize, 2005).

Moreover, the role of international human rights frameworks in shaping national abortion policies has been a focal point of academic discussion. The European Court of Human Rights (ECHR) and international treaties, such as the Convention on the Elimination of All Forms of Discrimination Against Women (CEDAW), have played significant roles in challenging restrictive abortion laws and advocating for reproductive rights as fundamental human rights (Zampas & Gher, 2008). However, the enforcement of these international standards often encounters resistance at the national level, particularly in countries where religious and cultural values strongly oppose liberal abortion policies.

The primary objective of this chapter is to explore how strengthening abortion-centric laws from an all-inclusive, comprehensive perspective can cater to the evolving needs of society. By examining both liberal and restrictive approaches, this analysis seeks to address key concerns about the accessibility, safety, and legality of abortion in various EU countries. A critical examination of existing laws is essential to understanding how these frameworks either support or hinder reproductive rights. The chapter will investigate how liberal approaches highlight the importance of individual freedom and autonomy in reproductive health decisions, while restrictive policies often emphasize societal, religious, or moral concerns about the sanctity of life.

The chapter also aims to investigate how a balanced approach one that incorporates the strengths of both liberal and restrictive policies can potentially prevent the abuse of reproductive health rights while ensuring that individuals retain their fundamental freedoms. Moreover, it will examine how the intersection of legal, cultural, and social factors influences the enforcement and success of these laws, and how global perspectives on reproductive health can shape future legislative developments within the EU. The ultimate goal is to offer insights into the ways in which the legal landscape of abortion in Europe can be improved to better serve both individual and societal needs.

The scope of this chapter extends beyond a purely legal analysis to include the cultural, social, and ethical dimensions that shape abortion laws across the EU. The chapter will examine the historical evolution of these laws, with a focus on key legislative milestones that have either expanded or restricted access to abortion services. It will also consider contemporary debates surrounding reproductive health, including the role of the judiciary, healthcare policies, and international human rights obligations. Furthermore, the chapter will explore the significance of an all-inclusive legal perspective that considers not only the legal text but also the practical implementation of laws in diverse social and cultural contexts. In particular, attention will be given to how regional disparities, such as those between Northern, Southern, Eastern, and Western EU countries, contribute to differing interpretations and applications of abortion laws. The chapter will emphasize the need for an integrated legal framework that accommodates the diversity of EU member states while ensuring the protection of reproductive rights for all individuals.

At the international level, the chapter will address how EU abortion laws serve as a model for other countries and regions that are grappling with similar reproductive health issues. By examining the EU's approach to balancing individual rights with societal values, this chapter will provide a comparative perspective that highlights the global implications of European abortion laws.

To achieve these objectives, the chapter will be organized into several key sections. The first section will provide a historical overview of abortion laws in Europe, tracing their evolution from ancient times to the present day. This will include a discussion of major legislative milestones, such as the UK's Offences Against the Person Act (1861) and the legalization of abortion in Sweden (1975) and Ireland (2018). The section will also examine the influence of feminist movements, religious institutions, and social reformers in shaping public opinion and legal frameworks surrounding abortion.

The second section will delve into contemporary abortion laws in various EU countries, offering a comparative analysis of liberal and restrictive approaches. This will include case studies from countries such as France, Spain, Italy, and Poland, providing insight into how different legal frameworks impact access to reproductive healthcare. The section will also explore the role of the judiciary in interpreting and enforcing abortion laws, with a focus on recent rulings from the European Court of Human Rights and the EU Commission.

The third section will focus on the social and economic factors that influence reproductive health and abortion, including access to healthcare, geographical disparities, and the role of healthcare professionals. It will also address the impact of economic inequality and cultural attitudes on the availability and quality of abortion services. Finally, the chapter will conclude with a comparative analysis of abortion laws within the EU and beyond, drawing lessons from countries such as the USA, Japan, China, and India. This global perspective will highlight the similarities and differences in how nations approach reproductive rights, offering recommendations for future reforms in the European legal landscape.

Overall, this chapter will provide a thorough examination of abortion-related reproductive health laws in the European Union, offering a nuanced understanding of the complex legal, social, and cultural factors that shape these laws. By drawing on historical, legal, and international perspectives, the chapter will contribute to ongoing discussions about the future of reproductive rights in Europe and beyond.

## HISTORICAL PARADIGM OF HEALTH CARE LAWS RELATING TO ABORTION

In search of the traces of Abortion or related activities, the farthest that we can go down the historical lane is up to the pre-historic Europe. For reference, history of Europe is generally divided into four parts, that is, the pre-historic Europe which dates back to the period prior to 800 BC; the Classical Antiquity period, that is, the period from 800 BC to 500 AD; The Middle Ages, that is, the period from 500 AD to 1500 AD and finally the Modern Era, that is, the period commencing from 1500 AD to the present day.

In the ancient civilizations of Europe being the Minoan and Mycenaean civilizations, the evidences found by the archeologists show that certain practices like physical removal of the fetus, use of herbs, oils or drugs, surgical methods and use of Abortion wine i.e. a drink prepared from several components of drugs, were prevalent as pregnancy abortive measures among the people (Ostergren & Bossé, 2004). These were not merely accidental discoveries meaning thereby that they highlight the prevalence of concept of abortion either in form of a natural circumstance or as a measure for a medical necessity. It was only in the $19^{th}$ century that the definite evidence of abortion being a practice condemned by the religious and legal fraternities is available (David, 1992).

As we trace the scenario pertaining to the history of abortion in Europe, we observe that gradually, the concept of abortion which was initially a recognized practice became restricted and later on banned in the different times. Initially the restrictions were in the form of selective abortion but later on considered illegal and complete ban due to it being associated to crime of homicide, and/or health issues.

### Abortion in Pre-Historic Europe

The pre-historic Europe (prior to 800 BC) was the period when 'Early Man' or the 'Stone Age Man' used to live. In these times, no direct evidence of abortion was identified however, the stone tools and the other related evidences found by the archeologists suggest that abortion related procedures were conducted in the pre-historic times as well. Various burial sites and the skeletal remains found therein from Europe suggest that still birth deserved equal respect as ordinary death and it in turn indicates that they accorded personality to the child in womb. The cave paintings, ancient stone scriptures and age-old texts indicate images of woman giving birth and the archeologists and historians indicate that certain practices similar to surgical child birth and related practices were prevalent in those times (Pagden, 2000).

In this period, many migrations from the European regions to the different parts of the world took place and these migrations show that information of medical use and practices also spread to different parts of the world. The stone inscriptions from the Egyptian tombs depict a woman nursing a child etc., which is indicative of an authority of a woman or rather a mother over such decisions. The social structure was matriarchal and thus women held authoritative positions in the society which gave spiritual and religious importance to all practices related to childbirth including abortion.

Papyrus is regarded as an ancient Egyptian text written at around 1500 BC which is suggestive of practices of induced abortion i.e. abortion with human intervention. It makes it clear that apart from the natural miscarriages, practices of using dates and honey mixed with drugs, tampons, plant based medicines, etc. were known procedures prevalent for abortion.

In pre- historic Europe, abortion was treated to be a part of healing practices. The aim of using the medical procedures, etc. was either to safeguard the mother and the child or to imply such measures so as to cure them or there was a need of medical emergency. It is also important to mention here that nothing is indicative of the fact that there was a difference in how the society saw women who had induced abortion or who had naturally miscarried.

## Abortion in the Period of Classical Antiquity: 800 BC to 500AD

This period is characterized by flourishing ancient Greece and Rome. This period ends with the end of Western Roman Empire (Carr-Saunders, 1922). During this period, the ancient societies moved towards moral and ethical issues of abortion. The religious beliefs of the people were on equal pedestal with the medical knowledge possessed by them and as a result both were given due credence while formulation of laws and accepted behavioral norms of the individuals in the society.

In these times, a paradigm shift was seen in the society, that is, it was moving from a matriarchal to a patriarchal one. The Greek and Roman philosophers accorded an inferior position to the female in the society. The daily lives of the females were much restricted. The age-old laws pertaining to the Greek and Romans highlight the fact that personality in law is accorded to a person only after birth and thus they did not regard the embryo to be alive (Yarmohammadi et al., 2013). The fetus was merely considered as a part of the woman's body. The concept that embryo also has life was included in the catholic teaching only about 150 years ago and is depictive of how technology can influence way of life and teachings. The philosophers and historians are divided on this belief as to at what stage the embryo would attain life.

According to Plato, abortion was necessary to keep the population in control but as per Aristotle, abortion should not be conducted once the fetus acquires soul. The Athenian laws allowed abortion of women who were sick and their life was at risk but this too was subjected to rounds of cumbersome social, ethical and religious scrutiny.

The Greek plays such as '*Lysistrata*' written by Aristophanes depicted that certain plant based drugs were used to induce abortion in young women. In Rome, *Silphium* was used to terminate an unwanted pregnancy, however, it got extinct due to its overuse. With lack of scientific evidence in this regard, it cannot be said with certainty as to how effective these practices were in proper termination of unwanted pregnancy. There are instances where use of these drugs have rather turned the course towards infertility which though may not have been intended.

In ancient Greece, abortion of a developing child in mother's womb was a legally recognized right of the father of the child and mother had no say in this as she was not allowed to abort the child without the permission of her husband (Georges, 1996). In case a woman was a slave, she had to seek permission of her master and at times, such abortions were forcefully imposed upon the women as well. Plato and Aristotle have regarded abortion as a means of birth control or rather population control. They believed that the state should be of a constant population size and thus with the permission of the father of the child, who was politically superior to the mother, the child could be aborted so that there would be less mouths to feed. In ancient Rome, practices such has physical strains on the body, poison like substances, pressure belts, etc. were used to induce abortion. It is not in contradiction with the Hippocratic Oath as well.

## Middle Ages (500AD TO 1500 AD) and Abortion

This period marks the beginning from collapse of the Roman Empire and is characterized of the Era of the Crusades, Rise of the Ancient church and the foundation stone of the idea of Modern day Europe (Cline, 2015). This was the period which marks the relationship between religion and Law and as to how both these had impact over each other and the society at large.

In the medieval times, the concept of abortion was not what it means today. It mostly referred to a miscarriage that occurred suddenly or without any reason after what was called 'quickening'. 'Quickening' refers to early signs of movement of the fetus experienced by a mother which fortifies the presence of a child in the womb and is often linked to potential beginning of a human life (Taylor, 2024). It was only after quickening being achieved that the embryo would be said to have a personality.

The historians, often regard the illegal abortions to be preferred by the people than the legalized abortions in the middle ages because the illegal ones were less expensive, quick and hassle- free as opposed to the legalized ones which non only striped the person of their respect in the eyes of the society but also took a lot of time for approval, were unsafe and caused them to undergo various procedures for purification, etc. that followed. They however posed risk of infections and hemorrhage due to absence of anesthesia and sterilization. Herbal drinks such as *Rue*, *Pennyroyal* and *Sage* were found to be useful in abortive practices. In these times, legal time periods of age of embryo were prescribed for abortion and it was an established norm that the sooner it is done, the better.

## Influence of Religion and culture

During these times, family held an important position in the society over personal or individual capacity. Bearing a child out of wedlock was shunned by the society and people had stricter views upon accepted norms and traditions. In these times various crimes such as infidelity or adultery, prostitution, etc. were on the rise. In order to hide their possible crimes, illegal abortions were conducted by the women. Islamic medicine as well to a certain extent impacted the European medicine.

The ancient Pope texts depict that in these times, any woman who would intentionally terminate her pregnancy post quickening, would be said to have committed a sin and would be guilty of crime and deserved punishment (McDougall, 2021). This punishment was only applicable on Christians and the women who had previously undergone abortion were also banned from entering religious places because of the ideology that they had the burden of their ill- doings which was not considered auspicious and rather polluting. Quickening was considered to play an important role in these matters as it would determine whether it was intentional act of the parties or a natural circumstance.

Soranus apart from Hippocrates supported abortion. As per his thought, abortion was possible within thirty days from acquiring pregnancy. He supported abortive practices such as herbal drinks, physical activities, etc. to be safer methods of abortion. The Byzantine Code was influenced by the religious teachings but supported the abortion and its focus was on protecting the fetus and the mother.

Since legal restrictions were employed in these times, people developed their own local practices and cultural norms. Apart from the pre-existing religious rituals for pregnancy and fertility, local remedies in form of potions and herbs for regular consumption were used by people to maintain their reproductive health. However, these often led to chronic illnesses and due to established taboos in the society, women had a lack of access to reproductive health care.

## Abortion in Modern Era (1500 AD to Present)

In this era, the society evolved with the technological advancements that were taking place. It changed the paradigm of Reproductive Health Rights as new laws pertaining to Anti- abortive measures were on the rise.

In 1500's the Church penalized and classified the concept of abortion to be a homicide irrespective of the stage of the fetus it was conducted on. In 1588, Pope Sixtus V officially classified it to be homicide however after his death, Pope Gregory XIV overturned this mandate and held that it would be homicide only if it was conducted on fetuses who would said to have acquired souls.

### Emergence of Anti- Abortion Laws in the 17th to 19th Century and Industrial Revolution

The Industrial Revolution which brought with it, a fast-paced life and the hectic work life impacted the social lives of the people to great extent. The modern ideas that were flowing in the realm of industrial revolution placed women to a somewhat higher pedestal as they were allowed to take up jobs and work outside. Though the wages were less, however still women could now break stereotypes and progress. This impacted the personal lives of the people as well. The society was divided into the working class and the elite and as a result, 'out of wedlock' relationships were on the rise which in turn gave rise to unwanted pregnancies.

Towards the End of 16th and 17th centuries, any child that was born alive was regarded as a person and all the laws of crime relating to homicide were said to apply to child born alive only. Separate laws pertaining to abortion were thus developed to accord illegality to abortion in different part of Europe.

### Sweden's Infanticide Act

In 1778, Sweden for the first time passed the Infanticide Act which granted the mothers, a right to go for 'anonymous birth'. The aim of this law was to accord legality to childbirth outside of marriage so that abortion and infanticide could be stopped. It was a complete maneuver from the already established societal norms in most of the Europe. It was later on restricted to mere 'confidential births' in 1856. The difference between anonymous birth and confidential births was that in confidential births, the child had a choice to know his lineage or biological ancestry through mother's name kept sealed by the nurses that had aided in delivery of the child. Child born out of anonymous or confidential birth would be later on be placed in an orphanage. As per the Act, the midwives were prohibited from enquiring about or investigating into the name of the father of the child. It was upon the mother to keep the details sealed in the envelope and make a request for urgent delivery in a prescribed manner. Thereafter in 1793, France in its Civil Code (Napoleonic Code), legalized the anonymous as well as confidential births.

## UK's Lord Ellenborough Act, 1803

UK passed the Lord Ellenborough Act in 1803, which made abortion after quickening, a felony, that is, a crime of a serious nature and penalized it with Death Penalty. It penalized actions of persons administering poison etc. to the women with capital punishment. Abortion prior to quickening was also penalized to some extent (Keown, 1988). This not only led to curbing of Abortions to some extent but it completely banned the procedures of abortion upon women in general.

## The Offences Against Persons Act, 1861

The Offences Against the Person Act of 1861 criminalized abortion in the UK, imposing severe penalties on both women attempting self-abortive practices and those aiding them. The law made it illegal to administer substances or use instruments to induce a miscarriage, punishable by life imprisonment. It did not allow exceptions for cases like rape, incest, or threats to the woman's health, creating a harsh legal environment that forced many women into unsafe, clandestine procedures. This legislation remained in place for over a century, shaping abortion law until reforms like the Abortion Act of 1967 addressed women's reproductive rights and health more progressively.

In 1827, Illinois passed the act of "An Act to Prevent the Administering of Medicines, Drugs or Substances to Produce Abortion," which criminalized any attempt to induce abortion by declaring that such medicines or substances were to be considered poisons. This law aimed to prevent not only medical professionals but also individuals from administering any harmful substances to terminate pregnancies, marking an early attempt in the U.S. to regulate abortion through criminal law.

## Role of Feminist Movements of 1960 and 1970 in Abortion

The 1960s and 1970s witnessed a dramatic shift in societal attitudes toward women's reproductive rights, including abortion. Feminist movements, fueled by the broader civil rights and sexual liberation movements of the time, brought the issue of abortion to the forefront of public debate. Women began to assert more control over their bodies and reproductive choices, challenging traditional legal and moral frameworks that criminalized abortion.

The feminist movement, particularly in the West, argued that abortion laws disproportionately affected poor women and women of color, as wealthier women often had access to safer, albeit illegal, abortion services. These activists pushed for reforms that would decriminalize abortion and grant women the legal right to make decisions about their pregnancies. The slogan "My Body, My Choice" became emblematic of the struggle for reproductive freedom.

This growing pressure led to significant legal reforms across various countries. For instance, in the U.S., the landmark Supreme Court case *Roe v. Wade* (1973) recognized a woman's constitutional right to choose an abortion, setting a precedent for reproductive rights globally. Similarly, Slovenia legalized abortion in 1952, with further updates to its laws in 1977 to ensure more accessible reproductive healthcare.

In many countries, the feminist push for reform resulted in the establishment of more liberal abortion laws, allowing women to terminate pregnancies within specific time frames, subject to medical advice. The 1960s and 1970s movements laid the foundation for modern debates on reproductive rights, shifting the conversation from criminalization to choice, autonomy, and access to safe healthcare. These movements emphasized that reproductive rights are a critical aspect of gender equality and human rights.

## CONTEMPORARY ABORTION LAWS ACROSS THE EUROPEAN UNION

Abortion laws across the European Union (EU) reflect deep-seated regional differences, shaped by a combination of cultural, religious, political, and social influences. These variations are stark, with some countries embracing liberal, progressive policies that prioritize women's autonomy and health, while others impose severe restrictions, often rooted in religious doctrine and conservative ideologies. Understanding the regional dynamics of abortion laws requires a closer examination of how different parts of Europe approach reproductive rights.

### Northern Europe

In Northern Europe, countries such as Sweden, Denmark, and the Netherlands exemplify some of the most liberal and accessible abortion frameworks within the EU. These countries generally allow abortion on request within a gestational limit, typically up to 12 to 18 weeks. After this period, abortion is still permitted under certain conditions, such as when the pregnancy poses a risk to the woman's physical or mental health or in cases of severe fetal abnormalities.

Sweden is often regarded as a model for liberal abortion laws. The Abortion Act of 1974 grants women the right to terminate a pregnancy up to 18 weeks without providing any specific reason. After 18 weeks, abortion is permitted only under exceptional circumstances, such as significant health risks to the woman or serious fetal malformations. In 2022, Sweden reported an abortion rate of 18.6 per 1,000 women of reproductive age (15-44 years). The Swedish system emphasizes accessibility, with abortion services fully integrated into the public healthcare system, making the procedure available at no cost to women (Lennerhed, 2019). This approach ensures that socio-economic factors do not hinder access to reproductive healthcare, contributing to Sweden's reputation as a leader in gender equality and reproductive rights.

Denmark's abortion law, enacted in 1973, allows abortion on demand up to the 12th week of pregnancy with 90% of abortions occurring within the first trimester. Beyond this period, exceptions are made for cases involving health risks to the woman, fetal impairments, or other serious conditions. Like Sweden, Denmark prioritizes easy access to abortion services through its public healthcare system. A notable feature of Denmark's approach is the emphasis on confidentiality and patient-centered care, ensuring that women have access to counseling and support without fear of stigma or judgment (Skalts & Norgaard, 1965). This reflects broader societal attitudes in Northern Europe, where there is a strong cultural emphasis on individual autonomy, secularism, and social welfare.

The Netherlands also maintains a progressive stance on abortion. The Netherlands has one of the lowest abortion rates in the EU, with an abortion rate of 8.5 per 1,000 women of reproductive age in 2021, owing to a robust system of contraception access and comprehensive sex education. The Termination of Pregnancy Act, passed in 1984, permits abortion up to 24 weeks of gestation. However, in practice, most abortions are performed within the first 12 weeks. The Dutch model emphasizes both prevention and care, with a strong focus on comprehensive sex education, access to contraception, and high-quality reproductive healthcare. Abortion services in the Netherlands are covered under the national health insurance system, ensuring that all women have equitable access, regardless of their financial situation. The Dutch approach, which combines liberal abortion laws with robust social support systems, is often cited as a model for other countries seeking to balance reproductive rights with public health goals.

## Eastern Europe

In stark contrast to the liberal approaches seen in Northern Europe, Eastern European countries, particularly Poland and Hungary, exhibit some of the most restrictive abortion laws in the EU. These restrictive policies are heavily influenced by religious and conservative cultural values, often rooted in the region's strong Catholic and Orthodox Christian traditions.

Poland represents one of the most extreme examples of restrictive abortion laws in the EU. The country's abortion law, governed by the Family Planning, Human Embryo Protection, and Conditions of Permissibility of Abortion Act of 1993, initially allowed abortion in cases of severe fetal impairment, risk to the woman's life or health, and pregnancy resulting from rape or incest. However, in 2020, Poland's Constitutional Tribunal ruled that abortion due to fetal abnormalities was unconstitutional, effectively banning almost all legal abortions in the country. This ruling sparked widespread protests, both domestically and internationally, as it significantly curtailed reproductive rights. The ruling left Polish women with very limited legal options for abortion, leading many to seek procedures abroad, particularly in neighboring Germany and the Czech Republic, or to resort to unsafe, illegal abortions. The ruling also exposed the deep divide between the conservative government, supported by the Catholic Church, and a growing segment of the population advocating for greater reproductive freedoms.

Hungary, while not as restrictive as Poland, has implemented a series of measures that complicate access to abortion. The Hungarian abortion law, dating back to 1956 and amended several times, allows abortion up to 12 weeks of pregnancy, with extensions permitted under specific circumstances, such as health risks or cases of rape. However, recent government policies under Prime Minister Viktor Orbán's administration have made accessing abortion more challenging. Mandatory counseling and a three-day waiting period are required, which critics argue are designed to discourage women from proceeding with the abortion. Hungary's approach reflects the government's broader pro-family, pro-natalist policies, which seek to encourage higher birth rates and traditional family structures. These policies often intersect with broader political agendas, where reproductive rights are framed within the context of national identity and demographic concerns.

## Southern Europe

Southern European countries, such as Italy, Spain, and Greece, present a more mixed legal landscape when it comes to abortion, often influenced by the strong presence of the Catholic Church and conservative societal values. However, recent years have seen notable liberalization in some areas, reflecting a gradual shift in public attitudes and political priorities.

Italy legalized abortion in 1978 with the passage of Law 194, which permits abortion up to 90 days (12 weeks) of pregnancy. After this period, abortion is allowed only when the woman's life is at risk or when there are serious fetal abnormalities. Despite the legal framework, access to abortion services in Italy remains uneven due to the high rate of conscientious objection among medical professionals. In some regions, as many as 70% of doctors refuse to perform abortions, forcing women to travel long distances or seek private, often costly, alternatives. This regional disparity in access is particularly pronounced in more conservative southern parts of Italy, where religious influence is stronger. The tension between legal rights and actual access remains a critical issue in the country, highlighting the need for policy reforms that ensure the law's full implementation (Caruso, 2023).

Spain, traditionally a Catholic stronghold, has undergone significant legal changes in recent decades. The 2010 law on sexual and reproductive health and voluntary interruption of pregnancy allows abortion on demand up to 14 weeks, with extensions up to 22 weeks in cases of severe fetal abnormalities or risks to the woman's health. Recent reforms under the government of Prime Minister Pedro Sánchez have further expanded access to abortion, including removing requirements for parental consent for minors and improving access to abortion services in public hospitals. These changes reflect a broader trend in Spain towards secularization and the strengthening of women's rights, despite ongoing opposition from conservative and religious groups.

Greece's abortion law, enacted in 1986, allows abortion on demand up to 12 weeks, with extensions for health reasons or cases of rape. While the law is relatively liberal, access to abortion services can be inconsistent, particularly in rural areas where healthcare infrastructure is weaker. Additionally, societal stigma around abortion persists in some conservative segments of Greek society, particularly among older generations. However, younger generations and urban populations tend to hold more progressive views on reproductive rights, leading to a gradual shift in public discourse and policy implementation. The abortion rate in Greece is estimated at 6.7 per 1,000 women, but data reporting is inconsistent due to societal stigma.

## Western Europe

Western European countries like France, Germany, and Belgium offer a blend of liberal and regulated approaches to abortion, balancing women's rights with societal concerns about the procedure. While access to abortion is generally protected, legal frameworks often include certain restrictions, such as mandatory counseling or waiting periods, reflecting ongoing debates about the moral and ethical dimensions of abortion.

France is a leading example of progressive reproductive health policies. The country's abortion law, first enacted in 1975 with the Veil Law, has undergone several reforms, most recently in 2022, when the gestational limit for abortions was extended from 12 to 14 weeks. France's public healthcare system covers the cost of abortions, ensuring that financial barriers do not prevent women from accessing services. Additionally, the government has taken steps to combat the spread of misinformation about abortion and to support women who face barriers to accessing reproductive healthcare. France's approach reflects its strong commitment to secularism and gender equality, which are central tenets of the country's legal and political framework.

Germany, while also committed to ensuring access to abortion, takes a more regulated approach. Abortion is legal within the first 12 weeks of pregnancy, but women are required to undergo mandatory counseling and observe a three-day waiting period before the procedure. The counseling is intended to ensure that the decision is well-considered and that women are informed about available alternatives, such as adoption. After 12 weeks, abortion is permitted only under specific circumstances, such as medical necessity or serious fetal abnormalities. Germany's approach reflects its historical and cultural context, balancing reproductive rights with concerns about the sanctity of life, which are deeply rooted in the country's post-war legal and ethical framework.

Belgium has a similar approach to Germany, allowing abortion on request up to 12 weeks of pregnancy, with mandatory counseling and a waiting period. Recent efforts in Belgium have focused on improving access to abortion services, particularly for vulnerable populations such as migrants and low-income women. The country's healthcare system ensures that abortion is accessible and affordable, but ongoing debates about the moral implications of the procedure continue to shape public policy and discourse.

## The Role of Judiciary

The judiciary plays a pivotal role in shaping and interpreting abortion laws across the European Union (EU). As individual member states maintain their sovereignty over reproductive rights, national courts are often called upon to balance these rights with broader societal values, including religious, cultural, and ethical considerations. At the supranational level, the European Court of Human Rights (ECHR) has also been instrumental in influencing abortion laws through landmark rulings that emphasize the protection of fundamental human rights. This section explores the judiciary's role in defining abortion laws in the EU, highlighting key cases and legal principles that have shaped the reproductive rights landscape.

## National Courts

National courts across the EU have been at the forefront of interpreting and applying abortion laws within their respective legal frameworks. In many instances, these courts have been tasked with reconciling conflicting interests, such as the protection of prenatal life, the rights of the pregnant woman, and societal values rooted in religious and cultural traditions.

One of the most notable examples of judicial influence on abortion laws can be seen in Germany. The German Federal Constitutional Court has played a central role in shaping the country's abortion regulations. In a 1975 ruling, the court declared that the fetus has a right to life, and as such, the state has a duty to protect it. However, the court also acknowledged the pregnant woman's right to self-determination, leading to the establishment of a legal framework that permits abortion within the first 12 weeks of pregnancy, provided that mandatory counseling and a waiting period are observed. This balancing act between protecting fetal life and respecting women's rights has become a defining feature of Germany's abortion laws, reflecting broader societal values that emphasize both life and personal autonomy (MacDonnell & Hughes, 2013).

In Spain, the judiciary has also played a crucial role in advancing reproductive rights. The Spanish Constitutional Court has upheld the legality of abortion within the framework established by the 2010 law on sexual and reproductive health, which allows abortion on demand up to 14 weeks of pregnancy. The court has reinforced the view that the law strikes an appropriate balance between the protection of prenatal life and the rights of women. Recent challenges to the law, particularly from conservative groups, have been rejected by the court, signaling a judicial commitment to maintaining reproductive freedoms in the face of ongoing political and societal debates.

Similarly, in Italy, the Constitutional Court has had a significant impact on the interpretation and application of the country's abortion laws. In several rulings, the court has reinforced the legality of abortion as established by Law 194 of 1978, while also addressing the contentious issue of conscientious objection. The court has emphasized that while doctors have the right to refuse to perform abortions on moral or religious grounds, this right cannot undermine women's access to the procedure. As a result, the court has called for the state to ensure that sufficient medical personnel are available to provide abortion services, particularly in regions where conscientious objection rates are high.

## European Court of Human Rights (ECHR)

At the supranational level, the European Court of Human Rights (ECHR) has significantly influenced abortion laws across the EU by interpreting the European Convention on Human Rights in the context of reproductive rights. Although the ECHR does not impose a uniform abortion policy on member states, its rulings have established important principles that member states must consider when crafting their abortion laws.

One of the most prominent ECHR cases related to abortion is A, B and C v. Ireland (2010). In this case, the court considered a challenge to Ireland's then highly restrictive abortion laws, which effectively prohibited abortion except in cases where the woman's life was at risk. The court ruled that while states have a "margin of appreciation" in regulating abortion, they must ensure that their laws do not violate the rights protected under the European Convention on Human Rights. In particular, the court found that Ireland's legal framework was insufficiently clear and accessible, resulting in uncertainty for women and healthcare providers. This ruling highlighted the importance of clear and coherent legal frameworks for abortion that respect women's rights while acknowledging the diversity of national approaches (Staunton, 2011).

In another landmark case, R.R. v. Poland (2011), the ECHR ruled that Poland's failure to provide timely access to diagnostic prenatal testing and subsequent access to legal abortion violated the applicant's right to respect for private life under Article 8 of the Convention. The court emphasized that legal abortion must be effectively accessible and that procedural barriers should not obstruct women from exercising their rights under domestic law. This ruling underscored the ECHR's commitment to ensuring that states not only provide legal avenues for abortion but also ensure that these avenues are practically accessible to women in need.

The ECHR's rulings have set important precedents that influence national abortion laws by reinforcing the principle that reproductive rights are integral to the broader framework of human rights. These rulings compel states to ensure that their abortion laws are compatible with the rights enshrined in the European Convention on Human Rights, particularly the rights to privacy, health, and non-discrimination.

## International Obligations and EU Influence

Although abortion remains a matter of national law within the European Union, member states are subject to a range of international obligations that shape their legal frameworks on reproductive rights. Global human rights instruments and EU-level initiatives both play influential roles in guiding member states toward ensuring access to safe and legal abortion services. This section explores how international obligations and EU policies intersect with national abortion laws, highlighting the tension between international norms and national sovereignty.

International human rights frameworks have become increasingly relevant in the context of abortion laws, particularly through the work of the United Nations and global health organizations. The Convention on the Elimination of All Forms of Discrimination Against Women (CEDAW), adopted by the United Nations in 1979, is one of the most significant international treaties influencing abortion laws in the EU. CEDAW calls on state parties to eliminate discrimination against women in all areas, including healthcare, and to ensure access to reproductive health services, including safe and legal abortion.

The CEDAW Committee has repeatedly emphasized that restrictive abortion laws constitute discrimination against women and has urged states to decriminalize abortion and ensure access to safe and legal procedures. For example, in its concluding observations on Poland in 2014, the CEDAW Committee expressed concern about the country's restrictive abortion laws and recommended that Poland liberalize its legislation and remove barriers to accessing abortion services. Such international scrutiny places pressure on member states to align their abortion laws with global standards on gender equality and reproductive health.

The World Health Organization (WHO) also plays a critical role in setting international standards for reproductive health, including abortion. The WHO's guidelines emphasize that access to safe abortion is a fundamental aspect of women's health and rights. The organization advocates for the removal of legal and policy barriers to abortion and highlights the public health risks associated with unsafe abortion practices. Member states are encouraged to adopt WHO guidelines as part of their broader commitment to improving reproductive health outcomes, which in turn influences national policy-making within the EU.

While the European Union itself does not have a unified policy on abortion, several EU institutions and initiatives have increasingly recognized reproductive rights, including access to abortion, as essential to gender equality and human rights. The European Parliament and the European Commission have taken active roles in promoting reproductive rights within the EU, often in the face of opposition from conservative member states.

In 2021, the European Parliament adopted the Matić Report, a landmark resolution that called for universal access to safe and legal abortion within the EU. The resolution framed reproductive rights, including abortion, as fundamental human rights and urged member states to ensure that women have access to these services without facing legal, financial, or procedural barriers. The report also highlighted the importance of comprehensive sexual education and access to contraception as key components of reproductive health. While the Matić Report is non-binding, it reflects the growing recognition within EU institutions of the need to protect and promote reproductive rights across the union.

The European Commission, through its work on gender equality, has also supported initiatives aimed at improving access to reproductive health services, including abortion. The EU Gender Equality Strategy 2020-2025 emphasizes the need to ensure that all women in the EU have access to the full range of reproductive health services, including safe abortion. The strategy recognizes that reproductive rights are central to gender equality and calls on member states to address barriers that prevent women from exercising these rights.

Despite these efforts, the EU faces significant challenges in harmonizing abortion laws across its member states. The principle of subsidiarity, which grants member states autonomy over certain policy areas, including health, means that the EU's influence on abortion laws is limited. As a result, the EU's role is often one of advocacy and support rather than direct intervention. This creates a tension between the EU's commitment to human rights and gender equality and the diverse legal frameworks that exist across its member states.

## COMPARATIVE ANALYSIS OF ABORTION LAWS IN THE EUROPEAN UNION

This chapter provides a detailed comparative analysis of abortion laws across European Union (EU) member states. It delves into the differences in legal frameworks, gestational limits, grounds for abortion, healthcare access, and the impact of EU regulations. By examining these factors, this section highlights the disparities that exist within the EU, while also considering the common principles that guide abortion-related laws across the region.

### Gestational Limits

Gestational limits are one of the most significant aspects of abortion laws across the European Union, as they define the period during which a woman can legally obtain an abortion. The variations in these limits reflect the diverse legal, cultural, and ethical perspectives within the EU.

In France and Germany, abortion is generally allowed up to 12 weeks of pregnancy, with some exceptions for cases where the woman's health is at risk or in instances of fetal abnormalities. This 12-week limit is fairly standard across many EU countries, representing a compromise between the protection of prenatal life and the recognition of women's rights to autonomy and reproductive health. In these countries, the law typically requires that abortions be performed under medical supervision and after a consultation process, which often includes mandatory counseling and a waiting period.

On the other hand, Sweden stands out as one of the most liberal countries in the EU concerning gestational limits. In Sweden, abortion is permitted on request up to 18 weeks of pregnancy. After 18 weeks, abortion is still possible but requires authorization from the National Board of Health and Welfare, which assesses the reasons for the request, such as serious fetal anomalies or threats to the woman's physical or mental health. Sweden's approach reflects its strong commitment to reproductive rights and the principle of bodily autonomy, as well as its emphasis on ensuring that women have access to safe and legal abortion throughout a significant portion of their pregnancy.

By contrast, some EU countries have much more restrictive gestational limits. In Poland, abortion is now only permitted under very limited circumstances, such as cases of rape, incest, or when the woman's life is at risk. The near-total ban on abortion, which was reinforced by a 2020 ruling by Poland's Constitutional Tribunal, has led to widespread protests and international condemnation. Poland's abortion laws are among the most restrictive, with fewer than 1,100 legal abortions reported annually before the 2020 ruling. Following this, only 107 legal abortions were performed in 2021, while an estimated 150,000 women sought abortions abroad. Similarly, Malta maintains a complete ban on abortion, with no exceptions, making it the most restrictive EU member state in terms of abortion rights. This absolute prohibition highlights the significant cultural and religious influence on abortion laws in certain parts of the EU.

In other countries, such as Italy and Spain, the legal gestational limit for abortion generally aligns with the 12-week standard but may extend under certain conditions. For example, in Italy, abortion is permitted up to 90 days (approximately 13 weeks) from conception, while in Spain, abortion is allowed up to 14 weeks. Both countries allow for exceptions beyond these limits in cases of severe fetal anomalies or risks to the woman's health.

These disparities in gestational limits illustrate the complex interplay between legal standards, societal values, and political influences across the EU. While many countries seek to balance women's reproductive rights with the protection of prenatal life, the diversity of approaches highlights the ongoing challenges in achieving a more harmonized framework for abortion across the EU.

## Grounds for Abortion

The grounds on which abortion is permitted vary significantly across EU member states, reflecting differing legal, ethical, and cultural considerations. These grounds often include factors such as the woman's physical or mental health, fetal anomalies, and socio-economic conditions.

In countries with more liberal abortion laws, such as Sweden and Denmark, abortion is available on request during the early stages of pregnancy, and women are not required to provide a specific reason for seeking the procedure. These countries prioritize women's autonomy and reproductive choice, recognizing that women are best placed to make decisions about their own bodies and lives. This approach reflects broader societal attitudes that emphasize gender equality and individual rights.

In France and Germany, while abortion is generally available on request within the first trimester, the law also permits abortion under specific circumstances beyond the gestational limit. For example, in France, abortion can be performed later in pregnancy if there is a risk to the woman's health or if the fetus is diagnosed with a severe and incurable condition. Similarly, in Germany, abortions beyond 12 weeks are allowed if there are medical indications, such as risks to the woman's physical or mental health or serious fetal abnormalities (Huss & Kaiser, 2022). These provisions reflect a more nuanced approach that seeks to accommodate exceptional circumstances while maintaining certain restrictions.

By contrast, in countries with more restrictive abortion laws, such as Poland and Hungary, the grounds for abortion are much more limited. In Poland, following the 2020 Constitutional Tribunal ruling, abortion is only allowed in cases of rape, incest, or when the woman's life is at risk. The removal of fetal abnormality as a ground for abortion has sparked significant controversy, as it severely limits access to the procedure and places Poland among the most restrictive countries in the EU in terms of reproductive rights. Hungary's abortion laws are also relatively restrictive, allowing the procedure only under certain conditions, such as medical necessity or cases of severe distress.

The differences in the grounds for abortion across the EU underscore the tension between individual rights and societal values. While some countries prioritize women's autonomy and reproductive health, others impose more restrictive conditions based on cultural, religious, or moral considerations. These variations highlight the ongoing debate over the role of the state in regulating reproductive rights and the challenges of reconciling diverse perspectives within a common European framework.

## Healthcare Access

Healthcare access is a critical factor in determining the practical availability of abortion services across the European Union. While the legal framework provides the foundation for abortion rights, the actual ability to access these services varies greatly depending on several factors, including geography, healthcare infrastructure, and the presence of legal or procedural barriers. This section explores the disparities in healthcare access across the EU and how they impact women's ability to exercise their reproductive rights.

## Geographic Disparities

One of the most significant factors affecting access to abortion services in the EU is geographic disparity. Women living in urban areas generally have better access to healthcare facilities that provide abortion services compared to those in rural or remote regions. In countries like Sweden and France, where abortion is legal and widely accessible, women in major cities have relatively easy access to hospitals and clinics that offer abortion services. However, women in rural areas may face difficulties in obtaining timely care due to the limited availability of healthcare providers, longer travel distances, and in some cases, the absence of abortion services altogether in their local regions.

In Italy, this issue is exacerbated by the high rate of conscientious objection among healthcare providers. Although abortion has been legal since 1978, more than 70% of Italian gynecologists refuse to perform the procedure on moral or religious grounds, with this number exceeding 90% in some southern regions. This makes access to abortion extremely challenging, particularly for women in rural or conservative areas where alternative providers are scarce. The Italian government has faced criticism for failing to ensure that the right to abortion is meaningfully accessible, despite its legal status (Caruso, 2020).

Similarly, in Poland, where abortion laws are highly restrictive, access to legal abortion services is severely limited, even in cases where the procedure is permitted under law. Many hospitals refuse to perform abortions, citing conscientious objection, and women seeking legal abortions often face significant delays, lack of information, or outright refusals from healthcare providers. As a result, many Polish women are forced to seek abortion services abroad, particularly in neighboring countries like Germany or the Czech Republic, further highlighting the impact of geographic disparities on access to reproductive healthcare.

## Healthcare Infrastructure and Resources

Healthcare infrastructure and resources also play a crucial role in determining access to abortion services across the EU. In countries with well-developed healthcare systems, such as Germany and the Netherlands, abortion services are integrated into the broader healthcare framework, ensuring that women can access safe and legal abortions without significant barriers. These countries have well-established networks of healthcare providers and facilities that offer abortion services, along with comprehensive reproductive health services, including contraception and post-abortion care.

However, in countries with less developed healthcare infrastructure, such as Romania and Bulgaria, access to abortion can be more challenging. In Romania, for example, while abortion is legal and widely available, the healthcare system struggles with underfunding, resource shortages, and unequal distribution of healthcare services. Women in rural areas may face difficulties accessing abortion services due to a lack of facilities and trained providers, as well as financial barriers. Additionally, the prevalence of informal payments and corruption within the healthcare system can further restrict access to reproductive healthcare for disadvantaged populations.

In Ireland, following the repeal of the 8th Amendment in 2018, abortion services were legalized and integrated into the public healthcare system. However, there have been challenges in ensuring widespread access, particularly in rural areas where healthcare facilities are limited. Moreover, a significant number of general practitioners have opted out of providing abortion services, citing personal or professional reasons. While the Irish government has taken steps to address these gaps by providing funding and training for healthcare providers, access to abortion remains uneven across the country.

## Legal and Procedural Barriers

In addition to geographic and infrastructure-related challenges, legal and procedural barriers also play a significant role in limiting access to abortion services. Mandatory waiting periods, counseling requirements, and parental consent laws are some of the common procedural barriers that can delay or complicate access to abortion. These barriers often disproportionately affect marginalized groups, including young women, low-income women, and women from minority communities.

In Hungary, for example, the law requires women seeking an abortion to undergo mandatory counseling sessions and observe a mandatory waiting period of three days before the procedure can be performed. Critics argue that these requirements create unnecessary delays and can be psychologically burdensome for women, particularly those who have already made their decision. Furthermore, the requirement for minors to obtain parental consent can create additional obstacles for young women who may not have supportive families or who fear stigma or violence.

In Spain, while abortion is legal and generally accessible, certain regions have introduced procedural barriers that complicate access. For example, in some conservative regions, women seeking an abortion must navigate complex bureaucratic processes, including obtaining multiple medical certifications or facing delays due to administrative hurdles. These barriers can create significant delays, forcing women to travel to other regions or even abroad to obtain the care they need in a timely manner.

## Cross-Border Access

Cross-border access to abortion services has become a crucial option for women in countries with restrictive abortion laws. In the EU, the principle of free movement of people allows women to travel to other member states where abortion is legal and more accessible. For example, many women from Poland and Malta travel to neighboring countries, such as Germany, the Netherlands, or the UK, to obtain abortion services that are unavailable in their home countries. Women also travel for late abortion from France to countries like the UK, where regulations may be more lenient regarding gestational limits (Jubert et al., 2023).

However, cross-border access is not without its challenges. Travel costs, language barriers, and the need to navigate foreign healthcare systems can create significant obstacles for women seeking abortions abroad. Additionally, the COVID-19 pandemic has highlighted the vulnerability of cross-border access, as travel restrictions and lockdown measures severely limited women's ability to seek care in other countries. This underscores the importance of ensuring that abortion services are accessible within national borders and that women do not have to rely on cross-border travel to exercise their reproductive rights.

In conclusion, healthcare access remains a significant determinant of women's ability to obtain safe and legal abortion services across the EU. Geographic disparities, healthcare infrastructure, legal barriers, and cross-border access all contribute to the uneven landscape of reproductive healthcare. Addressing these challenges requires a comprehensive approach that prioritizes equitable access to abortion services for all women, regardless of their location, socio-economic status, or personal circumstances.

## Impact of EU Regulations

While abortion law remains primarily within the jurisdiction of individual member states, the European Union's legal framework and regulatory mechanisms play an increasingly important role in shaping national abortion policies and ensuring compliance with broader human rights standards. This section explores the impact of EU regulations on national abortion laws, focusing on the role of EU institutions, human rights frameworks, and the influence of EU policies on reproductive health.

The European Union is built on a foundation of human rights, as enshrined in the Charter of Fundamental Rights of the European Union and the Treaty on the European Union. These legal instruments emphasize the protection of human dignity, the right to healthcare, and gender equality, all of which are relevant to the issue of abortion. While the EU does not have a unified policy on abortion, its commitment to human rights has implications for member states' abortion laws, particularly when these laws conflict with fundamental rights guaranteed by EU law.

The European Court of Human Rights (ECHR) has played a significant role in influencing abortion laws across the EU, particularly through its rulings on cases related to reproductive rights. As discussed earlier, the ECHR has established important legal precedents that require member states to ensure that abortion laws are clear, accessible, and in line with human rights obligations. These rulings compel member states to align their national laws with the broader human rights framework of the EU, particularly in areas where restrictive abortion laws may violate women's rights to privacy, health, and non-discrimination.

The European Court of Justice (ECJ) also plays a role in ensuring that member states comply with EU law, including regulations related to healthcare and human rights. While the ECJ has not directly ruled on abortion cases, its jurisprudence on issues related to gender equality and healthcare access has implications for national abortion laws. For example, the ECJ's rulings on discrimination in healthcare and employment have reinforced the principle that member states must ensure equal access to reproductive healthcare services, including abortion, as part of their broader obligations under EU law.

EU policies on gender equality, healthcare, and social inclusion also have an indirect impact on national abortion laws. The EU Gender Equality Strategy 2020-2025, for example, emphasizes the importance of ensuring equal access to healthcare services for women, including reproductive health services. While the strategy does not specifically mandate changes to national abortion laws, it sets a broader framework for member states to improve access to reproductive healthcare and address barriers that prevent women from exercising their reproductive rights.

Similarly, the European Pillar of Social Rights, adopted in 2017, calls for universal access to quality healthcare, including sexual and reproductive healthcare services. This policy initiative encourages member states to take concrete steps to ensure that all women have access to safe and legal abortion services as part of their right to healthcare. The Pillar of Social Rights also emphasizes the need to address healthcare inequalities, including those related to reproductive health, and calls for targeted measures to reduce disparities in access to abortion services across the EU.

In addition to these policy initiatives, EU funding mechanisms, such as the EU-4Health program, support member states in improving healthcare infrastructure and access to services, including reproductive healthcare (Hervey & Banerjee, 2023). Through financial assistance and capacity-building initiatives, the EU can indirectly influence national abortion laws by helping member states strengthen their healthcare systems and ensure that abortion services are accessible to all women.

## SOCIAL AND ECONOMIC FACTORS AFFECTING REPRODUCTIVE HEALTH AND ABORTION

This chapter explores the social and economic factors that significantly impact reproductive health and access to abortion across the European Union. These factors include disparities in healthcare access, economic inequality, health and legal risks associated with abortion, and the influence of social norms and cultural attitudes. Understanding these elements is crucial for analyzing how various EU member states address or fail to address the needs of women seeking reproductive healthcare.

### Access and Availability

Access to abortion services across the European Union is deeply influenced by geographical disparities and the availability of healthcare facilities. Women living in urban areas generally enjoy better access to comprehensive healthcare services, including abortion, while those in rural or remote areas face significant challenges.

In countries like Sweden and France, where abortion is legally accessible and healthcare infrastructure is well-developed, urban centers boast numerous clinics and hospitals that provide abortion services. However, rural areas often suffer from a lack of healthcare providers, which can force women to travel long distances to obtain care. This situation is exacerbated in countries where healthcare resources are unevenly distributed, such as Romania and Bulgaria, where women in rural regions often encounter severe difficulties in accessing abortion services due to a scarcity of healthcare professionals and facilities.

In Ireland, following the legalization of abortion in 2018, efforts were made to ensure that abortion services were available across the country (Calkin & Berny, 2021). However, regional disparities persist, with rural areas still facing significant gaps in service provision. The availability of abortion services in rural areas is also influenced by the number of healthcare providers willing to perform the procedure, which remains limited in some parts of the country due to personal or religious objections.

These geographical disparities in access to abortion services not only affect the immediacy and quality of care but also place a disproportionate burden on women in less accessible regions, who may face delays, increased costs, and additional stress in seeking abortion care. The situation is further complicated in countries with more restrictive abortion laws, where women may need to travel abroad to obtain legal abortion services, as is the case for many women from Poland and Malta.

## Economic Inequality

Economic inequality is another major factor that affects access to reproductive healthcare and abortion services. Women from lower socio-economic backgrounds often face greater barriers to accessing abortion, including the cost of the procedure, travel expenses, and lost wages from taking time off work.

In countries where abortion is legally available but not fully covered by public healthcare systems, such as Italy and Spain, women may be required to pay for the procedure out of pocket. This can be prohibitively expensive for low-income women, leading to delays in obtaining an abortion or forcing them to seek unsafe alternatives. Even in countries where abortion is covered by public healthcare, additional costs related to travel, accommodation, and childcare can create significant financial obstacles for disadvantaged women.

Economic inequality also intersects with other forms of discrimination, such as race and immigration status, further compounding the barriers to accessing abortion. For instance, migrant women and women from ethnic minority communities in the EU often face multiple layers of disadvantage, including limited access to information about their rights, language barriers, and fear of deportation or legal repercussions. These factors can deter them from seeking legal abortion services or force them into unsafe or illegal procedures.

The economic barriers to abortion are particularly stark in countries with restrictive laws, where women may need to travel abroad to access legal abortion services. For example, women from Poland and Ireland (before the 2018 legalization) often had to travel to the UK or other EU countries to obtain an abortion, incurring significant financial costs. This situation creates a stark divide between those who can afford to travel and those who cannot, effectively limiting access to safe abortion for economically disadvantaged women.

## Health and Legal Risks

Health and legal risks associated with abortion vary widely across the EU, depending on the legal framework and the availability of safe, regulated services. In countries where abortion is legal and accessible, such as Sweden and the Netherlands, women are generally able to obtain abortions in a safe and regulated environment, minimizing health risks. However, in countries with restrictive abortion laws, such as Poland and Malta, women face significant health risks if they resort to illegal or unsafe abortions. The lack of legal and safe options drives some women to seek abortions in clandestine conditions, where the risk of complications, including infection, hemorrhage, and even death, is much higher (Ishola et al., 2021). These health risks are exacerbated by the fear of legal repercussions, which may deter women from seeking necessary post-abortion care if complications arise.

The legal risks associated with abortion also vary significantly across the EU. In Poland, for example, the near-total ban on abortion has led to increased legal risks for both women seeking abortions and healthcare providers. Women who seek illegal abortions risk criminal charges, while healthcare providers who perform abortions outside the narrow legal exceptions face severe penalties, including imprisonment. This legal environment creates a climate of fear and uncertainty, which can have a chilling effect on access to abortion and reproductive healthcare more broadly.

In addition to the direct legal risks, restrictive abortion laws also have broader implications for women's health and well-being. In countries like Hungary and Slovakia, where restrictive abortion laws are combined with mandatory counseling and waiting periods, women may experience increased stress and anxiety as they navigate complex legal and procedural hurdles. These barriers not only delay access to care but can also have long-term psychological effects, particularly for women who are already vulnerable due to socio-economic or personal circumstances.

## Social Norms and Cultural Factors

Social norms and cultural attitudes towards abortion play a crucial role in shaping reproductive health laws and access to abortion services across the EU. These norms and attitudes are deeply rooted in the religious, cultural, and historical contexts of each member state, leading to significant variations in public opinion and policy.

In countries with strong Catholic traditions, such as Italy, Spain, and Poland, cultural and religious opposition to abortion remains a powerful force. In these countries, the influence of the Catholic Church has historically shaped abortion laws and continues to affect public opinion and policy-making. For example, in Poland, the Catholic Church played a key role in advocating for the 2020 Constitutional Tribunal ruling that further restricted access to abortion. Public support for restrictive abortion laws is also higher in these countries, reflecting the deep cultural and religious opposition to abortion.

In contrast, countries with more secular and progressive social norms, such as Sweden and Denmark, tend to have more liberal abortion laws and higher levels of public support for reproductive rights. In these countries, abortion is widely accepted as a fundamental aspect of women's healthcare, and there is a strong emphasis on gender equality and individual autonomy. These cultural attitudes are reflected in the legal frameworks, which prioritize women's rights to access safe and legal abortion services.

Generational differences also play a significant role in shaping attitudes towards abortion (Scott, 1998). In many countries, younger generations are more likely to support liberal abortion laws and view access to abortion as a basic human right. This generational shift is particularly evident in countries like Ireland, where the 2018 referendum to repeal the 8th Amendment was driven by strong support from younger voters. However, in more conservative societies, older generations may continue to hold more traditional views on abortion, contributing to ongoing political and social tensions.

Social norms and cultural factors also influence the stigma associated with abortion, which can have a profound impact on women's access to care. In countries where abortion is heavily stigmatized, women may face social ostracism, discrimination, or even violence for seeking an abortion. This stigma can deter women from accessing legal services, leading them to seek unsafe or clandestine abortions instead. Efforts to reduce abortion stigma, through public education and advocacy, are therefore critical to ensuring that all women can access safe and legal abortion services without fear of social or cultural repercussions.

## CONCLUSION AND RECOMMENDATIONS

The legal landscape governing abortion in the European Union reflects a wide array of approaches, from progressive frameworks to restrictive regimes. This diversity is rooted in the distinct historical, cultural, religious, and political contexts of each EU member state. Throughout this chapter, the analysis has revealed how these different legal frameworks impact women's access to safe and legal abortion services. While more liberal countries such as Sweden, France, and Germany provide robust access to reproductive healthcare, restrictive laws in countries like Poland and Hungary pose significant barriers, leading many women to seek services abroad or resort to unsafe procedures. These disparities highlight the critical role that legal structures play in determining reproductive health outcomes and ensuring the protection of women's rights.

Judicial intervention has proven to be a key factor in shaping abortion laws across the European Union. National courts and the European Court of Human Rights have influenced the interpretation and enforcement of abortion-related laws, often acting as a counterbalance to political forces attempting to either expand or limit access to reproductive healthcare. Judicial decisions in this realm have shown the importance of safeguarding reproductive rights, even in environments where political and societal pressures threaten to curtail them. The ability of the judiciary to uphold human rights standards, particularly in countries with restrictive abortion policies, remains a vital component of the legal landscape.

Social and economic factors also play a significant role in determining access to abortion within the EU. Even in countries with more liberal legal frameworks, disparities in healthcare infrastructure and socio-economic conditions can limit access, particularly for marginalized populations and those living in rural areas. These challenges demonstrate that legal reforms alone are insufficient to ensure equitable access to reproductive healthcare. Addressing underlying social and economic barriers is essential to realizing the full promise of legal rights and ensuring that all women, regardless of their socio-economic status or geographic location, have access to safe abortion services.

Looking ahead, there are several key recommendations for enhancing abortion-related reproductive health laws across the European Union. First, the EU should take steps to strengthen its role in promoting minimum standards for abortion access across member states. While reproductive health remains primarily a national competence, the EU can provide guidance on best practices, enforce human rights frameworks more effectively, and support member states in reforming restrictive laws. Second, judicial protection of reproductive rights must continue to be a priority. The European Court of Human Rights and national courts should remain vigilant in ensuring that national laws align with international human rights obligations, particularly in cases where political forces seek to undermine women's access to abortion.

In addition to these legal recommendations, addressing socio-economic barriers to abortion access is crucial. National governments should work to expand healthcare infrastructure, particularly in underserved rural areas, and ensure that abortion services are accessible to all women, regardless of their financial situation. Providing comprehensive healthcare coverage for abortion services, as well as targeted financial support for low-income women, will be essential to closing gaps in access. Furthermore, public education and awareness campaigns can play a pivotal role in shifting social attitudes toward abortion. By promoting a better understanding of reproductive rights, public health implications, and the importance of access to safe abortion, such campaigns can help to build public support for legislative changes and foster a more supportive environment for reproductive healthcare.

Advocacy efforts must continue to push for progressive reforms that expand access to abortion and protect women's reproductive rights. Civil society organizations, activists, and advocacy groups should collaborate across borders, share successful strategies, and build alliances to counteract conservative movements that seek to roll back these rights. By working together and learning from the successes and challenges within the EU, these groups can contribute to creating a more unified and equitable legal framework for reproductive rights.

The future of abortion-related reproductive health laws in the European Union will depend on a combination of legal reforms, judicial oversight, and efforts to address social and economic disparities. By adopting a holistic approach that integrates legal, social, and economic considerations, the EU and its member states can ensure that all women have access to the care they need, regardless of their location or circumstances. The European Union, as a leader in human rights, has the opportunity to set a global example by upholding and advancing reproductive freedoms for all its citizens.

## REFERENCES


Berer, M. (2017). Abortion law and policy around the world: In search of decriminalization. *Health and Human Rights*, 19(1), 13–27. https://www.hhrjournal.org/2017/06/abortion-law-and-policy-around-the-world-in-search-of-decriminalization/ PMID: 28630538

Calkin, S., & Berny, E. (2021). Legal and non-legal barriers to abortion in Ireland and the United Kingdom. *Medicine Access @ Point of Care*, 5, 23992026211040023. Advance online publication. DOI: 10.1177/23992026211040023 PMID: 36204506

Carr-Saunders, A. M. (1922). *The population problem: A study in human evolution*. Clarendon Press.

Caruso, E. (2020). The Ambivalence of Law: Some Observations on the Denial of Access to Abortion Services in Italy. *Feminist Review*, 124(1), 183–191. DOI: 10.1177/0141778919894965

Caruso, E. (2023). The hyper-regulation of abortion care in Italy. *International Journal of Gynaecology and Obstetrics: the Official Organ of the International Federation of Gynaecology and Obstetrics*, 163(1), 1036–1042. DOI: 10.1002/ijgo.15150 PMID: 37724041

Cline, E. H. (2015). *1177 B.C.: The year civilization collapsed*. Princeton University Press.

David, H. P. (1992). Abortion in Europe, 1920-91: A public health perspective. *Studies in Family Planning*, 23(1), 1–22. DOI: 10.2307/1966824 PMID: 1557791

Georges, E. (1996). Abortion policy and practice in Greece. *Social Science & Medicine*, 42(4), 509–519. DOI: 10.1016/0277-9536(95)00174-3 PMID: 8643977

Hervey, T., & Banerjee, T. (2023). Abortion rights in EU law: Recent developments. BioLaw Journal – Rivista di BioDiritto, 1, 331-341.

Hogan, L. (2021). Women's reproductive rights and the legacy of religion in Ireland: The Eighth Amendment and its repeal. *Religion & Human Rights*, 16(2-3), 143–172. DOI: 10.1163/18710328-bja10021

Huss, B., & Kaiser, F. (2022). Induced abortion and life satisfaction in Germany: The role of selection processes and short-term effects. *Zeitschrift für Soziologie*, 51(4), 404–419. DOI: 10.1515/zfsoz-2022-0022

Ishola, F., Ukah, U. V., & Nandi, A. (2021). Impact of abortion law reforms on women's health services and outcomes: A systematic review protocol. *Systematic Reviews*, 10(1), 192. DOI: 10.1186/s13643-021-01739-w PMID: 34183064

Jubert, A., Bayen, M., Serman, F., Robin, G., Catteau-Jonard, S., Ollivon, J., Tilly, A., Messaadi, N., & Bayen, S. (2023). Medical tourism for late abortion: Women's profile and circumstances. A quantitative study among women who travelled within Europe for late abortion. *Sexual & Reproductive Healthcare : Official Journal of the Swedish Association of Midwives*, 36, 100824. DOI: 10.1016/j.srhc.2023.100824 PMID: 36893521

Keown, J. (1988). Anti-abortion legislation 1803–1861 and medical influence thereon. In *Abortion, doctors and the law: Some aspects of the legal regulation of abortion in England from 1803 to 1982* (pp. 26–48). Cambridge University Press. DOI: 10.1017/CBO9780511563683.004

Lennerhed, L. (2019). No backlash for Swedish women? The right to abortion on demand, 1975–2000. *Journal of Modern European History*, 17(3), 326–336. https://www.jstor.org/stable/26832829. DOI: 10.1177/1611894419854681

MacDonnell, V., & Hughes, J. (2013). The German abortion decisions and the protective function in German and Canadian constitutional law. *Osgoode Hall Law Journal*, 50(4), 999–1050. DOI: 10.60082/2817-5069.1008

McDougall, S. (2021). Pardoning infanticide in late medieval France. *Law and History Review*, 39(2), 229–253. DOI: 10.1017/S0738248020000267

Mishtal, J. (2014). Reproductive Governance in the New Europe: Competing Visions of Morality, Sovereignty and Supranational Policy. *Anthropological Journal on European Cultures*, 23(1), 59–76. DOI: 10.3167/ajec.2014.230104

Ostergren, R., & Bossé, K. (Eds.). (2004). *The Europeans: A history* (pp. 79–80). Guilford Press.

Pagden, A. (Ed.). (2000). *The Oxford illustrated history of prehistory*. Oxford University Press.

Pheterson, G., & Azize, Y. (2005). Abortion practice in the northeast Caribbean: "Just write down stomach pain.". *Reproductive Health Matters*, 13(26), 44–53. DOI: 10.1016/S0968-8080(05)26201-8 PMID: 16291485

Scott, J. (1998). Generational Changes in Attitudes to Abortion: A Cross-National Comparison. *European Sociological Review*, 14(2), 177–190. https://www.jstor.org/stable/522633. DOI: 10.1093/oxfordjournals.esr.a018233

Sedgh, G., Singh, S., & Hussain, R. (2016). Intended and unintended pregnancies worldwide in 2012 and recent trends. *Studies in Family Planning*, 45(3), 301–314. DOI: 10.1111/j.1728-4465.2014.00393.x PMID: 25207494

Skalts, V., & Nørgaard, M. (1965). Abortion legislation in Denmark. *Case Western Reserve Law Review*, 17(2), 498–556. https://scholarlycommons.law.case.edu/caselrev/vol17/iss2/10

Staunton, C. (2011). As easy as A, B and C: Will A, B and C v. Ireland be Ireland's wake-up call for abortion rights? *European Journal of Health Law*, 18(2), 205–220. DOI: 10.1163/157180911X564589 PMID: 21644438

Taylor, S. (2024). Abortion was a crime: Three medievalists respond to English cases dating back to the 13th century. Law and History Review. https://lawandhistoryreview.org/article/abortion-was-a-crime-three-medievalists-respond-to-english-cases-dating-all-the-way-back-to-the-13th-century-corroborate-the-treatises-statements-that-abortio/

Yarmohammadi, H., Zargaran, A., Vatanpour, A., Abedini, E., & Adhami, S. (2013). An investigation into the ancient abortion laws: Comparing ancient Persia with ancient Greece and Rome. *Acta Medico-Historica Adriatica : AMHA*, 11(2), 291–298. PMID: 24304111

Zampas, C., & Gher, J. M. (2008). Abortion as a human right: International and regional standards. *Human Rights Law Review*, 8(2), 249–294. DOI: 10.1093/hrlr/ngn008

## KEY TERMS AND DEFINITIONS

**Reproductive Rights:** Legal and human rights that enable individuals to make autonomous decisions about their reproductive health, including access to contraception, abortion, maternal health services, and assisted reproductive technologies.

**Contraception:** Methods or devices designed to prevent pregnancy by either inhibiting fertilization or implantation, encompassing hormonal, barrier, and permanent solutions.

**Maternal Health:** The health and well-being of women during pregnancy, childbirth, and the postpartum period, including access to essential medical care and measures to reduce maternal mortality.

**Abortion:** A medical procedure to terminate a pregnancy, with legal frameworks ranging from unrestricted access to severe restrictions, influencing the safety and legality of the procedure.

**Reproductive Autonomy:** The right of individuals to make independent and informed decisions about their reproductive lives, free from coercion, discrimination, or external pressure.

**Legal Frameworks:** The body of laws and regulations that govern reproductive health and rights within a given jurisdiction, including national, regional, and international legal instruments.

**Socio-Economic Factors:** Social and economic conditions that influence access to reproductive healthcare, including disparities in income, education, and geographic location that affect the availability and quality of services.

# Chapter 4
# Reproductive Rights as a Human Rights Challenge With Special Focus on Abortion:
## Insights From Poland and Slovenia

**Magdalena Matusiak-Frącczak**
*University of Lodz, Poland*

**Maja Pucelj**
https://orcid.org/0009-0001-9063-9080
*EMUNI University, Slovenia*

## ABSTRACT

*Women's right to abortion has recently been disputed after the judgment of the Polish Constitutional Tribunal of 22nd October 2020 and the judgment of the Supreme Court of the United States of 24th June 2022. These two decisions are regarded as restricting the right to abortion with the aim to protect the right to life of a foetus. Especially the Polish judgment resulted in massive protests in Poland, however in 2022 there was another attempt to limit women right to abortion by making it equal to murder. Therefore, it needs to be analysed what actually is the current status of women's right to abortion as part of reproductive rights, comparing the experiences of Poland and Slovenia. The research analyses the new developments regarding women's right to abortion and it strongly concentrates on the most recent case law and its impact on global understanding of basic human rights.*

DOI: 10.4018/979-8-3693-7837-3.ch004

## INTRODUCTION

According to the recent data, it is estimated that about 55,7 million abortions occurred worldwide each year in years 2010-2014. Out of these around 25,1 million abortions were unsafe, with 97% of them took place in developing states (Gantara et al., 2017, p. 2372; Margolin, 2007, pp. 29, 71; Mitra, 2017, p. 178). The WHO statistics show that the number of abortions each year has risen in the recent years to 73 million worldwide, out of which 45% is unsafe, with 97% still occurring in the developing states (WHO, 2015a; WHO, 2021). While Guttmacher Institute (2022) added that from 2015 to 2019, there were an estimated 121 million unplanned pregnancies per year worldwide, out of which about 61% resulted in abortions, regardless of the economic situation or legal position on abortion in the respective country.

Abortions are mostly permitted due to the risks of a threat to the woman's life or health, if the pregnancy is a result of incest or rape or in case of foetal impairment. Nowadays only 30% of states permit abortion on woman's request during a specified period of gestation (WHO, 2015a; Blagojević, 2020, p. 137-138, 147; Davis, 2018, p. 34). Yet there are jurisdictions, in which abortion is fully penalized regardless of any reasons (CEDAW, Costa Rica; CEDAW, Honduras; CRC, Malta), with the flagrant example of El Salvador that punishes women severely even in cases of miscarriages (El Salvador, Decreto Legislativo N° 1030 Código Penal, 26.4.1997, D.O. 105 of 10 June 1997, Articles 133-137; CEDAW, El Salvador; UN HRC, El Salvador). There are also states that theoretically permit abortion, however they set up such conditions therefor that lead to almost a complete abortion ban. For example, in Indonesia abortion can be provided up to the sixth week of pregnancy and only if the woman concerned furnishes a consent from the husband or, in the case of rape, a doctor's letter and an official statement from an expert concerning the alleged rape (CEDAW, Indonesia). Many restrictions are introduced by different states, like Somalia, Saudi Arabia, Afghanistan, El Salvador, or Malaysia, for religious reasons (Margolin, 2007, p. 80, 90-91; Davis, 2018, p. 36-37).

The direct incentive to revisit the right to abortion were two recent anti-abortion judicial decisions. One of them was the judgment of the Polish Constitutional Tribunal delivered in 2020 (Constitutional Tribunal (Poland), judgment of 22 October 2022, K 1/20) that declared unconstitutionality of the Polish law on abortion in the case of a serious foetus' abnormality (Article 4(1)(2) Statute of 7 January 1993 on the family planning, protection of human foetus and conditions of pregnancy termination, Dz. U. 2022, poz. 1575). This decision was followed by massive anti-governmental protests in Poland and was criticised by the European Parliament as a new attack on the rule of law (European Parliament resolution of 26 November 2020).

The other one was the judgment of the Supreme Court of the United States of 2022 in *Dobbs vs. Jackson* (SCOTUS, Dobbs, State Health Officer of the Mississippi Department of Health, et al. vs. Jackson Women's Health Organization et al. 597 U. S. ___ (2022)), overruling the SCOTUS' judgments in *Roe vs. Wade* (SCOTUS, Roe vs. Wade 410 U.S. 113 (1973)) and in *Casey* (SCOTUS, Planned Parenthood vs. Casey 505 U.S. 833 (1992)). The SCOTUS concluded that the right to abortion is not enshrined in the US Constitution and therefore it is the competence of the legislatures of the Federal States to regulate this issue independently.

These rulings permitted to ask a question whether the right to abortion is in rise or in decline. To answer this question, different laws and case-law, both international and national, will be analysed in the article. First, it will be deliberated, whether abortion can be considered to be a human right and what is the nature of this right. Then it will be explored, which human rights might potentially collide with the right to abortion. This examination will permit to form conclusion on which of the rights should prevail in the situation of conflict and answer the question that constitute the article's title, whether the women's right to abortion is in rise or in decline.

The aim of this paper is to explore and analyse the right to abortion in a broad international context from the legal perspective. That is why the deliberations will be based on legal texts, including judgments of international courts and tribunals, as well as decisions of international bodies. The human rights perspective will permit to establish the rights that stand behind the women's right to abortion and indicate those rights that oppose abortion. The deliberations in this area will allow to form conclusions on the balance of the conflicting rights at stake and to indicate which rights and why should prevail. The analysis in this chapter will be helpful especially to officials (like judges, policymakers, legislators) and lawyers to deal with the cases concerning abortion both in the area of law-making as well as during the process of the application of law. Having established the international standards, the authors will also offer some insights from their respective jurisdictions: Poland and Slovenia.

## ABORTION AS A HUMAN RIGHT

International law conventions as a rule do not mention expressly abortion as a separate human right. The only legal instrument that does so is art. XIV (2)(c) of the Protocol to the African Charter on Human and Peoples' Rights on the Rights of Women in Africa (Maputo, 1 July 2003):

> *"States Parties shall take all appropriate measures to protect the reproductive rights of women by authorising medical abortion in cases of sexual assault, rape, incest, and where the continued pregnancy endangers the mental and physical health of the mother or the life of the mother and the foetus".*

This protocol entered into force on 25.11.2005 and was signed by 49 states, yet until now it reached only 42 ratifications.

A comparative analysis, that will be the subject of this part of the article, shows that women's right to abortion needs to be regarded as a bundle of interrelated rights that need to be viewed as an entirety. Therefore, those rights will be deliberated in detail to show the variety of aspects that the right to abortion covers.

## Freedom from Cruel, Inhuman, or Degrading Treatment

The crucial human right for women's right to abortion is the freedom from torture or other cruel, inhuman or degrading treatment, which is a *jus cogens* norm of international law. A violation of this right encompasses both physical and mental suffering of a victim (Zureick, 2015, pp. 103-104; UN HRC, L.M.R. vs. Argentina (1608/2007), Views, CCPR/C/101/D/1608/2007, at para 9.2). Women denied abortion are subjected to abnormal suffering, they are forced to accept changes to their bodies and psychics regardless their physical and mental abilities (Sifris & Belton, 2017, p. 210; High Court of Kenya, *PAK & another v Attorney General & 3 others* (Constitutional Petition E009 of 2020) [2022] KEHC 262 (KLR); IA-CommHR, Beatriz vs. El Salvador, report No 9/20, decision of 3 March 2020; UN Committee on Economic, Cultural and Social Rights, General Comment No. 22). This breach of human rights occurs especially in, but is not limited to, the cases of minors being pregnant, of fatal foetus' abnormalities or of rape (Zureick, 2015, pp. 135-137; UN HRC, *Amanda Jane Mellet vs. Ireland* (2324/2013), Views, CCPR/C/116/D/2324/2013, at para 7.4; UN HRC Karen Noelia Llantoy Huamán vs. Peru (1153/2003), Views, CCPR/C/85/D/1153/2003 (2005); UN HRC, L.M.R. vs. Argentina, at para 9.2; UN HRC, General Comment No. 36).

The collision between abortion restrictions and the freedom from torture or other cruel, inhuman, or degrading treatment was noticed by the Committee Against Torture in its observations on Nicaragua. The CAT underlined that for women, especially for victims of gender-based violence, a complete abortion ban entails constant exposure to the violation committed against them and causes serious traumatic stress and a risk of long-lasting psychological problems such as anxiety and depression (CAT, Nicaragua).

In its views in *Mellet vs. Ireland* the UN HRC indicated the factors that determined a violation of the prohibition of cruel, inhuman, or degrading treatment by abortion ban in case of foetus' unviability. The applicant's rights were breached because she was not able to continue receiving medical care and health insurance coverage for her treatment from the Irish health care system, she was forced to travel to another country while carrying a dying foetus, at personal expense and separated from the support of her family, and to return while not fully recovered, she faced the shame and stigma associated with the criminalization of abortion of a fatally ill foetus, she left the foetus' remains in another country and then had them unexpectedly delivered to her by courier. In the end the state refused her to provide her with necessary and appropriate post-abortion and bereavement (at para 7.4). This position was reaffirmed by the in views in *Whelan vs. Ireland,* as the Committee took into consideration the facts that Ms. Whelan: was unable to continue to receive medical care and health insurance coverage for her treatment from the Irish health-care system, was abandoned by the Irish health-care system and had to gather information on her medical options alone, was forced to choose between continuing her non-viable pregnancy or travelling to another country while carrying a dying foetus, at personal expense and separated from the support of her family, suffered the shame and stigma associated with the criminalization of abortion of a fatally ill foetus, had to leave the baby's remains in a foreign country and did not receive necessary and appropriate bereavement counselling in Ireland (at para 7.5).

The ECtHR found a violation of Article 3 ECHR in *P. and S. vs. Poland* in which the minor P. was pregnant as a result of a rape. Due to this fact and the applicant's age the Court found her to be in a state of great vulnerability. Despite these circumstances, doctors tried to impose on her their religious views, in hospital she was even obliged to talk to a priest without asking, if she wanted to see one at all. As the information about the applicant seeking abortion leaked to anti-choice movements, i.e. through the media, the applicant was harassed by numerous unknown people and received many unwanted and intrusive text messages. All this led the Court to a conclusion that the applicant was treated by the authorities in a deplorable manner and that her suffering reached the minimum threshold of severity under Article 3 (ECtHR, *P. and S. vs. Poland,* Application No 57375/08, Merits and Just Satisfaction, 30 October 2012, at paras 157-169). However, in other instances the ECtHR was reluctant to find a breach of this human right (ECtHR, A, B, C vs. Ireland, Application No 25579/05, Merits and Just Satisfaction, 16 December 2010, at paras 160-165).

As it can be seen from the above-mentioned case law, restrictions on abortion can be regarded as a violation of the prohibition of cruel, inhuman or degrading treatment. It happens mostly when a woman is placed in a situation of great vulnerability due to her age, her state of health, the severe foetus' impairment, rape or incest. As the prohibition of cruel, inhuman or degrading treatment is a peremptory norm, states cannot derogate thereof, so at least in the above-mentioned situations abortion should be permissible without any exceptions and should not be subjected to any further conditions.

## Right to Life

Limitations or bans on abortion might result in violations of the right to life, as there exist a corelation between lack of abortion or unsafe abortions and maternal mortality, whereas women have right to survive pregnancy, childbirth and motherhood (Sifris & Belton, 2017, pp. 210, 217; WHO, 2015a; WHO, 2015b; Ngwena, 2013, p. 406; CEDAW, Congo; CEDAW, Honduras; CEDAW, Nicaragua; CRC, Argentina; International Conference on Population and Development, Resolutions adopted by the Conference, A/Conf.171/13. UN, Report of the Fourth World Conference on Women, Beijing, A/CONF.177/20/Rev.1. UN Committee on Economic, Cultural and Social Rights, General Comment No. 22). In 2020 about 287 000 women died during and following pregnancy and childbirth. 95% of these deaths occurred in low and lower-middle income states. 87% (253 000) of these deaths happened in Sub-Saharan Africa (202 000) and Southern Asia (47 000). In low income states the maternal mortality rate was 430 per 100 000 live births whereas at the same time in high income states it was only 13 per 100 000 live births (WHO, 2024a).

An unsafe abortion is a procedure for terminating an unwanted pregnancy either by persons lacking the necessary skills or in an environment lacking the minimal medical standards, or both (International Conference on Population and Development, Resolutions adopted by the Conference, A/Conf.171/13; African Commission on Human and People's Rights, General Comment no. 2 on Article 14.1 (a), (b), (c) and Article 14.2 (a) and (c) of the Protocol to the African Charter on Human and Peoples' Rights on the Rights of Women in Africa).

In international law sphere it is emphasized that states should ensure that women do not have to undergo clandestine abortions that constitute threat for their lives (CEDAW, Concluding comments, Chile; CEDAW, Kenya; CEDAW, Report, Twentieth Session, High Court of Kenya, *PAK & another v Attorney General & 3 others*; IACommHR, *Beatriz vs. El Salvador*; Supreme Court of India, Meera Santosh Pal and Ors vs Union of India and Ors [2017] AIR SC 787; UN HRC, Concluding Observations, Senegal; UN HRC, General Comment no. 28; UN HRC, General Comment no. 36). That is why almost all jurisdictions (95%) permit abortion when the pregnancy poses a risk to the life of the woman (WHO, 2015a). The CAT presents even the view that maternal deaths caused by the lack of timely medical intervention (abortion) to safe women's lives are in clear violation of numerous ethical standards of the medical profession (CAT, El Salvador; CAT, Nicaragua).

## Right to Health

Within women's right to abortion also women's right to physical and mental health is at stake as pregnancy, especially if unwanted, affects physical and psychological integrity of a woman and it is the woman who solely bears consequences of pregnancy in her body and mind (Davis, 2018, p. 40; Sifris & Belton, 2017, p. 210; Supreme Court of Canada, R. vs. Morgentaler 1988 CanLII 90 (SCC), [1988] 1 SCR 30; Supreme Federal Tribunal (Brazil), judgment of 29 November 2016 No 84.025-6/RJ; UN Economic and Social Council, Costa Rica). Right to health, meaning the right to the enjoyment of the highest attainable standard of physical and mental health, in confirmed in international law conventions (Article 12(1) International Covenant on Economic, Social and Cultural Rights, 1966, UN GA resolution 2200A (XXI)) and understood as including right to reproductive health (Margolin, 2007, p. 82; WHO, 2015b; CEDAW, Saint Lucia; Constitutional Court (Colombia), C-355/06, judgment of 10 May 2006; Constitutional Court (Colombia), D-13.956, judgment of 21 February 2022; European Parliament resolution of 26 November 2020; High Court of Kenya, *PAK & another v Attorney General;* Supreme Court of India, *Suchita Srivastava & Anr vs Chandigarh Administration,* (2009) 9 SCC 1; Supreme Federal Tribunal (Brazil), No 84.025-6/RJ; UN Human Rights Council, Resolution on Elimination of all forms of discrimination against women and girls) encompassing the freedom to make informed, free and responsible decisions on reproductive behaviour. The Constitutional Court of Colombia stressed expressly that women's right to health involves the right to abortion that is indispensable to safeguard to women a dignified life (Constitutional Court (Colombia), D-13.956; High Court of Kenya, *PAK & another v Attorney General*).

A detailed description of women's right to reproductive health was given by the UN Human Rights Council in its resolution of 2018. It pointed out that every individual, including women, has the right to have full control over and decide freely and responsibly on all matters relating to their sexuality and sexual and reproductive health, free from discrimination, coercion and violence. Bodily autonomy and universal access to sexual and reproductive health services should be respected (UN Human Rights Council, Resolution on Elimination of all forms of discrimination against women and girls).

The importance of right to reproductive health was also emphasized by the UN Committee on Economic, Cultural and Social Rights in its *General Comment no. 22* of 2016:

> *"The right to sexual and reproductive health is also indivisible from and interdependent with other human rights. It is intimately linked to civil and political rights underpinning the physical and mental integrity of individuals and their autonomy, such as the rights to life; liberty and security of person; freedom*

*from torture and other cruel, inhuman or degrading treatment; privacy and respect for family life; and non-discrimination and equality. For example, lack of emergency obstetric care services or denial of abortion often leads to maternal mortality and morbidity, which in turn constitutes a violation of the right to life or security, and in certain circumstances can amount to torture or cruel, inhuman or degrading treatment" (UN Committee on Economic, Cultural and Social Rights, General comment No. 22).*

Within this right it is postulated that medicines for abortion and post-abortion care should be made available to women (UN Committee on Economic, Cultural and Social Rights, General comment No. 22). Even if someone does not regard ban on abortion as a violation of the prohibition of torture or other cruel, inhuman or degrading treatment, it is undisputable that pregnancy might constitute a threat to women's health. Therefore, this risk is one of commonly approved situations in which abortion can take place (Sifris & Belton, 2017, p. 211), as it is accepted by 64% of jurisdictions (WHO, 2015a). It is worth noticing that a constant opponent of regarding abortion as a dimension of reproductive health is the Holy See (UN, Report of the Fourth World Conference on Women, Beijing, A/CONF.177/20/Rev.1).

Within the right to health the IACommHR decided that the rights of victims of sexual abuse are of utmost importance. These rights encompass not only access to appropriate medical services, including abortion, but also information and education in the discussed area (IACommHR, *Paulina del Carmen Ramírez Jacinto vs. Mexico*, report No 21/07, friendly settlement of 9 March 2007, at 19. European Parliament resolution of 26 November 2020). Another aspect on the right to health in relation to abortion is that unsafe abortions, to which women are forced by abortion restrictive laws, may cause serious illnesses like uterine perforation, sepsis, peritonitis, haemorrhage and even infertility (Ngwena, 2013, p. 406).

Therefore, women's right to health is connected to abortion in multiple ways. Termination of pregnancy is an element of reproductive health. If a woman chooses an abortion, she should have access to safe and professional medical services. Both, clandestine abortions and unwanted pregnancies influence negatively women's physical and mental health and integrity. We have to be aware of one crucial fact, that is that:

*"Global estimates from 2010–2014 demonstrate that 45% of all induced abortions are unsafe. Of all unsafe abortions, one third were performed under the least safe conditions, i.e. by untrained persons using dangerous and invasive methods. More than half of all these unsafe abortions occurred in Asia, most of them in south and central Asia. In Latin American and Africa, the majority (approximately 3 out of 4) of all abortions were unsafe. In Africa, nearly half of all abortions occurred under the least safe circumstances". (WHO, 2024b)*

## Non-Discrimination of Women

Next important source of women's right to abortion is the right to equality or in other words, the prohibition of discrimination in exercising the right to sexual and reproductive health. It is undisputable, that health needs of women differ from the needs of men and this divergence should be taken into consideration when regulating availability and legality of health services. Abortion restrictions or bans constitute gender-based discrimination and further undermine women's already unequal status in the society based on stereotypes related to women being subordinates of men and their role being solely as caregivers and mothers. As termination of pregnancy is a medical procedure that is related solely to women, it needs to be underlined that no medical procedures connected to men are banned or restricted in a way abortion is (Blagojević, 2020, p. 143; Margolin, 2007, p. 81; Sifris & Belton, 2017, p. 210; Ngwena, 2013, p. 401-402; Constitutional Court (Colombia), C-355/06; High Court of Kenya, *PAK & another v Attorney General*. Supreme Federal Tribunal (Brazil), No 84.025-6/RJ; UN Committee on Economic, Cultural and Social Rights, General Comment No. 22; UN HRC, *Mellet vs. Ireland*, at paras 7.10-7.1).

In fact, abortion bans make of a woman a mere object, an incubator, a vessel, a simple instrument of reproduction of human race, placing the woman and her body under "the use and control of others". It would constitute for women a deprivation of their human dignity. No such dehumanizing law is enacted with reference to male reproductive capacities (Blagojević, 2020, p. 143; Constitutional Court (Colombia), C-355/06 (the Court uses even the word "a receptacle"); High Court of Kenya, *PAK & another v Attorney General*). As the High Court of Kenya indicated, women's bodies were instrumentalized for cultural, political and economic purposes rooted in patriarchal traditions (High Court of Kenya, *PAK & another v Attorney General*).

To this regard Article 12 (1) of the Convention on the Elimination of All Forms of Discrimination against Women (New York, 18 December 1979, 1990 UNTS 1249) should be taken into consideration as the States are obliged to eliminate discrimination against women in the field of health care in order to ensure, on a basis of equality of men and women, access to health care services, including those related to family planning. The CEDAW in its *General Recommendation 24* concluded that limitations on abortions, especially the penalization thereof, is contrary to Article 12 (CEDAW, General Recommendation 24). This was subsequently confirmed in the CEDAW's views in *L.C. vs. Peru* (CEDAW, *L.C. vs. Peru* (22/2009), Views, CEDAW/C/50/D/22/2009). In this case the minor applicant's health was at stake, as she was 13 years old and pregnant due to sexual abuse. As a result, thereof, the applicant attempted to commit a suicide and afterwards required a surgery to avoid serious complications for her health in the future. The CEDAW emphasized that L.C. was discriminated, because the decisions on her health were postponed and influenced by the stereotype that protection of the foetus should prevail over the health of the mother. As a result of the delay L.C. was paralysed from the neck down save for some partial movement in her hands.

A firm conclusion on the violation of the right to non-discrimination on the basis of sex was declared by the UN HRC in *Whelan vs. Ireland* regarding the penalization of women for having an abortion. The Committee highlighted that the Irish penal regulations subjected the applicant to a gender-based stereotype according to which the primary role of women is reproductive and maternal. The Committee determined additionally that Ms. Whelan was denied, on the basis of her sex, access to medical services that she needed in order to preserve her autonomy, dignity, and physical and psychological integrity. *A contrario*, male patients and patients in other situations in Ireland are not expected to disregard their health needs and travel abroad in relation to their reproductive functions (UN HRC, *Whelan vs. Ireland,* at paras 7.11-7.12).

An interesting issue was decided by the ECtHR in *Evans vs. the United Kingdom* – a case that concerned embryos stored for an IVF procedure. Ms. Evans and her partner J. ended their relationship and afterwards he wrote to the clinic to notify it of the separation and to state that the embryos should be destroyed. The applicant opposed to his decision and looked for a judicial redress. The ECtHR determined that Article 8 incorporates the right to respect for both the decisions to become and not to become a parent. Taking that into consideration the Court concluded that the United Kingdom by respecting Mr. J.'s decision not to have a child with Ms. Evans and to destroy embryos obtained from his gametes has not transgressed the margin of appreciation (ECtHR, Evans vs. the United Kingdom, Application No 6339/05, Merits 10 April 2007, at paras 71, 90-92. Similarly on the right of gamete-donor to decide on embryos: Supreme Court of Tennessee, *Davis vs. Davis* 842 S.W.2d 588 (1992)). Therefore, if a man's right to decide on having or not having a child should be respected by destroying embryos, the same logic should be equally applied to a woman.

A similar logic is presented by the CEDAW in its *General Recommendation no. 21*. The Committee indicated that the number and spacing of their children have impact on women's lives and affect their physical and mental health. That is why women are entitled to decide on the number and spacing of their children (CEDAW, General Recommendation 21).

The right to anti-discrimination in the case of abortion is multidimensional. Prohibition or severe limitation of abortion might lead not only to discrimination on the basis of sex, but it can form a racial discrimination as well. In the United States its sources might be tracked to slavery period after 1808 (USA, An act to prohibit the importation of Slaves into any port or place within the jurisdiction of the United States, from and after the first day of January, in the year of our Lord one thousand eight hundred and eight, 2 March 1807, 2 Stat. 426), when international slave trade became prohibited and the only way for getting new slaves for slave owners was reproduction of enslaved persons. A more modern data in the United States show that due to costs of the medical services, anti-abortion laws influence heavily mostly poor women. Many of them are women of colour, who simply cannot afford neither contraception, nor abortion (Murray, 2021, pp. 2046-2048, 2030-2035, 2055).

A discrimination on social and race grounds may also stem from regulations providing that abortion medical services are not financed from public resources (as decided by the SCOTUS in Harris vs. McRae 448 U.S. 297 (1980). Similarly: United Kingdom Supreme Court, *R (on the application of A and B) (Appellants) v Secretary of State for Health (Respondent)* [2017] UKSC 41) or the necessity to travel abroad or to distant cities to look for a gynaecologist who does not object to abortion on the grounds of their religion (conscientious objection), so women are treated differently depending on the area in which they live (European Committee of Social Rights, *Confederazione Generale Italiana del Lavoro ((CGIL) vs. Italy*, complaint No 91/2013, decision of 12 October 2015, 190, at paras 204-213; European Committee of Social Rights, *International Planned Parenthood Federation – European Network (IPPF EN) vs. Italy*, complaint No 87-2012, decision of 10 March 2014, at paras 189-194). This might cause that abortion will be inaccessible to specific groups of women, placing their life and health at risk as mothers' mortality is higher among women in poor social and economic conditions (Sifris & Belton, 2017, pp. 212, 217; Ngwena, 2013, p. 406; Murray, 2021, pp. 2091-2093; Supreme Federal Tribunal (Brazil), No 84.025-6/RJ; Constitutional Court (Colombia), D-13.956). For example, in Texas abortions are not only excluded from public financing, but also private health insurers cannot cover abortion care, unless it is offered under a separate premium and signed for separately. On the contrary, in Canada abortion is largely covered by public finances (Davis, 2018, pp. 35, 37).

It results from the preceding deliberations that abortion bans and restrictions are discriminative. In the first place, women are limited in available medical services in a way men never were. Secondly, mostly poor women in difficult socio-economic situations are affected in protecting their most basic rights.

## Right to Privacy

One of the affected rights can be eventually right to privacy and personal liberty (Blagojević, 2020, pp. 142-143; Sifris & Belton, 2017, p. 210; Constitutional Court (Croatia), U-I-60/1991, judgment of 21 February 2017. High Court of Kenya, *PAK & another v Attorney General*; Supreme Court of Canada, *R. vs. Morgentaler*; UN HRC, *Mellet vs. Ireland*, at para 7.7), which was the right on which the *Roe vs. Wade* judgment was based, omitting anti-discrimination claims raised in other proceedings (Those claims were raised by the applicants in: *Hall vs. Lefkowitz* 305 F. Supp. 1030

(SDNY), *Abele vs. Markle* 342 F. Supp. 800 (D. Conn. 1972). Nevertheless, the *Roe vs. Wade* case preceded these cases in the SCOTUS, so finally *Hall vs. Lefkowitz* and *Abele vs. Markle* have never reached the Supreme Court). Naturally, abortion reflects women's private life and their private choices to have or not to have a child. Women have also right to freely decide on their own bodies (Sifris & Belton, 2017, p. 210). However, this right is not absolute and might be a subject to limitations. Due to this fact, the *Roe vs. Wade* logic could be undermined (Blagojević, 2020, p. 143; Murray, 2021, pp. 2048-2049, 2052, 2055), what finally happened in 2022 in *Dobbs vs. Jackson*.

The right to privacy was also discussed in other jurisdictions. The UN HRC decided on an arbitrary interference in the applicant's right to privacy (Article 17 ICCPR) in *Llantoy Huamán vs. Peru*. In this case the life of a minor mother was threatened by a fatal foetus' abnormality – anencephaly and the abortion was legally available in Peru, yet the applicant was refused the medical service by medical professionals. In *L.M.R. vs. Argentina* the Committee added that the right to privacy is also breached if judiciary intervenes in exercising women's right to abortion, which is a matter that should be decided by a woman and her physician (at paras 9.3-9.4).

The UN HRC confirmed its interpretation of the right to private life in *Whelan vs. Ireland* and decided that the Irish law penalizing women for having an abortion violated Article 17 ICCPR, as well as the limitations of the right to privacy stemming from the Irish regulations breached the principle of proportionality and did not balance the rights at stake properly, and were therefore arbitrary (UN HRC, *Whelan vs. Ireland,* at paras 7.8-7.9).

Within the ECHR the right to private life is a broad concept, encompassing, inter alia, the right to personal autonomy and personal development, whereas the notion of personal autonomy is an important principle underlying the interpretation of its guarantees. Moreover the notion of private live applies to decisions both to have or not to have a child or to become parents (ECtHR, *A, B, C vs. Ireland*, at para 212; ECtHR, *R.R. vs. Poland,* Application No 27617/04, Merits and Just Satisfaction 26 May 2011, at para 180; ECtHR, Tysiąc vs. Poland Application No 5410/03, Merits and Just Satisfaction, 20 March 2007, at para 107).

In the analysed area the ECtHR indicated that right to privacy (Article 8 ECHR) does not encompass a right to abortion on one hand, but on the other the decision of a pregnant woman to continue her pregnancy or not, as well as the prohibition of abortion when sought for reasons of health and/or well-being falls within the sphere of private life and autonomy (ECtHR, *A, B, C vs. Ireland*, at para 214; ECtHR, *P. and S. vs. Poland*, at para 96; ECtHR, *R.R. vs. Poland*, at para 181). On the basis of Article 8 ECHR States are under a positive obligation to secure to its citizens their right to effective respect for their physical and psychological integrity (ECtHR, *R.R. vs. Poland*, at para 185).

After analysing the laws of the member states of the Council of Europe, the ECtHR reached a conclusion that there is a consensus amongst the majority of these states towards allowing abortion and that most of them have in their legislation resolved the conflicting rights of the foetus and the mother in favour of greater access to abortion. Some limitations of women's access to abortion are permissible, however in individual cases the Court will assess, whether a fair balance between individual rights of a woman and the public interest in the protection of a foetus has been maintained (ECtHR, A, *B, C vs. Ireland*, at paras 213, 235; ECtHR, *R.R. vs. Poland*, at para 186).

Within positive obligations of states stemming from Article 8 ECHR, the ECtHR pointed at a right closely connected to abortion. States should effectively ensure to pregnant women access to diagnostic services which would make it possible for them to establish or dispel a suspicion that the foetus may be affected with ailments. To this regard the Court underlined that during pregnancy the foetus' condition and health constitute an element of the pregnant woman's health (ECtHR, R.R. vs. Poland, at paras 192-214).

Also, IACommHR referred to right to privacy by concluding, that this right is connected to reproductive autonomy of a person and access to medical services relating to reproductive health. For this reason, women should have access to the full scope of medical services without discrimination on the basis of sex (IACommHR, *Beatriz vs. El Salvador*).

Another area in which the right to privacy of women might be violated is the doctor-patient confidentiality, especially when treating women for abortion complications. This right may mostly be breached in states that have very strict penal provisions on abortions (CEDAW, Paraguay). Sometimes, as in the ECtHR's case in *P. and S. vs. Poland,* those data leaked from medical clinics to the general public. In this case anti-choice movements were sending letters to clinics in which a pregnant minor P. was trying to get an abortion, and some of their representatives organized protests at the entrance to the clinics, causing P.'s fear and intimidation. Confidentiality of medical data is a vital principle in democratic systems. The disclosure of such data may dramatically affect an individual's private and family life, as well as his or her social and employment situation, by exposing that person to opprobrium and the risk of ostracism. Moreover, this confidentiality is essential for the maintenance of that person's confidence in the medical profession and in the health services in general. As a result, affected persons might be reluctant to look for appropriate treatment (ECtHR, P. and S. vs. Poland, at para 128). In the discussed matter, women might be forced to look for unsafe, but secret, abortions, risking their life and health.

A similar view was adopted by the Constitutional Court of Colombia. The Court highlighted that the decision on abortion for reason of risk to woman's life and health is the decision of a woman and her doctor. For these purposes, the information about woman's identity and other sensitive data should not be revealed in relevant public decisions, including judicial ones (Constitutional Court (Colombia), T-841/11, judgment of 3 November 2011).

According to the African Commission on Human and People's Rights women's rights to privacy and confidentiality are violated if they are subjected by health care providers, police and/or judicial authorities to an interrogation on the reasons why they want to interrupt a pregnancy or when they are charged or detained for suspicion of illegal abortion when they seek post-abortion care. States should remove the obligation imposed by law to physicians and other health care providers to denounce cases of women who have undergone abortions (African Commission on Human and People's Rights, General Comment no. 2 on Article 14.1 (a), (b), (c) and Article 14.2 (a) and (c) of the Protocol to the African Charter on Human and Peoples' Rights on the Rights of Women in Africa).

It results from the above considerations that abortion is connected to the right to privacy in several ways. In the first place, the decision to have or not to have a child belongs to one's private life. An abortion itself, as part of women's health, is also covered by a patient-doctor confidentiality and the information about it should not be unreasonably revealed.

## Right to Effective Remedy

Regarding the above-mentioned rights, it is also emphasized that states should provide sufficient procedural guarantees and effective remedy for the protection of these rights. Currently in many states, despite partial legalization of abortion in cases of threat to maternal life or rape, women still have problems with availability of legal abortion services as they are lacking clear regulations that would ensure an effective implementation of the right to abortion (CEDAW, Mauritius; CRC, Argentina; ECtHR, *A, B, C vs. Ireland*, at paras 264, 267, UN HRC, *Mellet vs. Ireland*). A lack of an effective remedy is considered to be a separate human rights violation in abortion cases (ECtHR, *R.R. vs. Poland*, at paras 215-218; Supreme Court of Canada, *R. vs. Morgentaler*; UN HRC, *Llantoy Huamán vs. Peru*, where the Committee decided on a violation of Article 2 ICCPR) and states are under an obligation to establish an appropriate legal framework that allows women to exercise their right to abortion under conditions that guarantee the necessary legal security, including a rapid decision-making and the right to appeal in order to diminish the probability of complications and risk for women's health and life caused by delayed abortions (CEDAW, *L.C. vs. Peru* (22/2009); Supreme Court of Canada, *R. vs. Morgentaler*).

As it was concluded by the ECtHR, state's obligations cover both the provision of a regulatory framework of adjudicatory and enforcement machinery protecting individuals' rights, and the implementation, where appropriate, of specific measures. This legal framework should be shaped in a coherent manner which allows the different legitimate interests involved to be taken into account adequately and in accordance with the provisions of the Convention. The relevant procedure should guarantee to a pregnant woman at least the possibility to be heard in person and to have her views considered (ECtHR, *P. and S. vs. Poland,* at paras 96, 99). In the proceedings on abortion the time factor is of critical importance. That is why these procedures should ensure that such decisions are timely so as to limit or prevent damage to a woman's health which might be occasioned by a late abortion or by a coercion to give birth (ECtHR, *Tysiąc vs. Poland*, at para 118).

It needs to be underlined that a mere civil action for compensation and claiming damages in tort as a result of a breach of one's personal rights in various situations connected with unwanted pregnancies and access to abortion does not constitute an effective and accessible procedure allowing the victims of abortion refusals to vindicate their rights. These are retrospective measures that are not sufficient to protect personal rights of vulnerable women seeking for abortion (ECtHR, *P. and S. vs. Poland*, at paras 110-111; ECtHR, *R.R. vs. Poland*, at para 209; ECtHR, *Tysiąc vs. Poland*, at paras118-128). The available remedy should permit women a timely access to abortion.

On these grounds it can be concluded that women's right to abortion is multidimensional and it is formed by an interplay between different human rights. It encompasses freedom from cruel, inhuman, or degrading treatment, right to life and health, prohibition of discrimination and right to privacy. In order to safeguard an effective protection of these rights, they should be followed by procedural guarantees and right to effective remedy. They should also be seen as an entirety when confronted with the colliding rights.

## RIGHTS POTENTIALLY COLLIDING WITH THE WOMEN'S RIGHT TO ABORTION

The opponents of women's right to abortion often refer to several colliding rights. In this part of the paper following rights will be analysed: the foetus' right to life, non-discrimination of specific foetuses, women's right to health, rights of a potential father, conscientious objection and even freedom of expression.

## The Foetus' Right to Life

The right usually opposed to women's right to abortion is the foetus' right to life (Federal Constitutional Court (Germany), 1 BvF 1/74, 1 BvF 2/74, 1 BvF 3/74, 1 BvF 4/74, 1 BvF 5/74, 1 BvF 6/74, judgment of 25 February 1975, BVerfGE 39, 1; Constitutional Court (South Korea), 2017Hun-Ba127, judgment of 11 April 2019; Constitutional Tribunal (Poland): judgment of 28 May 1997, K 26/96; K 1/20; SCOTUS, *Dobbs vs. Jackson*) and the supporters of this view claim that a foetus is a person. The German Federal Constitutional Court has even declared that in general a woman has an obligation to carry "the child" until it is born and abortion might be permissible only in strictly exceptional situations. A woman is namely required to sacrifice her rights except of the point in which she would be requested to give up her own existential values like: her own human dignity, her life, her physical inviolability and her right to free development of her personality (Federal Constitutional Court (Germany), 2 BvF 2/90, 2 BvF 4/92, 2 BvF 5/92, judgment of 28 May 1993, BVerfGE 88, 203).

The foetus' right is *expressly* included in only one international convention – Article 4 (1) of the American Convention on Human Rights, according to which the protection of the right to life starts, in general, from the moment of conception. Yet this wording was the result of a compromise between catholic states of Latin America and those American states that permit abortion (Mitra, 2017, pp. 154-157). It was confirmed by the Inter-American Commission on Human Rights in *White and Potter (Baby Boy) vs. United States*. The Supreme Judicial Court of Massachusetts acquitted a doctor charged with manslaughter for performing an abortion. According to the Commission, this acquittal did not constitute a violation of Article 4 (1) AmCHR, as the wording "in general" used in framing the text of Article 4 (1) was aimed at granting states a discretion in formulating national laws on abortion and does not grant an absolute protection of a foetus (IACommHR, *White and Potter (Baby Boy) vs. United States*, case 2141, resolution 23/81 of 6 March 1981. Similarly: Constitutional Court (Colombia), C-355/06).

There are yet jurisdictions in which it is accepted that the right to life does not protect a foetus at all (Constitutional Tribunal (Austria), case no. G8/74, judgment of 11 October 1974) and in others it is highlighted that the right to life is not absolute and the protection of the right to life of a foetus does not reach the same level as the protection of a human person as higher protection is granted to life already formed than to life in formation (Constitutional Court (Colombia), C-355/06; Constitutional Court (Colombia), T-209-08, judgment of 28 February 2008; Constitutional Court (South Korea), 2017Hun-Ba127). To this regard the Supreme Court of Canada analysed in detail different stages of a foetus' development and stated that the value to be placed on the foetus as potential life is directly related to the stage of its development during gestation. The undeveloped foetus starts out as a newly fertilized ovum; the fully developed foetus emerges ultimately as an infant. A developmental progression takes place between these two extremes, and it has a direct bearing on the value of the foetus as potential life. Accordingly, the foetus should be viewed in differential and developmental terms. For these reasons, an abortion should be permissible in the early stages where the woman's autonomy would be absolute and restricted in the later stages where the states' interest in protecting the foetus would justify its prescribing conditions (Supreme Court of Canada, *R. vs. Morgentaler*). Also in the discussion on the foetus' right to life it is emphasized that although in some situations the foetus' rights might be even granted protection, its rights are subjected to and do not prevail over the rights of the woman (Blagojević, 2020, pp. 148-149; Constitutional Court (Colombia), C-355/06; Similarly: Constitutional Court (Croatia), U-I-60/1991; ECtHR, *Paton vs. United Kingdom*, Application No 8416/78, Admissibility, 13 May 1980; ECtHR, *Boso vs. Italy*, Application No 50490/99, Merits, 5 September 2000; ECtHR, *Vo vs. France*, Application No 53924/00, Merits, 8 July 2004, at paras 81-95).

As *A. Blagojević* and *I. Tucak* ironically but correctly point out, regarding of a foetus as a person is far from any kind of rational discussion. A foetus will become a person, once born. Moreover, these authors emphasize that abortion does not constitute a murder but a denial of the use of one body to provide sustenance to another (Blagojević, 2020, p. 142).

That is why, taking into consideration violations of prohibition of torture or other cruel, inhuman or degrading treatment, which is a peremptory norm of international law and states cannot derogate thereof regardless any reasons (IACommHR, *Beatriz vs. El Salvador*), the foetus' right to life cannot be legitimately claimed to be prevailing over women's rights. This interpretation was confirmed especially in cases in which the pregnancy was not viable, and the foetus' had fatal abnormalities, and the interference with women's right in those cases was decided to be unreasonable and arbitrary (UN HRC, *Mellet vs. Ireland*; UN HRC, *Whelan vs. Ireland*). A denial of an abortion in cases of a serious foetal impairment with little to no chance that the child survives long after birth neither serves the protection of life, nor constitutes a respect for life. In such cases women's rights always prevail (Zureick, 2015, p. 134; Constitutional Court (Colombia), C-355/06).

## Non-Discrimination of Foetus

Those connecting abortion with eugenics claim that abortion violates right to non-discrimination on the basis of sex, disability or race. They raise that these features of a foetus might be decisive factors in the decision-making process on abortion

(SCOTUS, *Kristina Box, Commissioner, Indiana Department of Health, et al. vs. Planned Parenthood of Indiana and Kentucky, Inc., et al.* 587 U. S. ___ (2019)).

Yet, these deliberations are based on randomly selected data and facts, as well as opportunistic and disregarding the data on systemic race inequities with the availability of abortion to women of different social classes and races (Murray, 2021, pp. 2088-2090). As it was shown in the previous part of the paper, termination of pregnancy affects right to non-discrimination of women as opposed to men and among women in different socio-economic situations. Therefore, abortion is a realisation of the women's equality rights, not their violation.

## Women's Right to Health

As an argument against abortion some opponents raise women's right to health and the protection of women against "post-abortion syndrome". Yet, the eventual existence of this "syndrome" is not based on any reliable evidence (SCOTUS, *Kristina Box, Commissioner, Indiana Department of Health, et al. vs. Planned Parenthood of Indiana and Kentucky, Inc., et al.* 587 U. S. ___ (2019)). A real threat to women's health is unsafe abortion provided by unqualified persons, what is proven by maternal deaths statistics discussed at the beginning of this article. Also the development of science needs to be taken into consideration, as nowadays it is possible to avoid surgical abortions and offer women safer pharmacological abortions with the use of substances like misoprostol or mifepristone (Sifris & Belton, 2017, p. 212), which currently in some jurisdictions are either unavailable or are restricted or prohibited by law (WHO, 2015b) despite the fact that they are enumerated by the WHO as essential medicines (WHO, 2021). The French Constitutional Council expressly rejected the argument that abortion within first 12 weeks of pregnancy threatens women's health (Constitutional Council (France), decision No 2001-446 DC of 27 June 2001).

## Potential Father's Right

Rights of a woman also prevail over rights of a man being a potential father. This issue was discussed by the European Commission on Human Rights. In *H. vs. Norway* the Commission indicated that when considering rights of a father under Article 8 ECHR one should take into account the rights of the woman being the person primarily concerned with the pregnancy and whose interests should be protected first of all (ECtHR, *H. vs. Norway*, Application No 17004/90, Admissibility, 19 May 1992. Similarly: ECtHR, *X. vs. Austria*, Application No 7045/75, Admissibility, 10 December 1976). Moreover, abortion is a private decision of a woman and nothing in the ECHR encompasses a man's right to be consulted or to apply to a court about an abortion which his wife or partner intends to have performed on her (ECtHR, *Paton vs. United Kingdom*; ECtHR, *Boso vs. Italy*. Similarly: Council of State (France), decision no. 13028 of 31 October 1980).

During pregnancy, the entire health burden rests on women not men. In addition, men's decisions on their bodies are never subjected to women's approval. There exist therefore no medical, moral nor logical arguments, why women's decisions on their bodies should be subjected to men's views.

## Conscientious Objection

Some states approve a conscientious objection to a doctor, as a part of their right to freedom of religion (WHO, 2015b; Constitutional Tribunal (Poland), judgment of 7 October 2015, K 12/14. UN HRC, Colombia). It permits doctors to refuse providing abortions at all or outside a case of emergency. At the same time this doctors' right should be followed by an obligation to provide women with information about her other options and places in which they can undergo abortions (Zureick, 2015, p. 134; Sifris & Belton, 2017, pp. 215-216; Constitutional Court (Colombia), C-355/06; Ontario Court of Appeal, *Christian Medical and Dental Society of Canada vs. College of Physicians and Surgeons of Ontario* 2019 ONCA 393; High Court of New Zealand, *NZ Health Professionals' Alliance v Attorney-General* [2021] NZHC 2510). States should impose strict justification rules to prevent blanket use of the conscientious objection by doctors, in particular when a minor is pregnant and ensure that these rules are applied both in public and private sectors (CEDAW, Concluding observations, Chile). Another prerequisite of the application of the objection is that a person concerned should make it expressly in writing (Constitutional Court (Colombia), T-388/09, judgment of 28.5.2009).

The Constitutional Court of Colombia raised important issues regarding the conscientious objection. Only natural persons, so doctors and other medical personnel, can refer to this objection. Legal persons and public entities, like states, hospitals, clinics, cannot deny abortion on religious grounds. Moreover, an objection should not be arbitrary, that is why it should be subsequently determined through mechanisms established for medical profession, whether it was in fact appropriate and pertinent (Constitutional Court (Colombia), C-355/06; Constitutional Court (Colombia), T-388/09, judgment of 28.5.2009). In another judgment the Court highlighted that conscientious objection cannot be raised by natural persons other than the medical staff directly responsible for the medical intervention necessary to terminate the pregnancy. Therefore, it is excluded for members of administrative staff or employees engaged in pre-abortion and post-abortion care. The Court added as well that the right to conscientious objection is not absolute. If there is no another health provider available in a due time to avoid risks to a woman's life or health, woman's rights should have priority over the doctor's religious rights (Constitutional Court (Colombia), T-388/09, judgment of 28.5.2009. Similarly: Constitutional Council (France), decision No 2001-446 DC).

The negative results of conscientious objection were enumerated by the European Committee on Social Rights. As a consequence of the introduction of this objection in Italy decreased the number of hospitals that carry out abortions, in many of the hospitals there are no or there is just one non-objecting gynaecologist, what causes problems with replacements during their illness, holiday or retirement, a relationship between the number of available non-objecting personnel and the number of abortion requests is disproportionate, the waiting time for abortion is excessive and there appear unfounded refusals of pre-abortion and post-abortion medical care. According to the Committee, conscientious objection has discriminative effect not only on women seeking abortion, but also it is an arbitrary discrimination of workers, namely the medical personnel. Moreover, in Italy doctors providing abortions were very often victims of mobbing so state failed to protect those medics from illegal harassment at work (European Committee of Social Rights, *Confederazione Generale Italiana del Lavoro ((CGIL) vs. Italy*, at paras 174, 235-246, 289-298. Similarly: European Parliament resolution of 26 November 2020).

Nevertheless, it cannot be omitted that freedom of religion is not an absolute right and can be subjected to limitations. If it is confronted with freedom from torture and other cruel, inhuman or degrading treatment, with women's right to life or health, these are the women's right that should prevail, as some of them are even of *jus cogens* nature. Due to the conscientious objection the realization of women's rights is at least delayed, and it might be completely jeopardized. According to the UN HRC states should completely remove this barrier for women in access to a safe abortion (UN HRC, General Comment No. 36).

This view seems to be partially adopted by the ECtHR in *P. and S. vs. Poland*. This case concerned numerous obstacles of a raped minor P. in having a legal abortion made by several hospitals. The Court determined that the right of physicians to refuse certain services on grounds of conscience, relying on Article 9 of the Convention, does not denote each and every act or form of behaviour motivated or inspired by a religion or a belief. Polish law has acknowledged the need to ensure that doctors are not obliged to carry out services to which they object and put in place a mechanism by which such a refusal can be expressed. This mechanism also includes elements allowing the doctor's right to objection to be reconciled with the patient's interests, by making it mandatory for such refusals to be made in writing and included in the patient's medical record and by imposing on the doctor an obligation to refer the patient to another physician competent to carry out the same service. None of this happened in the case of the applicant P. (ECtHR, *P. and S. vs. Poland*, at paras 106-107. Similarly: ECtHR, *R.R. vs. Poland*, at para 206). Actually currently, as it was correctly stated by the European Parliament, doctors create additional non-statutory obstacles, such as unnecessary medical examinations, psychological consultations or additional consultations with experts, that prevent women from obtaining a timely abortion (European Parliament resolution of 26 November 2020).

An interesting issue was raised in the Canadian jurisprudence. The Supreme Court of Canada presented an opinion that decision whether or not to terminate a pregnancy is essentially a moral decision belonging to woman's freedom of conscience and religion (Supreme Court of Canada, *R. vs. Morgentaler*. Similarly: Constitutional Court (Croatia), U-I-60/1991). Therefore doctors should not impose their own religion on a woman-patient seeking for medical treatment.

The above considerations lead to a conclusion that even if a state accepts the conscientious objection, women's right to abortion should be effectively guaranteed by procedural safeguards. On the other hand, there exist better places than hospital or other health units to perform religious beliefs, for example churches. In the author's personal view, the conscientious objection should be abandoned by states. If a doctor cannot provide all medical services solely due to religion, he or she should choose other medical specialisations than gynaecology or simply choose other profession.

## Freedom of Expression

Finally, women's right to privacy was also opposed to right to free speech of protesters manifesting against abortions at medical premises and preventing women the entry into the clinics. This use of right to free speech constitutes an intimidation and harassment of women that are already stressed by the medical service they want to undergo and to which they are entitled to (Sifris & Belton, 2017, p. 214). That was the reason underlying the adoption by the Victoria Parliament (Australia) *the Public Health and Wellbeing Amendment (Safe Access Zone) Act 2015 (Vic.)*. (no. 66 of 2015, 1 December 2015). For these reasons the women's right to abortion precedes claims based on freedom of expression of pro-choice activists.

It can be concluded that women's right to abortion might be in collision with several fundamental rights enumerated above. Taking into consideration the women's rights at stake, especially freedom from cruel, inhuman or degrading treatment, these are women's rights that should have priority in protection. Even the foetus' right to life is subjected to women's rights of fundamental character.

## INSIGHTS

## Abortion in Poland

Abortion is regulated in Poland by the statute on family planning, protection of human foetus and conditions of admissibility of abortion (ustawa z dnia 7 stycznia 1993 r. o planowaniu rodziny, ochronie płodu ludzkiego i warunkach dopuszczalności przerywania ciąży, Dz. U. 2022, poz. 1575, ze zm.). In its article the above-mentioned statute indicates that the right to life is protected also in the prenatal phase within the limits set forth in the statute.

The amendment of the statute made in 1996 (ustawa z dnia 30 sierpnia 1996 r. o zmianie ustawy o planowaniu rodziny, ochronie płodu ludzkiego i warunkach dopuszczalności przerywania ciąży, Dz. U. 1996, Nr 139, poz. 646) precised the conditions under which women could undergo abortion. It inserted Article 4a into the statute on family planning, protection of human foetus and conditions of admissibility of abortion permitting the abortion in the following situations:

a) when the pregnancy constitutes a threat to life or health of the pregnant woman;
b) prenatal examination or other medical indications show a high probability of severe and irreversible impairment of the foetus or an incurable disease that threatens its life;
c) there exists a reasonable suspicion that the pregnancy resulted from a crime;
d) the pregnant woman is in difficult living conditions or a difficult personal situation.

Already in 1997, the Polish Constitutional Tribunal annulled Article 4a (1)(d) permitting an abortion if the pregnant woman is in difficult living conditions or a difficult personal situation (Constitutional Tribunal (Poland), K 26/96, judgment of 28 May 1997). The Tribunal emphasized that the right to life of a foetus since conception is protected by the Polish Constitution and cannot be restricted by a statute, although the intensity of the protection might depend on the phase of life of the foetus and specific circumstances of the given case. The protection of the life of the foetus was also interpreted by the Tribunal from Article 24 UN Convention on the Rights of the Child (UNGA resolution 44/25 of 20 November 1989) and Article 79 (1) of the Polish Constitution protecting marriage, maternity, and family.

The next judgment of the Polish Constitutional Tribunal referred to the conscientious clause (Constitutional Tribunal (Poland), K 12/14, judgment of 7 October 2015) and in this judgment the Tribunal decided that every medical doctor has a constitutional right to the aforementioned objection, however it went a bit further. Before the judgment Article 39 of the statute on medical doctors and dentists' professions (ustawa z dnia 5 grudnia 1996 r. o zawodach lekarza i lekarza dentysty, Dz. U. 2022, poz. 1731, ze zm.) obliged doctors refusing abortions to present to the pregnant woman a real possibility of having an abortion made by another doctor or another health entity. The Constitutional Tribunal declared that this obligation violates Article 53 of the Polish Constitution providing for the right to freedom of conscience and religion. Ever since then on the basis of Article 39 of the statute on medical doctors and dentists' professions obliges medical doctors refusing an abortion only to make a note in the patient's medical records and to inform their employer in writing that they apply the conscientious clause.

Another huge blow to the women's right to abortion was brought by the judgment of the Polish Constitutional Tribunal of 2020 (Constitutional Tribunal (Poland), K 1/20), as it annulled art. 4(1)(b) of the statute on family planning, protection of human foetus and conditions of admissibility of abortion permitting for an abortion if prenatal examination or other medical indications show a high probability of severe and irreversible impairment of the foetus or an incurable disease that threatens its life. Once again, the judgment focus on the right to life of the foetus and repeated broadly the justification of the judgment of 1997. However, it needs to be emphasized that this very judgment was issued by an organ that cannot be considered to be an impartial and independent tribunal established by law (ECtHR, *Xero Flor w Polsce sp. z o.o. vs. Poland,* Application No. 4907/18, judgment of 7 May 2021). This was confirmed to be a violation of procedural guarantees protecting against arbitrariness as enshrined in Article 8 ECHR by the European Court of Human Rights in 2023 (ECtHR, *M.L. vs. Poland,* app. no. 40119/21, judgment of 14 December 2023).

A careful analysis of the Polish Constitution and the preparatory works thereof suggests however, that the Polish Constitutional Tribunal erred in law in several aspects. It was an intention of the Polish legislator not to insert into the constitution the protection of the right to life from the moment of conception, such possibility was subjected to voting during the legislative works and it was finally rejected. Moreover, the legislator itself used words like "foetus" or "nasciturus", whereas the work "human" was reserved only to those who were already born. The deliberations in all of the abovementioned judgments were very general and vague what might lead to a conclusion that it was not a dogmatic analysis of existent law, but rather an ideological one. Thus, the Tribunal instead of judging, imposed a self-created regulation on the entire society, so it acted arbitrarily not like a court but like a legislator in clear violation of the division of powers (Kozub-Ciembroniewicz, Szumiło-Kulczycka, 2022, pp. 33-34, 39-45; Adamus, 2020, p. 97).

In all of the above-mentioned judgments of the Constitutional Tribunal there is one issue missing, namely the rights of women colliding with the foetus' right to life and with the medical doctors right to freedom of conscience and religion. This problem has become apparent especially after the judgment in K 1/20 on the embryo-pathologic reasons for abortion. The decision of a woman to interrupt the pregnancy in such a case cannot be considered differently than a serious moral decision adherent to the woman because of her own human dignity. In the judgment of 2020, the Polish Constitutional Tribunal decided in place of every Polish woman. This leads to the violation of the prohibition of torture or other inhuman, cruel or degrading treatment, the right of women that has not been taken by the Tribunal into consideration. Yet, in the current state of the Polish constitutional law, as well as international law, the right to life and the freedom of conscience and religion are not an absolute right and can be limited, whereas the prohibition of torture or other inhuman, cruel or degrading treatment is a *jus cogens* norm. Additionally, it has to be mentioned that the legal system in Poland provides for no sociological and psychological support to women in such situations (Adamus, 2020, p. 103-104; Gutowski, Kardas, 2020, pp. 5, 8, 11).

In August 2024 the CEDAW delivered its report on abortion in Poland, in which it confirmed that the restrictive laws on abortion lead to numerous violations of women's rights, leading also to deaths of pregnant women. It emphasized that it is difficult for women to obtain abortion even in the cases provided for by the Polish law, and this concerned especially difficulties faced to access abortion based on a threat for the woman's mental health. The criminal code penalizing help in abortion causes a chilling effect among medical staff. A very important barrier in accessing abortion by women in Poland are refusals of medical personnel to carry out abortion based on conscientious objection. Poland was called i.a. to ensure effective, timely and accessible procedures for abortion and to recognize the right to abortion as a human right (CEDAW, Inquiry concerning Poland...).

## Abortion in Slovenia

As Jerebič noted the legalization of abortion in the Soviet Union in 1955 had a positive impact on most communist countries. Women in Yugoslavia obtained the right to undergo abortion in a progressive manner. Starting in 1952, it was permissible during the initial trimester, but only with the consent of the commission, which typically granted approval due to the pregnant woman's social misery. Otherwise, it was formally prohibited. The official authorization for abortion was granted in 1977, but women were still required to obtain consent from a specialized panel (Jerebič, 2018).

The procedure of artificial termination of pregnancy is free for everyone who has compulsory health insurance in Slovenia. Mentioned possibility is (looking at European territory) beside Slovenia available only in Belgium and Denmark. Slovenia permits artificial termination of pregnancy by the woman's request up to the 10th week of pregnancy (counted from the 1st day of the last menstrual period). The free decision on the birth of children is given by the Constitution of the Republic of Slovenia in the Article 55, where it is stated: "Deciding on the birth of your children is free. The state provides opportunities for the realization of this freedom and creates conditions that allow parents to make decisions about the birth of their children. (URS, 1991, Article 55) If an individual residing in Slovenia lacks compulsory health insurance or is a non-resident foreigner, they are required to pay for the service themselves. The cost of an elective abortion can significantly differ based on factors such as gestational age, termination method, anesthesia type, length of hospitalization, and other variables. The duration of the hospital stays and recovery after an artificial termination of pregnancy is uncertain due to infrequent but potential complications.

All conditions and additional information regarding artificial termination of pregnancy are stated in the Health Measures in Exercising Freedom of Choice in Childbearing Act (ZZNPOB, 1977). In first article of the mentioned act, it is stated: "A person has the right to freely decide on the birth of children. Women and men must have access to all the options that help them realize this right in the context of health care." (ZZNPOB, 1977). Despite the fact that reproductive rights are declared in Slovenia, these rights are still being called into question by conservative organizations. Their argumentation is focused on the aspects that they object to abortion as they prioritize the sanctity of life. Abortion is regarded as a sin or moral transgression in numerous religious systems. They also argument that opting for abortion might result in enduring adverse psychological, emotional, and occasionally physical repercussions for women. Some opponents support their argument against abortion with the help of reference on the scientific information regarding the development of unborn babies, including factors such as heartbeat and pain sensibility. This diametral opinion is reflected also in public gatherings, where for example in 2023, we could see the March for Life in Ljubljana, where opponents of the right to abortion gathered and advocated that human life begins at conception and ends at natural death. At the same time, a countermarch under the slogan "My body, my decision" took place in the same city, which defended the importance of the right to abortion for a woman. (N1info.si, 2023).

On the other hand, Ministry of Labor, Family, Social Affairs and Equal Opportunities emphasizes the importance of the right to an abortion:

> *"is not only a right to medical intervention, but in its essence is the right to self-determination, to bodily autonomy and to the ability to decide about one's own future. /.../ The right and access to safe termination of pregnancy is a civilizational achievement that enables a choice in one of the key decisions in the lives of many women and /.../ is an achievement that primarily recognizes the freedom, autonomy, integrity and dignity of every woman. In a world where*

*women are still fighting for equality, it is imperative that we defend and preserve these rights." (Gov.si, 2023).*

When looking at statistical data in Slovenia, we can see that the number of permitted abortions in Slovenia is decreasing due to the availability of contraceptives. (Intihar, 2023) In 1997 (up to the tenth week), according to data from the National Institute of Public Health, 9,273 abortions were performed, in 2007 4,801, and in 2022 only 2,760 abortions were performed. The number of abortions per thousand women between the ages of 15 and 49, i.e. of reproductive age, is seven, which ranks Slovenia alongside the most developed countries. (Pust, 2023) Specialist in gynecology and obstetrics from the Gynecological Clinic of the University Hospital Ljubljana assoc. prof. dr. Bojana Pinter, Ph.D. med., spec. noted that: "In 2011, the permitted abortion rate was 9.0/1000, and in 2021 it was 6.9/1000, which means that the permitted abortion rate in Slovenia has decreased by 30% in the last ten years. This is extremely good. The data show that the permitted abortion rate in Slovenia is constantly decreasing, while the birth rate is still high. We have 6.3 births per one permitted abortion" (Pinter in: Pust, 2023) The continues effort of Slovenia to ensure the right to abortion for women has surpassed its inner boarders, when 8 March Institute from Slovenia within the framework of the My Voice, My Decision campaign, submitted a European citizens' initiative in 2024 with a clear request - that the European Union must prepare a financial mechanism that would support member states in ensuring safe and accessible abortion rights (N1info.si, 2024). But nevertheless, even though constitution gives the right to women to safely, legally, and without cost terminate an undesired pregnancy through abortion, we can still note a presence of major stigmatization of mentioned practice in the society. Slovenia still exhibits a disparity between its legislative framework and community views, emphasizing the necessity for continuous public education and dialogue to rectify misunderstandings and foster a more comprehensive comprehension of reproductive rights.

## CONCLUSION

To sum up, despite the judgments of the Polish Constitutional Tribunal and of the SCOTUS, it can be concluded that women's right to abortion is in rise (Davis, 2018, pp. 37-38) and more positive changes should be seen in that area. Recently, on the 5.1.2023 the Supreme Court of South Carolina decided that the Constitution of South Carolina grants protection to right to privacy and an abortion ban after 6$^{th}$ week of the pregnancy constitutes an unreasonable intrusion into a person's private reproductive health decisions (Supreme Court of South Carolina, *Planned Parenthood et al. vs. State of South Carolina et al.*, appellate case no. 2022-001062, opinion no.

28127 of 5 January 2023), so it interpreted the state Constitution contrary to the way the SCOTUS interpreted the US Constitution.

When examining abortion regulations in Slovenia and Poland, important differences can be observed that are shaped by societal, legal, and political factors. Slovenia permits abortion upon request until the 10th week, affirming women's autonomy in making decisions regarding delivery, as emphasised by its Constitution and healthcare policy. Poland's abortion regulations are rigorous and have been influenced by recent decisions from the Constitutional Tribunal. These laws strictly limit abortion, allowing it only in limited situations, such as when the woman's life or health is at risk, or when there are specific prenatal abnormalities. The legislative frameworks in Slovenia and Poland are a reflection of the cultural and political attitudes towards reproductive rights in each nation. Slovenia has implemented more inclusive policies, while Poland has imposed restrictive ones. These distinct approaches have sparked public debate and demonstrations, highlighting the contrasting societal views on the topic.

In international area it is emphasized that abortion laws should be liberalized and that a mere decriminalisation of abortion is not enough to safeguard women's rights properly (Sifris & Belton, 2017, p. 214; WHO, 2015a; CEDAW, Brazil; CEDAW, Concluding comments, Chile; CEDAW, Lichtenstein; CEDAW, Mauritius; IACommHR, *Beatriz vs. El Salvador*; UN Economic and Social Council, Peru; UN Committee on Economic, Cultural and Social Rights, General Comment No. 22). States should ensure that legal abortion is available and enforced by medical professionals in due time without intervention by the courts (CEDAW, Monaco; CEDAW, Sri Lanka; Constitutional Court (Colombia), T-841/11; CRC, Argentina). It should be followed by guarantees of universal and equitable access to affordable, acceptable and quality sexual and reproductive health services, goods and facilities, as well as measures to prevent unsafe abortions (Constitutional Court (Colombia), D-13.956; High Court of Kenya, *PAK & another v Attorney General*; UN Committee on Economic, Cultural and Social Rights, General Comment No. 22). Women should be also promptly and correctly informed about their reproductive rights and the procedures for their vindication and protection (Constitutional Court (Colombia), T-627/12, judgment of 10 August 2012).

Moreover, states should as well prevent and address stigma and discrimination against women who seek abortion services or treatment for abortion complications (WHO, 2015a; UN HRC, General Comment No. 36). Additionally, if a pregnancy is the result of rape, states should not subject women to excessive questioning and invasive measures for securing forensic or medico-biological proof (CEDAW, Monaco; CEDAW, Hungary).

In case of a pregnant minor, states are obliged to provide for safe abortion and post-abortion services irrespective of whether abortion itself is legal at all (CRC, General Comment no. 15 (2003)). They should also ensure that the minor's views are always heard and given consideration as part of the decision-making process (CRC, Malta), so that the decision is not based solely on the minor's parents' or state representative's opinion.

It needs to be pointed out that neither legal restrictions result in fewer abortions, nor they result in significant increases in birth rates. Therefore, it is doubtful, whether abortion restrictions and bans protect "life in gestation" effectively. To the contrary, the removal of barriers in the access to abortion results in reduction of maternal mortality and serious illnesses stemming from unsafe abortion (WHO, 2015a, Constitutional Court (Colombia), D-13.956).

An attention should be also paid to a linguistic phenomenon. The analysis of different documents shows that the anti-abortion case-law as well as movements try to re-shape the language that is used in the public discussion on women's most basic rights. In the decisions and judgments that limit women's right to abortion the authors use "unborn", "unborn life", "child", "conceived child", "unborn child" or "unborn human being", which are emotive words, instead of the medical terms "foetus" or "*nasciturus*" (Constitutional Tribunal (Poland), K 1/20; ECtHR, *A, B, C vs. Ireland*, at para 233; Federal Constitutional Court (Germany): 1 BvF 1/74...; 1 BvR 2306/96, 1 BvR 2314/96, 1 BvR 1108/97, 1 BvR 1109/97, 1 BvR 1110/97, judgment of 27 October 1998, BVerfGE 98, 265; SCOTUS, *Dobbs vs. Jackson*; UN HRC, *Whelan vs. Ireland*, in which Ireland used the notion "the unborn", whereas the Committee used emotionally neutral notion of "a foetus"). Moreover, abortion itself, together with birth control movements, are associated with eugenics (SCOTUS, *Kristina Box vs. Planned Parenthood*), although these arguments are simplistic and based on a mere fact, that early abortion movements appeared at the same time when eugenic movements developed (2028, 2032-2033). Others associate abortion with euthanasia, assisted suicide or even a murder/killing of a foetus (Blagojević, 2020, pp. 142-143: The authors indicate that such views appear in the public debate on abortion, but they do not identify themselves with them; Federal Constitutional Court (Germany), 2 BvF 2/90...). At the same time anti-choice movements avoid mentioning women's rights. This policy aims at creating a negative atmosphere over abortion in public debate and stigmatizes women seeking protection of their most basic rights.

Nevertheless, discussion on abortion should be based on legal and scientific arguments, and not on the emotional ones, as only then making a proper balance of conflicting rights is possible. Moreover, these emotional arguments of the anti-choice movements can be denied for several reasons. The authors of these arguments usually forget that women are human beings with set of human rights inherent to them. With the moment of impregnation women do not lose their rights nor these rights are restricted. Thus, women enjoy full legal personhood and they are entitled to reproductive autonomy and bodily integrity. Depriving women of these rights would make them a mere object, maybe even only an incubator, that serves to safeguard foetus' rights irrespective of circumstances. Such a result would be unacceptable from the human rights perspective.

## REFERENCES


Adamus, R. (2020). Przesłanka eugeniczna (embriopatologiczna) jako przesłanka legalnego przerywania ciąży – glosa do wyroku Trybunału Konstytucyjnego z 22.10.2020 r. (K 1/20). *Palestra*, 11, 95–105.

Blagojević, A. (2020). Rethinking the Right to Abortion. *Balkan Social Science Review*, 15, 136–157. DOI: 10.46763/BSSR20150136b

CAT. Concluding observations of the Committee against Torture: Nicaragua. CAT/C/NIC/CO/1.

CAT. Concluding observations of the Committee against Torture: El Salvador. CAT/C/SLV/CO/2.

CEDAW. Report of the Committee on the Elimination of Discrimination against Women, Twentieth Session (19 January – 5 February 1999). A/54/38/Rev.1.

CEDAW. Concluding comments of the Committee on the Elimination of Discrimination against Women: Chile. CEDAW/C/CHI/CO/4.

CEDAW. Concluding comments of the Committee on the Elimination of Discrimination against Women: Congo. CEDAW/C/COG/CO/6.

CEDAW. Concluding comments of the Committee on the Elimination of Discrimination against Women: Costa Rica. CEDAW/C/CRI/CO/7.

CEDAW. Concluding comments of the Committee on the Elimination of Discrimination against Women: El Salvador. CEDAW/C/SLVCO/8-9.

CEDAW. Concluding comments of the Committee on the Elimination of Discrimination against Women: Honduras. CEDAW/C/HND/CO/7-8.

CEDAW. Concluding comments of the Committee on the Elimination of Discrimination against Women: Indonesia. CEDAW/C/IND/CO/8.

CEDAW. Concluding comments of the Committee on the Elimination of Discrimination against Women: Kenya. CEDAW/C/KEN/CO/7.

CEDAW. Concluding comments of the Committee on the Elimination of Discrimination against Women: Lichtenstein. CEDAW/C/LIE/CO/5/Rev.1.

CEDAW. Concluding comments of the Committee on the Elimination of Discrimination against Women: Mauritius. CEDAW/C/MUS/CO/8.

CEDAW. Concluding comments of the Committee on the Elimination of Discrimination against Women: Saint Lucia. CEDAW/C/LCA/CO/6.

CEDAW. Concluding comments of the Committee on the Elimination of Discrimination against Women: Nicaragua. CEDAW/C/NIC/CO/6.

CEDAW. Concluding comments of the Committee on the Elimination of Discrimination against Women: Paraguay. CEDAW/C/PRY/CO/6.

CEDAW. Concluding observations on the combined seventh and eight periodic reports of Hungary adopted by the Committee at its fifty fourth session. CEDAW/C/HUN/CO/7-8.

CEDAW. Concluding observations on the eight periodic report of Sri Lanka. CEDAW/C/LKA/CO/8.

CEDAW. Concluding observations on the seventh periodic report of Chile. CEDAW/C/CHLCO/7.

CEDAW. General Recommendation 21: Equality in Marriage and Family Relations. A/49/38.

CEDAW. General Recommendation 24: Article 12 of the Convention on the Elimination of All Forms of Discrimination against Women. A/54/38/Rev.1.

CEDAW. Inquiry concerning Poland conducted under article 8 of the Optional Protocol to the Convention. CEDAW/C/POL/IR/1.

CEDAW. Concluding comments of the Committee on the Elimination of Discrimination against Women: Brazil. CEDAW/C/BRA/CO/6.

CEDAW. Concluding observations on the combined initial to third periodic reports of Monaco. CEDAW/C/MCO/CO/1-3.

CRC. General Comment no. 15 (2013) on the right of the child to the enjoyment of the highest attainable standard of health (art. 24). CRC/C/GC/15.

CRC. Concluding comments of the Committee on the Elimination of Discrimination against Women: Malta. CRC/C/MLT/CO/3-6.

CRC. Consideration of reports submitted by States parties under article 44 of the Convention, Concluding observations: Argentina. CRC/C/Arg/CO/3-4.

Davis, M. F. (2018, August 1). *Truth is Truth: U.S. Abortion Law in the Global Context*. Retrieved September 18, 2024, from https://papers.ssrn.com/sol3/papers.cfm?abstract_id=3264833

European Parliament resolution of 26 November 2020 on the de facto ban on the right to abortion in Poland (2020/2876(RSP)), OJ C 425, 20.10.2021, pp. 147-154

Ganatra, B., Gerdts, C., Rossier, C., Johnson, B. R.Jr, Tunçalp, Ö., Assifi, A., Sedgh, G., Singh, S., Bankole, A., Popinchalk, A., Bearak, J., Kang, Z., & Alkema, L. (2017). Global, regional, and subregional classification of abortions by safety, 2010–14: Estimates from a Bayesian hierarchical model. *Lancet*, 390(10110), 2372–2381. DOI: 10.1016/S0140-6736(17)31794-4 PMID: 28964589

Gov.si. (2023, October 6). *Pravica do splava je civilizacijski dosežek.* Retrieved September 18, 2024, from https://www.gov.si/novice/2023-10-06-pravica-do-splava-je-civilizacijski-dosezek/

Gutowski, M., & Kardas, P. (2020). Trybunał Konstytucyjny nie mógł rozstrzygnąć gorzej, czyli o dewastacji systemu jednym rozstrzygnięciem. *Palestra*, 10, 5–12.

Guttmacher Institut. (2022). *Unintended Pregnancy and Abortion Worldwide.* Retrieved September 18, 2024, from https://www.guttmacher.org/fact-sheet/induced-abortion-worldwide

Intihar, A. (2023). *Možnost za varno prekinitev nosečnosti rešuje življenja. Delo.si.* Retrieved September 18, 2024, from https://www.delo.si/novice/slovenija/moznost-za-varno-prekinitev-nosecnosti-resuje-zivljenja/

Jerebič, T. (2018, May 28). *Pravica do splava. HomoCumolat.com.* Retrieved September 18, 2024, from https://homocumolat.com/2018/05/28/pravica-do-splava/

Kozub-Ciembroniewicz, K., & Szumiło-Kulczycka, D. (2022). Czy aborcja naprawdę jest sprawą Konstytucji? *Palestra*, 10, 33–49.

Margolin, T. A. (2007). Abortion as a Human Right. *Women's Rights Law Reporter*, 29(77), 77–98.

Mitra, A. (2017). "We're always going to argue about abortion" – International law's changing attitudes towards abortion. *New Zealand Women's Law Journal*, 1, 142–181.

Murray, M. (2021). Race-ing Roe: Reproductive Justice, Racial Justice, and the Battle for Roe v.vs. Wade. *Harvard Law Review*, 134(6), 2025–2102. Retrieved September 18, 2024, from https://harvardlawreview.org/print/vol-134/race-ing-roe/

N1info.si. (2023). V *Ljubljani so se zbrali podporniki in nasprotniki pravice do splava.* Retrieved September 18, 2024, from https://n1info.si/novice/slovenija/v-ljubljani-so-se-zbrali-podporniki-in-nasprotniki-pravice-do-splava-video/

N1info.si. (2024). *Institut 8. marec z vseevropsko kampanjo: Borili se bodo za pravico do splava*. Retrieved September 18, 2024, from https://n1info.si/novice/slovenija/institut-8-marec-z-vseevropsko-kampanjo-borili-se-bodo-za-pravico-do-splava/

Ngwena, C. G. (2013). *Reforming African abortion laws to achieve transparency : arguments from equality*. Retrieved September 18, 2024, from https://repository.up.ac.za/handle/2263/41812?show=full

Pust, S. (2023). *Zato se toliko splavov pri nas opravi samoplačniško. Žurnal24*. Retrieved September 18, 2024, from https://www.zurnal24.si/zdravje/zato-se-toliko-splavov-pri-nas-opravi-samoplacnisko-403232

Sifris, R., & Belton, S. (2017). Australia: Abortion and Human Rights. *Health and Human Rights Journal*, 19, 209–220. PMID: 28630553

UN Committee on Economic, Cultural and Social Rights. General Comment No. 22 (2016) on the right to sexual and reproductive health (article 12 of the International Covenant on Economic, Social and Cultural Rights). E/C.12/GC/22.

UN Economic and Social Council. Concluding observations on the fifth periodic report of Costa Rica. E/C.12/CRI/CO/5.

UN Economic and Social Council. Consideration of reports submitted by State parties under articles 16 and 17 of the Covenant, Peru. E/C.12/PER/CO/2-4.

UN HRC. Concluding observations on the seventh periodic report of Colombia. 17.11.2016. CCPR/C/COL/CO/7.

UN HRC. Concluding observations on the fifth periodic report of Senegal. CCPR/C/SEN/CO/5.

UN HRC. Concluding observations on the seventh periodic report of El Salvador. CCPR/C/SLV/CO/7.

UN HRC. General Comment No. 28, Article 3 (The equality of rights between men and women). CCPR/C/21/Rev.1/Add.10.

UN HRC. General Comment No. 36, Article 6: right to life. CCPR/C/GC/36.

UN Human Rights Council. Resolution on Elimination of all forms of discrimination against women and girls. UN Doc. A/HRC/38/L.1/Rev.1.

URS. (1991). *Constitution of the Republic of Slovenia*. Retrieved March 11, 2024, from https://pisrs.si/Pis.web/pregledPredpisa?id=USTA1

World Health Organization. (2015a) *Safe abortion: Technical & policy guidance for health systems*. Retrieved September 18, 2024, from https://apps.who.int/iris/bitstream/handle/10665/173586/WHO_RHR_15.04_eng.pdf

World Health Organization. (2015b) *Sexual health, human rights and the law*. Retrieved September 18, 2024, from https://apps.who.int/iris/bitstream/10665/175556/1/9789241564984_eng.pdf

World Health Organization. (2021) *Model list of essential medicines*, 22nd List.

World Health Organization. (2024a). *Maternal Mortality*. Retrieved October 6, 2024, from: https://www.who.int/news-room/fact-sheets/detail/maternal-mortality

World Health Organization. (2024b). *Abortion*. Retrieved October 9, 2024, from: https://www.who.int/news-room/fact-sheets/detail/abortion

Zureick, A. (2015, January 16). *(En)Gendering Suffering: Denial of Abortion as a Form of Cruel, Inhuman or Degrading Treatment*. Retrieved September 18, 2024, from https://papers.ssrn.com/sol3/papers.cfm?abstract_id=2579416

ZZNPOB. (1977). *Health Measures in Exercising Freedom of Choice in Childbearing Act*. Retrieved March 9, 2024, from https://pisrs.si/Pis.web/pregledPredpisa?id=USTA1

# Chapter 5
# Abortion and Women: Intersects of Religion, Law, and Society – A Perspective From Muslim Majority Countries

**Sana Ahmed**
https://orcid.org/0009-0003-4174-3660
*Henley Business School, University of Reading, UK*

## ABSTRACT

*Abortion is one of the most contentious and polarizing issues in contemporary society, invoking deep ethical, moral, legal, and emotional responses (Minkoff et al, 2024; Lewis, 2024; Petchesky, 2024; Chang et al, 2023). The practice of terminating a pregnancy has been present throughout human history, but its regulation and societal acceptance have varied widely across cultures and epochs (Cohen et al, 2023; Huzaimah et al, 2023; Pagoto et al, 2024; Petchesky, 2024). This chapter seeks to explore the multifaceted dimensions of abortion, examining its historical evolution, the influence of religious and ethical perspectives, the legal landscapes that govern its practice, and the implications for women's rights and health with a special focus on Muslim majority countries.*

## INTRODUCTION

Attitudes towards abortion have been shaped by a complex interplay of cultural, religious, and socio-political factors. However, with the advent of organized religions and the establishment of more formalized legal systems, the regulation of abortion began to take on new dimensions. Religious doctrines, particularly within Christianity, Islam, and Judaism, have had profound impacts on the societal and

DOI: 10.4018/979-8-3693-7837-3.ch005

legal views of abortion, often framing it within broader discussions of morality and the sanctity of life (Pagoto et al, 2024).

The legal landscape surrounding abortion is a tapestry of diverse and often conflicting regulations. In some countries, abortion is widely accessible and viewed as a fundamental aspect of women's healthcare and rights lives. Conversely, in Muslim majority countries, it is heavily restricted or outright banned, reflecting the influence of cultural, religious, and political forces (Huzaimah et al, 2023). The varying legal statuses of abortion worldwide highlight the contentious nature of the issue and the ongoing struggles to balance individual rights with societal norms. For example, several movements like #metoo have played crucial roles in shaping the discourse and policies on abortion, yet they also underscore the fragility of these rights in the face of political and ideological shifts (Lewis, 2024).

The impact of restrictive abortion laws on women's health and well-being cannot be understated (Minkoff et al, 2024). When legal avenues for safe abortion are blocked, as is in case of majority of Muslim countries, many women resort to unsafe and illegal procedures, posing significant risks to their health and lives. According to the World Health Organization (WHO), unsafe abortions are a major cause of maternal mortality and morbidity globally. This public health perspective emphasizes the necessity of ensuring access to safe abortion services as part of comprehensive reproductive healthcare, aligning with broader human rights principles that prioritize health, autonomy, and dignity (Francome, 2024).

At the heart of the abortion debate and political and ideological discourse lies the question of women's autonomy. The ability of women to make decisions about their own bodies and reproductive health is a cornerstone of gender equality and empowerment. Advocates for reproductive rights argue that access to safe and legal abortion is essential for women's health, economic stability, and social participation. Conversely, opponents often frame their arguments around the rights of the foetus and the moral implications of terminating a potential life (Tsai & Ziegler, 2023). The ethical tug-of-war highlights the deeply personal and complex nature of abortion, where individual rights and societal values frequently collide and are heavily backup by religion specially in the Muslim majority nations. Religious perspectives on abortion are particularly influential in shaping public opinion and policy. Many religious traditions emphasize the sanctity of life, which often translates into opposition to abortion. However, within these traditions, there is a spectrum of beliefs and interpretations. Some religious groups advocate for a more nuanced approach that considers the circumstances leading to abortion and supports women's autonomy. Understanding these diverse religious perspectives is crucial for a comprehensive analysis of the abortion debate, as they often provide the moral underpinnings for legal and policy decisions (Francome, 2024).

Technological advancements and medical innovations, however, have influenced the abortion landscape. From early surgical techniques to modern medical abortions using pharmaceuticals like mifepristone and misoprostol, the methods and safety of abortion have evolved significantly. These advancements have made abortion safer and more accessible, but they have also introduced new ethical and regulatory challenges. The increasing availability of telemedicine and online resources for self-managed abortions represents a new frontier in reproductive healthcare, raising questions about regulation, access, and the role of technology in personal health decisions (Sugarman et al 2023).

In conclusion, abortion is a complex and multifaceted issue that intersects with various aspects of society, including ethics, law, religion, and public health. This chapter aims to provide a comprehensive exploration of these dimensions, highlighting the historical evolution, current debates, and future directions in the discourse on abortion. By examining the diverse perspectives and experiences surrounding abortion in Muslim majority countries, we can better understand the profound implications it has for individual lives and societal structures. This nuanced approach is essential for fostering informed and empathetic discussions about one of the most enduring and contentious issues of our time.

## BACKGROUND

### Historical Context of Abortion

The historical context of women's autonomy and abortion reflects a long and tumultuous journey marked by shifting societal norms, legal frameworks, and ethical considerations. In ancient civilizations, such as Greece and Rome, abortion was relatively common and not heavily stigmatized (Lewis, 2024). Women had a certain degree of autonomy over their reproductive choices, although this autonomy was still influenced by societal expectations and gender roles. Methods to induce abortion were known and practiced, and there was little legal interference in these personal decisions (Tsai & Ziegler, 2023).

The advent of Christianity and its spread across Europe brought significant changes in attitudes towards abortion (Lewis, 2024). The early Christian church condemned abortion, viewing it as morally wrong and equating it to murder. This religious condemnation influenced legal practices, leading to the criminalization of abortion in many regions. During the Middle Ages, the control over women's reproductive choices became even more stringent, with harsh penalties for those who sought or provided abortions. Women's autonomy was severely restricted, as the patriarchal structures of both society and the church dictated reproductive roles and rights (Pagoto et al, 2024)

The Enlightenment period brought new philosophical ideas about individual rights and bodily autonomy, setting the stage for future debates on reproductive rights (Eskandar, 2024). However, it was not until the 19th and 20th centuries that significant legal and social changes began to occur. The women's suffrage movement, which fought for women's rights to vote and participate in public life, also laid the groundwork for discussions about reproductive autonomy. Activists started to challenge the restrictive laws on abortion, arguing that women should have the right to control their own bodies and reproductive choices.

In the 20th century, the feminist movement further advanced the cause of women's autonomy over their reproductive lives. The landmark Roe v. Wade decision by the U.S. Supreme Court in 1973 was a pivotal moment, recognizing a woman's constitutional right to choose an abortion (Lewis, 2024). This decision was a significant victory for women's rights activists, affirming the principle that women should have control over their reproductive decisions. However, this period also saw considerable backlash and the rise of pro-life movements, leading to ongoing legal and social battles over abortion rights.

Today, the historical context of women's autonomy and abortion continues to evolve. The legal status of abortion varies widely around the world, reflecting deep-seated cultural, religious, and political differences. While some countries have liberalized their abortion laws, recognizing women's rights to bodily autonomy, others have maintained or even increased restrictions, the historical struggle for reproductive rights underscores the ongoing challenges women face in achieving full autonomy over their bodies and highlights the importance of continued advocacy and legal protection for these fundamental rights.

The historical legal landscape surrounding abortion have also been marked by significant variability, reflecting the diverse cultural, religious, and political contexts within different countries. In some nations, such as Canada and the Netherlands, abortion is broadly legal and accessible, framed as a crucial aspect of women's healthcare and rights (Petchesky, 2024). Conversely, in Muslim majority countries, abortion remains heavily restricted or entirely prohibited, often resulting in significant legal and health risks for women seeking to terminate pregnancies. The contrast between these legal frameworks highlights the ongoing global struggle to balance women's rights with societal and ethical considerations Similarly, ethical debates surrounding abortion are equally multifaceted, often centering on fundamental questions about morality, personhood, and autonomy. Pro-choice advocates argue that women should have the right to control their reproductive lives, emphasizing the importance of bodily autonomy and gender equality. On the other hand, pro-life supporters contend that the foetus has an inherent right to life, which must be protected from the moment of conception. These ethical perspectives are deeply influenced by cultural, religious, and personal beliefs, making consensus challenging but dialogue essential throughout the history.

## To Do or Not to Do: A Social Perspective on Women's Right to Abort

The concept of women's autonomy, particularly in relation to abortion, is pivotal to understanding the broader discourse on reproductive rights and gender equality. Women's autonomy refers to the ability to make independent decisions about one's own body and life, free from external control or coercion. In the context of abortion, this autonomy is fundamentally about a woman's right to decide whether to continue or terminate a pregnancy. This right is seen as essential not only for individual freedom but also for broader social justice and equality.

Historically, women's autonomy over their reproductive lives has been heavily restricted by patriarchal systems and cultural norms. For centuries, women's bodies were seen as subjects of male control, with reproductive decisions often made by male family members or religious authorities (Lewis, 2024). The criminalization of abortion in many societies further entrenched this control, limiting women's ability to make choices about their own bodies. In countries like Canada, where abortion is legal and accessible, women's autonomy is supported by laws that recognize their right to make reproductive decisions. These legal protections ensure that women can access safe and legal abortion services without undue barriers. Conversely, in countries with restrictive abortion laws, women's autonomy is severely curtailed, often leading to dangerous and illegal abortion practices that jeopardize women's health and lives (Huzaimah et al, 2023).

Similar debates surrounding abortion often centre on the tension between a woman's autonomy and the rights of the foetus. Pro-choice advocates argue that respecting women's autonomy means acknowledging their capacity to make informed decisions about their own bodies and lives. They contend that a woman's right to choose is fundamental to her dignity and equality. On the other hand, pro-life advocates emphasize the foetus's right to life, arguing that this right should take precedence over a woman's autonomy (Cohen et al, 2023). These perspectives are deeply influenced by cultural, religious, and personal beliefs, making the debate highly complex and emotionally charged.

The impact of restrictive abortion on women's health and well-being cannot be overstated. When women are denied access to safe and legal abortion services, they are often forced to seek unsafe and illegal procedures. Unsafe abortions are a leading cause of maternal mortality and morbidity worldwide. Ensuring that women have access to safe abortion services is therefore a critical public health issue, as well as a matter of respecting women's autonomy and human rights. Women's autonomy in reproductive decisions is also closely linked to broader issues of gender equality. When women can control their reproductive lives, they are better able to participate in education, employment, and public life. Conversely, when their reproductive choices are restricted, their opportunities and freedoms are similarly constrained Ensuring that women can make autonomous decisions about their pregnancies is thus essential for achieving gender equality and empowering women to fully participate in society (Petchesky, 2024)

Women's autonomy in relation to abortion is a fundamental aspect of reproductive rights and gender equality. The ability to make independent decisions about one's own body is essential for personal freedom and dignity. Legal and ethical debates on abortion reflect broader societal struggles over power, control, and the recognition of women's rights. Ensuring that women have access to safe and legal abortion services is not only a matter of public health but also a critical issue of social justice. As societies continue to grapple with these complex issues, it is essential to prioritize women's autonomy and recognize their right to make informed and independent reproductive choices (Huzaimah et al, 2023).

## Religion and Women Abortion: A Broad-Spectrum Overview

Religion profoundly influences societal attitudes toward abortion, shaping ethical and moral frameworks that inform public policy and individual beliefs. The major world religions, including Christianity, Islam, Judaism, Hinduism, and Buddhism, each offer distinct perspectives on abortion, reflecting their diverse theological principles and cultural contexts (Adamczyk, 2022). These religious views significantly impact the legal and social landscapes of the countries where they are predominant, often driving both support and opposition to abortion rights.

Christianity, particularly in its Catholic and Evangelical branches, stands as one of the most vocal opponents of abortion The Catholic Church teaches that life begins at conception, and therefore, abortion is considered morally equivalent to murder (Schwartzman & Schragger, 2022). This belief is rooted in the principle of the sanctity of life, which asserts that human life is sacred from the moment of conception until natural death. Official Catholic doctrine, as articulated in papal encyclicals such as *Evangelium Vitae*, emphasizes the inviolability of the unborn and condemns any form of abortion without exception (Bhalotra et al, 2021). Similarly, many Evangelical Protestant denominations base their opposition to abortion on biblical interpretations that highlight the inherent value and sanctity of human life from conception.

Islamic perspectives on abortion are varied but generally lean towards restricting abortion except under specific conditions (Huzaimah et al, 2023). Islamic jurisprudence, or Sharia, typically permits abortion if the mother's life is at risk or in cases of severe foetal abnormalities. The timing and conditions under which abortion is permissible can vary significantly among different Islamic scholars and schools of thought. Some interpretations allow abortion within the first 120 days of pregnancy, based on the belief that ensoulment occurs at this point. However, other interpretations are more restrictive, reflecting the complexity and diversity of Islamic thought on this issue (Bhalotra et al, 2021;)

Judaism presents a more nuanced perspective on abortion, often prioritizing the health and well-being of the mother (Machalow, 2021). Jewish law, or Halacha, generally permits abortion if the mother's physical or mental health is at risk. The Talmud, a central text in Jewish law, discusses scenarios where the mother's life takes precedence over that of the foetus, particularly before birth. This pragmatic approach highlights a key difference from some Christian views, emphasizing the existing life of the mother over the potential life of the foetus, especially in cases of danger or significant hardship (Dorff, 2021).

Hinduism and Buddhism offer diverse views on abortion, often influenced by the cultural contexts in which these religions are practiced. Hinduism, with its emphasis on the principle of ahimsa (non-violence), generally views abortion as an act of violence against the unborn. However, interpretations can vary, and some Hindu communities may accept abortion in cases of significant maternal health risks or severe foetal anomalies (Dorff, 2021). Buddhism typically stresses the importance of intention and compassion, and while traditional teachings often discourage abortion, there is room for personal interpretation and situational ethics (Fidan et al, 2021). In both religions, the impact of local customs and social norms can significantly influence how abortion is perceived and practiced.

The influence of religious beliefs on abortion often translates into political action, shaping laws and policies in various countries. In many predominantly Catholic countries, such as Ireland (until recently) and Poland, strict abortion laws reflect the strong influence of the Church (Machalow, 2021). These laws often criminalize abortion with few exceptions, leading to significant legal and social ramifications for women seeking to terminate pregnancies. Similarly, in the United States, the political activism of Evangelical Christians has played a significant role in shaping the abortion debate, leading to numerous state-level restrictions and ongoing challenges to legal precedents like Roe v. Wade (Yadav, 2022).

Conversely, religious support for women's reproductive rights, though less prominent, also exists. Some religious groups advocate for a more compassionate and nuanced approach to abortion, emphasizing the importance of individual conscience and the need to consider the complex circumstances that lead women to seek abortions. For example, certain liberal Protestant denominations and Jewish organizations support women's autonomy in making reproductive choices, arguing that moral decisions should be made within the context of individual beliefs and situations. These groups often stress the importance of compassion, justice, and the recognition of women's rights (Francome, 2024).

The interplay between religion and abortion highlights broader tensions between individual rights and collective moral values. While religious beliefs provide essential ethical guidance for many individuals, they can also lead to policies that restrict women's autonomy and access to reproductive healthcare as mentioned earlier. Balancing these competing interests remains a contentious and challenging aspect of public policy and ethical discourse, necessitating ongoing dialogue and consideration of diverse perspectives. This balance is particularly crucial in multicultural and pluralistic societies where multiple religious beliefs coexist and influence the public sphere.

Religious teachings on abortion are not monolithic, and within each religious tradition, there is often a spectrum of beliefs and interpretations. For example, while the official stance of the Catholic Church is unequivocally against abortion, there are many Catholics who support reproductive rights and believe in the importance of personal conscience. Similarly, within Islam, there is a wide range of views on abortion, reflecting the diversity of thought within the Muslim world. This internal diversity within religious traditions underscores the complexity of the issue and the importance of considering multiple voices and perspectives (Corbin, 2023).

The impact of restrictive abortion laws on women's health and well-being cannot be overstated and often resulting in resorting to dangerous and prohibited procedures. Ensuring that women have access to safe abortion services is therefore a critical public health issue, as well as a matter of respecting women's autonomy and human rights. The opposition from religious groups often complicates efforts to improve access to reproductive healthcare, highlighting the need for dialogue and understanding.

The relationship between religion and abortion also underscores the broader issues of power and control over women's bodies. Religious doctrines that restrict abortion often reflect patriarchal values that seek to control women's sexuality and reproductive choices. As mentioned, Feminist critiques of these doctrines argue that true gender equality cannot be achieved without recognizing and supporting women's autonomy over their own bodies. This perspective highlights the need for a more inclusive and equitable approach to reproductive rights, one that respects both individual autonomy and diverse religious beliefs.

In conclusion, religion plays a profound and multifaceted role in shaping attitudes towards abortion and women's reproductive rights. The diverse religious perspectives on abortion reflect deep ethical and moral considerations, influencing both individual beliefs and public policies. While religious opposition to abortion often leads to restrictive laws and limited access to reproductive healthcare, there are also religious voices advocating for women's autonomy and compassionate approaches to abortion. The ongoing dialogue between these perspectives is crucial for addressing the complex and sensitive issues surrounding abortion, women's rights, and religious beliefs. As societies continue to grapple with these challenges, fostering mutual understanding and respect for diverse viewpoints will be essential in creating more just and equitable policies.

## Abortion and Islam: A Muslim World Perspective

Islam's perspective on abortion is nuanced, reflecting the diverse interpretations and schools of thought within the religion. The primary sources of Islamic jurisprudence, the ***Quran and Hadith*** (sayings and practices of the Prophet Muhammad), do not explicitly address abortion, leading scholars to extrapolate from related teachings on the sanctity of life, the protection of the foetus, and the health of the mother (Allotey et al, 2021). In general, Islamic scholars agree that life is sacred, and that the intentional termination of a pregnancy is a grave matter. The Quran emphasizes the sanctity of human life, stating in Surah Al-Ma'idah (5:32), "Whoever kills a soul unless for a soul or for corruption [done] in the land - it is as if he had slain mankind entirely." This verse underscores the gravity of taking a life, which includes the potential life of a foetus (Al-Bar, 2021; Bagheri, 2021).

### Scholarly Interpretations and Fiqh

There is a significant diversity of opinion regarding when the foetus is considered a living being with full human rights (Rahajeng, 2020). A central concept in Islamic discussions on abortion is "ensoulment," the moment when the soul is believed to enter the foetus. According to many scholars, this occurs at 120 days (around four months) of gestation, based on a Hadith from Sahih Muslim. Before this period, some jurists permit abortion under certain circumstances, such as to save the mother's life or in cases of severe foetal abnormalities (Outka, 2021).

The Hanafi school, one of the major Sunni schools of Islamic jurisprudence, is generally more lenient, allowing abortion up to 120 days for valid reasons (Osman, 2022). These reasons can include the well-being of the mother, both physical and psychological, and in some interpretations, economic hardship. The Maliki, Shafi'i, and Hanbali schools are generally more restrictive, with varying degrees of prohibition against abortion before ensoulment, except in dire circumstances (Rahajeng, 2020). Shia Islam also offers a nuanced view. Generally, Shia scholars permit abortion before ensoulment under specific conditions, such as when the pregnancy endangers the mother's life or in cases of severe foetal impairment (Outka, 2021). However, post-ensoulment, abortion is largely prohibited except to save the mother's life, reflecting a balance between the potential life of the foetus and the existing life of the mother.

The permissibility of abortion in cases of rape or incest varies among scholars. Some jurists allow it before ensoulment, considering the severe psychological and social impact on the woman. However, others oppose it, emphasizing the potential life of the foetus regardless of the circumstances of conception. This divergence reflects broader ethical debates within Islamic jurisprudence about balancing harm and benefit. In contemporary Muslim-majority countries, abortion laws vary widely, reflecting these diverse interpretations. Countries like Tunisia and Turkey have relatively liberal abortion laws, allowing the procedure for a variety of reasons, while others, such as Pakistan and Iran, are more restrictive, generally limiting abortion to cases where the mother's life is at risk or in instances of severe foetal deformities (Allotey et al, 2021)

Medical ethics within Islam also play a significant role in shaping perspectives on abortion (Ngo et al, 2024). Islamic bioethics emphasizes the principles of harm reduction and necessity. In situations where continuing a pregnancy poses significant harm to the mother or the foetus, these principles may support the permissibility of abortion. The debate over abortion in Islam is ongoing, with modern scholars and ethicists engaging with advances in medical science and changing social contexts. Issues such as prenatal screening and the potential for genetic disorders add complexity to the traditional frameworks of Islamic jurisprudence, prompting renewed discussion on the conditions under which abortion may be considered permissible.

Gender roles and the status of women in Islamic societies also intersect with the issue of abortion. Advocacy for women's rights and autonomy often includes the right to make decisions about one's body, including reproductive choices. Balancing these rights with religious and ethical considerations is a challenge faced by many Muslim women and communities. Ultimately, the Islamic discourse on abortion reflects broader themes of compassion, justice, and the protection of life. Scholars and communities continue to seek ways to uphold these values while addressing the realities and challenges faced by women. This ongoing dialogue illustrates the dynamic nature of Islamic jurisprudence and its capacity to respond to contemporary issues. Thus, the issue of abortion in Islam is characterized by a balance between the sanctity of life and the necessity of protecting the health and well-being of the mother. While there are divergent views among different Islamic schools of thought and across Muslim-majority countries, the emphasis on compassion and justice remains central to the discourse. As medical science and social contexts evolve, so too does the Islamic understanding and application of ethical principles relating to abortion but still it is a long way to go.

## The Social and Cultural Attitudes Towards Abortion in Muslim Majority Countries

Abortion in Muslim countries is a complex issue that intersects with social and cultural values, religious beliefs, and legal frameworks. The views and practices related to abortion vary significantly across different Muslim-majority countries, influenced by a combination of Islamic teachings, local traditions, and contemporary social dynamics thus Muslim women's experiences with abortion are influenced not only by religious teachings but also by cultural, social, and legal factors. In some societies, the stigma associated with abortion, particularly outside of marriage, can lead to significant social and psychological burdens. Access to safe and legal abortion services is also a critical issue, impacting women's health and well-being (Osman, 2022; Allotey et al, 2021).

One major factor shaping attitudes toward abortion in Muslim countries is the cultural emphasis on family and motherhood. In many societies, having children is considered a crucial aspect of a woman's identity and social status. This cultural value can lead to strong opposition to abortion, as terminating a pregnancy may be seen as rejecting a fundamental role of womanhood (Bhalotra et al 2021; Allotey et al, 2021). The cultural and social beliefs are heavily grounded in religious beliefs playing a central role in shaping attitudes toward abortion Islamic teachings, as interpreted by religious scholars, provide guidance on the permissibility and limits of abortion. The concept of ensoulment, as mentioned earlier, is crucial in this context. Before ensoulment, some flexibility may exist, but after this period, abortion is generally more restricted, except in cases where the mother's life is at risk.

Social stigma and cultural norms significantly impact women's experiences with abortion in Muslim countries. In conservative societies, abortion can be highly stigmatized, leading to social ostracism and psychological stress for women who undergo the procedure. This stigma often extends to unmarried women, who may face severe consequences for becoming pregnant out of wedlock. Access to safe and legal abortion services varies widely and as mentioned it is very common in Muslim majority countries, with restrictive laws and social stigma, women forced to seek unsafe, illegal abortions, risking their health and lives. The availability of healthcare services, including trained medical professionals and facilities, is also a crucial factor in determining the safety and accessibility of abortion which remain inadequate in Muslim majority countries because of the religious restrictions and social taboos surrounding the subject (Allotey et al, 2021; Huzaimah et al, 2023).

## Abortion Laws in Muslim World

Abortion laws in Muslim-majority countries vary significantly, reflecting diverse interpretations of Islamic jurisprudence and local cultural, social, and political contexts. In some countries, abortion laws are relatively liberal, allowing the procedure under a wide range of circumstances, while in others, laws are highly restrictive, permitting abortion only in cases where the mother's life is at risk or in instances of severe foetal abnormalities.

**Liberal Approaches.** Tunisia and Turkey have some of the most liberal abortion laws in the Muslim world. Tunisia allows abortion on demand up to the end of the first trimester, a policy established in 1973 as part of broader efforts to promote women's rights and reproductive health (Maffi & Tønnessen, 2023; Hatun & Yılmaz, 2020). Turkey's laws, established in 1983, also permit abortion up to ten weeks of gestation without restriction and beyond that in cases of severe health risks to the mother or fetal impairment. These laws reflect a more secular approach to governance and a commitment to women's health and rights (Fidan et al, 2021; Harris, 2020; Ansari, 2020). The abortion rate in Turkey has decreased over time. In 2018, the rate was approximately 14.8 abortions per 1,000 women aged 15-44.

**Restrictive Approaches.** In contrast, countries like Iran and Saudi Arabia have much stricter abortion laws rooted in conservative interpretations of Sharia (Islamic law). In Iran, abortion is generally prohibited except when the mother's life is in danger or in cases of severe foetal abnormalities, and even then, the procedure requires multiple medical approvals and religious authorization. Similarly, Saudi Arabia permits abortion only to save the mother's life or to prevent severe health complications, reflecting a strict adherence to religious doctrine that prioritizes the protection of potential life (Maffi & Tønnessen, 2023; Harris, 2020).

**Highly Restrictive and Prohibitive Approaches.** In some Muslim countries, abortion is highly restricted or outright prohibited, reflecting conservative interpretations of Islamic teachings and strong cultural opposition (Gomez, 2022). For example, in Iraq, abortion is generally prohibited except to save the mother's life (Inhorn, 2020). Cases of rape or incest are not typically considered valid reasons for abortion under Iraqi law. Official reports suggest 6,000 legal abortions annually, but unofficial estimates point to around 73,000 induced abortions, with many taking place clandestinely. Similarly in Yemen, abortion is illegal except in circumstances where the mother's life is at risk. Cultural and religious factors strongly influence the restrictive stance on abortion. Tunisia's abortion rate is one of the highest among Muslim-majority countries. A 2012 estimate placed the rate at approximately 20-25 abortions per 1,000 women. In Morocco, many women resort to unsafe procedures. According to a 2020 report, approximately 600 to 800 unsafe abortions occur daily in Morocco (Gomez, 2022).

## Lack of Legal Protection and The Spillover

In some countries, the legal framework allows for abortion under certain conditions, but the practical implementation is hampered by cultural stigma and limited access to medical services. For instance, in Pakistan, abortion is permitted to save the mother's life or to provide "necessary treatment" early in pregnancy, but social stigma and lack of healthcare infrastructure often force women to seek unsafe, illegal abortions. This gap between legal provisions and practical access highlights the challenges many women face in exercising their reproductive rights (Ansari, 2020). The evolving nature of abortion laws in Muslim-majority countries is influenced by ongoing debates about women's rights, health, and the role of religion in public life. As these countries navigate the balance between traditional values and modern imperatives, the discourse on abortion remains a contentious and dynamic issue, reflecting broader struggles over gender equality, health access, and individual autonomy. Understanding and addressing these legal complexities is essential for advancing women's health and rights in these societies.

## The Consequences: Impact of Restrictive Abortion Rights on Women's Health

Restrictive abortion laws have profound and often detrimental effects on women's health, contributing to significant medical, psychological, and social consequences which are specially pronounced in Muslim majority countries where the religion, laws and societal values inhibit women's right to safe abortion. These laws, which limit or completely prohibit access to safe and legal abortions, can force women to seek unsafe and illegal procedures, leading to increased rates of maternal morbidity and mortality. Unsafe abortions as a major public health issue, particularly in countries with stringent abortion restrictions, highlighting the urgent need for policy reform to protect women's health and rights (Sugarman et al 2023).

Unsafe abortions are a leading cause of maternal deaths globally, particularly in regions with restrictive abortion laws. When legal options are unavailable, many women resort to dangerous methods to terminate unwanted pregnancies. These methods include the use of unregulated medications, insertion of foreign objects, or seeking services from unqualified practitioners. Such practices can result in severe complications, including haemorrhage, infection, and injury to reproductive organs, often necessitating emergency medical treatment and leading to long-term health issues or death (Maffi & Tønnessen, 2023).

The health consequences of unsafe abortions extend beyond immediate physical harm. Women who undergo unsafe abortions may face long-term reproductive health problems, including chronic pain, pelvic inflammatory disease, and infertility. These conditions can have lasting impacts on a woman's quality of life, limiting her ability to participate fully in economic and social activities. Moreover, the stigma and secrecy associated with unsafe abortions can prevent women from seeking necessary medical follow-up, exacerbating health risks (Fidan et al, 2021).

Psychological impacts are also significant and multifaceted. Women denied safe and legal abortions often experience heightened levels of stress, anxiety, and depression. The trauma of undergoing an unsafe abortion or being forced to carry an unwanted pregnancy to term can have long-lasting mental health effects. Additionally, the fear of legal repercussions and societal judgment can compound these psychological stresses, creating a pervasive sense of isolation and helplessness (Bhalotra et al, 2021)

Restrictive abortion laws disproportionately affect marginalized and vulnerable populations. Women with limited financial resources, those living in rural areas, and adolescents are particularly impacted. These groups often lack access to safe medical care and accurate information about reproductive health, making them more likely to resort to unsafe abortion methods. The inequities in access to safe abortion services highlight broader issues of social and economic inequality, underscoring the need for inclusive and equitable healthcare policies (Fidan et al, 2021; Bhalotra et al, 2021).

Public health systems in Muslim countries with restrictive abortion laws face significant burdens (Schwartzman & Schragger, 2022). Treating complications from unsafe abortions requires substantial medical resources, including emergency care, surgery, and long-term treatment for reproductive health issues. These demands can strain already limited healthcare infrastructures, diverting resources from other essential health services. By contrast, legal and safe abortion services are relatively simple and cost-effective, reducing overall healthcare burdens and improving public health outcomes (Inhorn, 2020).

The societal impacts of restrictive abortion laws are also profound. Women who are unable to access safe abortions may be forced to continue unwanted pregnancies, leading to socioeconomic disadvantages. These disadvantages include interrupted education, diminished career opportunities, and increased financial dependency. Children born from unintended pregnancies are also at higher risk of adverse health and developmental outcomes, perpetuating cycles of poverty and inequality (Corbin, 2023)

Restrictive abortion laws also have broader implications for women's rights and gender equality. The ability to control one's reproductive health is fundamental to women's autonomy and empowerment. Laws that limit access to safe abortions undermine women's rights to make decisions about their own bodies and lives. These restrictions reinforce gender-based discrimination and control, perpetuating societal norms that subordinate women's health and choices to political and ideological agendas.

The global perspective on abortion rights underscores the variability in women's access to safe abortion services. While some countries have made significant strides in liberalizing abortion laws and improving access to reproductive health services, others have moved towards more restrictive measures. International human rights organizations, such as the United Nations and Amnesty International, advocate for the protection of reproductive rights as an essential aspect of human rights, urging governments to ensure safe and legal access to abortion.

In conclusion, restrictive abortion laws have far-reaching and detrimental effects on women's health. They drive women to seek unsafe procedures, leading to significant medical, psychological, and social consequences. The burden of these laws falls disproportionately on vulnerable populations, exacerbating existing inequalities. Public health systems and societal structures are also impacted, highlighting the need for comprehensive and equitable healthcare policies. Ensuring access to safe and legal abortion services is crucial for protecting women's health, rights, and well-being, and is an essential component of broader efforts to achieve gender equality and social justice.

## Islam, Ethics, and Women's Abortion Rights

The ethical considerations surrounding abortion within Islam are deeply rooted in the religion's teachings on the sanctity of life, the preservation of health, and the protection of individuals' rights (Ekmekci, 2017; Shapiro, 2014). Central to Islamic ethics is the principle that life is sacred and must be protected (Asman, 2004; Rahajeng, 2020). The Quran emphasizes the gravity of taking a life unjustly, as seen in the verse, "And do not kill the soul which Allah has forbidden, except by right" (Quran 17:33). This principle guides much of the Islamic discourse on abortion, making the deliberate termination of a pregnancy a serious moral issue.

However, Islamic jurisprudence also recognizes the complexities of life situations and the need for compassionate and pragmatic solutions. The concept of "maslahah" (public interest) and the principle of "darura" (necessity) play crucial roles in Islamic legal thought (Rahajeng, 2020). These principles allow for exceptions to general prohibitions when strict adherence to the law would result in harm or hardship. In the context of abortion, this means that while the default position is to protect the life of the foetus, exceptions are made when the mother's life is in danger or when there are severe foetal abnormalities.

Women's rights in Islam are multifaceted and encompass a wide range of entitlements, including the right to health, the right to life, and the right to dignity and personal autonomy (Asman, 2004). The Quran and Hadith emphasize justice, compassion, and the protection of individuals' rights, including those of women. For instance, Islamic teachings underscore the importance of maternal health and well-being, acknowledging that the mother's life takes precedence over the unborn foetus if her life is at risk. This perspective ensures that women's health and lives are protected and respected (Rahajeng, 2020; Ansari, 2020).

The debate over abortion within Islamic societies also reflects broader discussions on gender equality and women's autonomy. Advocates for women's rights argue that women should have the autonomy to make decisions about their own bodies, including the right to choose whether to continue a pregnancy. They contend that restricting access to safe and legal abortion services undermines women's health, rights, and social standing. This perspective is gaining momentum in many Muslim-majority countries, where movements for gender equality and women's empowerment are increasingly challenging traditional norms and advocating for reproductive rights (Demirel, 2011).

Islamic feminist scholars play a significant role in this discourse by reinterpreting religious texts through a gender-sensitive lens. They argue that many restrictive interpretations of Sharia law regarding abortion are influenced more by patriarchal cultural practices than by the religion itself. These scholars emphasize that Islam inherently supports women's rights and call for a re-examination of Islamic jurisprudence to ensure it upholds the dignity, rights, and health of women, including their reproductive rights (Ekmekci, 2017; Shapiro, 2014).

The issue of abortion also intersects with the ethical principle of balancing harm and benefit, a central tenet in Islamic thought. When a pregnancy poses a significant threat to a woman's physical or mental health, Islamic ethics may support the permissibility of abortion to prevent harm. This perspective aligns with the broader Islamic ethical framework that prioritizes the protection of human life and well-being, highlighting the religion's capacity for compassionate and pragmatic responses to complex moral issues (Demirel, 2011; Outka, 2021).

As discussed, legal frameworks in Muslim-majority countries reflect a range of interpretations of Islamic jurisprudence and local customs. These legal variations demonstrate the diverse ways in which Islamic teachings are interpreted and applied in different cultural and social contexts. The practical implementation of abortion laws is also shaped by social stigma and cultural norms. In conservative Muslim societies, abortion can be highly stigmatized, leading to social ostracism and psychological stress for women who undergo the procedure and as a result, women in these societies may be forced to seek unsafe, illegal abortions, risking their health and lives. Similarly, economic factors further complicate the issue of abortion in Muslim countries. In some contexts, economic hardship can be a compelling reason for seeking an abortion, particularly in settings where large families are financially unsustainable. However, this practical consideration often clashes with cultural and religious values that prioritize the sanctity of life and the importance of family. Addressing these economic realities requires a nuanced understanding of how financial pressures intersect with ethical and religious beliefs (Asman, 2004; Ansari, 2020).

In conclusion, the intersection of ethics, Islam, women's rights, and abortion is a complex and evolving area of discourse. Islamic ethics provide a framework that values life and health, allowing for nuanced interpretations that can accommodate the realities faced by women. The growing advocacy for women's rights and gender equality within Muslim societies is pushing for a more compassionate and just approaches and laws relating to reproductive health, including abortion. This ongoing dialogue highlights the dynamic nature of Islamic thought and its capacity to address contemporary issues while staying true to its core ethical principles. Understanding these complexities is essential for developing policies and practices that respect cultural values while promoting women's health and rights.

## Some Prominent Cases From the Muslim World

### *Case 1: Hajar Raissouni (Morocco) (www.amnesty.org)*

One of the most prominent cases of abortion in a Muslim-majority country occurred in Morocco in 2019, involving Hajar Raissouni, a journalist who was sentenced to prison for having an alleged illegal abortion and engaging in extramarital sex. This case sparked widespread outrage and debate across the Muslim world, bringing attention to the issue of abortion laws in conservative societies.

**Background.** Hajar Raissouni, a 28-year-old journalist for the independent newspaper Akhbar al-Yaoum, was arrested in August 2019, along with her fiancé, a Sudanese professor, as they were leaving a gynecologist's clinic in Rabat, Morocco. Moroccan authorities charged her with undergoing an illegal abortion and having sex outside of marriage, both of which are crimes under Moroccan law. Abortion is only permitted in Morocco if the mother's life is in danger, and even then, it requires spousal approval. Raissouni denied the charges, claiming that she had not undergone an abortion but had been seeking treatment for internal bleeding. Her doctor confirmed that he had treated her for complications related to a natural miscarriage, not an abortion. Despite this, she was sentenced to one year in prison, while her fiancé and the doctor were also given prison sentences.

**Public Outcry and Political Context.** Raissouni's case attracted massive attention both in Morocco and internationally. Critics argued that the trial was politically motivated, pointing to her work as a journalist for a newspaper known for criticizing the government and monarchy. Many saw her prosecution as part of a larger crackdown on freedom of expression and personal rights in Morocco. The case ignited a fierce debate about personal freedoms in the Muslim world, particularly regarding women's reproductive rights, abortion laws, and the criminalization of extramarital sex. Women's rights activists in Morocco condemned the prosecution, arguing that it violated Raissouni's privacy and autonomy. The case also highlighted the challenges faced by women in conservative Muslim societies where both cultural and legal restrictions significantly limit access to abortion and personal freedoms.

**Outcome.** The international outcry and pressure from human rights organizations led to Raissouni's release in October 2019, when King Mohammed VI of Morocco granted her a royal pardon. Her release was seen as a victory for women's rights advocates, but it also underscored the need for broader legal reforms. Despite Raissouni's pardon, Moroccan laws surrounding abortion and extramarital relations remain restrictive, sparking ongoing discussions about the balance between Islamic values and women's rights.

**Impact and Significance.** Hajar Raissouni's case became a symbol of the struggle for women's reproductive rights in the Muslim world, where abortion laws are often influenced by Islamic teachings and conservative social norms. While Islamic scholars have different interpretations of when and under what circumstances abortion is permissible, many Muslim-majority countries, like Morocco, have strict laws that restrict access to abortion except in extreme cases. The case highlighted the tension between personal freedoms and conservative values in many Muslim societies, raising questions about the need for reform and the role of religion in shaping laws related to women's health and reproductive rights. Raissouni's ordeal brought international attention to the issue, making it a landmark case in the ongoing debate over abortion in the Muslim world.

### *Case 2: Teenage Girl (Indonesia) (www.theguradian.com)*

Another prominent case of abortion in a Muslim-majority country occurred in Indonesia in 2020, involving a 15-year-old girl who was sentenced to six months in prison for having an illegal abortion after being raped by her brother. This case highlighted the complex intersection of abortion laws, sexual violence, and social stigma in the Muslim world, where restrictive abortion laws often fail to consider the vulnerabilities of women and girls in cases of rape or incest.

**Background.** In September 2020, a teenage girl from the Jambi province of Indonesia, one of the world's largest Muslim-majority nations, was sentenced to six months in prison for undergoing an abortion. The girl had become pregnant after being repeatedly raped by her older brother, who was 17 years old at the time. The case came to light after the foetus was discovered in a palm oil plantation, where it had been buried. Indonesia has strict laws governing abortion, allowing it only under certain conditions, such as if the woman's life is in danger or if the pregnancy is the result of rape, but only within the first six weeks. The law also requires that abortion must be carried out by a registered health professional and with the approval of the woman's family. In this case, the abortion was performed after the six-week window, making it illegal under Indonesian law.

Both the girl and her brother were charged with criminal offenses. The brother was sentenced to two years in prison for sexual assault, while the girl received a six-month sentence for having the illegal abortion.

**Public Reaction.** The case caused widespread outrage in Indonesia and internationally. Human rights groups, including Amnesty International, condemned the verdict, arguing that it punished a victim of sexual violence rather than addressing the root of the issue. The fact that the girl was a minor and had been raped by a family member further intensified the public outcry, as many believed the legal system had failed to protect a vulnerable child. Activists pointed out that the six-week limit for legal abortion in cases of rape is highly restrictive and unrealistic, particularly for young girls who may not even realize they are pregnant within such a short time frame. Additionally, the social stigma surrounding both abortion and sexual violence in Indonesia makes it difficult for victims to seek help or report their abuse.

**Legal and Cultural Context.** Indonesia's abortion laws are shaped by a combination of Islamic values, cultural conservatism, and legal restrictions. Abortion is generally prohibited except under specific conditions, such as when the pregnancy threatens the life of the mother or is the result of rape. Even in cases where abortion is legal, it is highly regulated, and access to safe abortion services remains limited, particularly in rural areas. The case also highlighted the broader issue of sexual violence in Indonesia, where victims often face significant barriers in seeking justice. Social and legal systems in many Muslim-majority countries, including Indonesia, can be punitive toward women and girls, particularly in cases involving sexual assault and abortion. Women's rights activists argue that laws need to be reformed to better protect victims of rape and incest, rather than subjecting them to further victimization through criminal charges.

**Outcome and Significance.** The girl's imprisonment sparked debates in Indonesia about the country's abortion laws and the treatment of rape victims. While there were no immediate legal reforms because of this case, it brought significant attention to the limitations of the country's abortion laws, particularly in cases involving minors and sexual violence. The case also underscored the need for greater awareness and education about sexual violence and reproductive rights in Indonesia. Internationally, the case was seen as part of a broader struggle for women's rights in Muslim-majority countries, where restrictive abortion laws and deeply entrenched social stigmas often prevent victims of sexual violence from accessing necessary medical care or legal protection.

**Impact.** The case in Indonesia became emblematic of the broader issues faced by women and girls in many Muslim-majority countries, where restrictive abortion laws fail to consider the complexities of situations involving rape and incest. It raised critical questions about the need for legal reforms and greater protections for victims of sexual violence, particularly minors, in societies where conservative values often shape laws around women's health and reproductive rights.

### *Case 3: Teenage Girl (Pakistan) (www.guttmacher.org)*

A significant case of abortion in a Muslim-majority country occurred in Pakistan in 2021, when a 14-year-old girl died after undergoing an unsafe abortion. This case brought attention to the issue of clandestine abortions, especially for victims of sexual violence, and the restrictive abortion laws in Pakistan, a country where access to safe abortion is limited due to social, religious, and legal barriers.

**Background.** In August 2021, a 14-year-old girl from a rural village in Pakistan tragically lost her life after undergoing a botched abortion. The young girl, who had been raped by a relative, became pregnant because of the assault. Fearing the social stigma and legal repercussions of carrying an illegitimate pregnancy, her family sought an unsafe, unregulated abortion. The procedure was performed by an unlicensed practitioner under poor medical conditions, leading to severe complications. Despite efforts to save her, the girl died shortly after the abortion due to infection and internal bleeding.

**Legal Context.** Abortion laws in Pakistan are restrictive and largely influenced by Islamic principles. According to the Pakistan Penal Code (Sections 338-338B), abortion is only permitted under limited circumstances. It is legal to terminate a pregnancy to save the life of the mother or for "necessary treatment" early in the pregnancy (within 120 days, or approximately four months), a timeframe that is derived from interpretations of Islamic law regarding when the foetus is considered to have "ensoulment." However, abortion is strictly prohibited for socioeconomic reasons or unwanted pregnancies. As a result, women and girls who find themselves in situations of rape, incest, or unintended pregnancies often resort to unsafe, clandestine abortions, performed by untrained individuals in unregulated settings. This is especially true in rural areas, where access to reproductive healthcare services is limited, and social stigma surrounding abortion remains strong.

**Public Reaction and Debate.** This case drew attention to the prevalence of unsafe abortions in Pakistan, particularly in situations where the victims are minors or victims of sexual violence. Women's rights groups and activists condemned the lack of access to safe abortion services and argued that the restrictive laws disproportionately harm vulnerable women and girls. The case also highlighted the significant social stigma surrounding both abortion and rape in Pakistan, which often prevents victims from seeking help or reporting sexual violence. The death of the young girl reignited debates about the need for legal reforms in Pakistan's abortion laws, as well as the importance of providing comprehensive sexual and reproductive healthcare services, including safe abortion. Activists also pointed to the need for better education and awareness about reproductive rights, as well as more robust legal protections for victims of sexual violence.

**Cultural and Religious Factors.** Pakistan, as a predominantly Muslim country, has abortion laws heavily influenced by Islamic teachings, which generally permit abortion only under very specific circumstances, such as to save the life of the mother or for health reasons before the foetus is "ensouled." Islamic scholars differ on when abortion is permissible, and the legal framework in Pakistan reflects a conservative interpretation of these teachings. Cultural factors also play a major role, with strong societal taboos against both abortion and extramarital pregnancies. For victims of rape or incest, the situation is even more complex. In Pakistan, rape is underreported due to the stigma surrounding sexual violence and the harsh societal judgments that victims often face. This, combined with restrictive abortion laws, puts many women and girls in extremely precarious situations, leading to unsafe and illegal abortions, often with fatal outcomes.

**Outcome and Significance.** While no immediate legal changes resulted from this specific case, it intensified discussions in Pakistan about the dangers posed by restrictive abortion laws and the lack of accessible reproductive health services. Women's rights groups in Pakistan continue to push for reforms that would expand access to safe abortions and provide more legal protections for victims of sexual violence, especially minors. However, progress has been slow, and deeply ingrained social and religious views continue to shape public discourse and policy on abortion. The case also drew international attention, with human rights organizations highlighting Pakistan's challenges regarding women's reproductive health and rights. The country has one of the highest rates of unsafe abortions in the world, with an estimated 2.2 million unsafe abortions occurring each year, according to the Guttmacher Institute. These unsafe abortions are a significant contributor to maternal mortality in the country.

**Impact.** This case became a focal point in the ongoing struggle for reproductive rights in Pakistan. It underscored the urgent need for comprehensive reforms to protect women's health, particularly in cases of sexual violence and unwanted pregnancies. The tragic death of the young girl symbolized the broader crisis of unsafe abortions in Pakistan and many other Muslim-majority countries where legal, social, and religious barriers prevent women from accessing safe reproductive healthcare.

## Contemporary Debates and Reform Movements in Muslim-Majority Countries: The Evolving Discourse on Abortion

In Muslim-majority countries, contemporary debates and reform movements around abortion reflect an evolving discourse shaped by diverse interpretations of Islamic law, cultural norms, and the changing socio-political landscape. As abortion in these countries is governed by a mix of religious, legal, and ethical considerations that vary significantly from one country to another, the ongoing debates highlight the dynamic nature of Islamic jurisprudence and its interaction with modern human rights frameworks, public health concerns, and women's rights movements (Scharp Brilly, 2021). Traditional Islamic teachings generally prohibit abortion, viewing it as a violation of the sanctity of life. However, there is considerable variation in how different schools of thought within Islam interpret these teachings. This diversity within Islamic thought provides a basis for nuanced debates and potential reforms (Shapiro, 2014; Huzaimah et al, 2023).

Public health considerations are increasingly becoming a critical aspect of the abortion debate in Muslim-majority countries. Unsafe abortions are a significant cause of maternal mortality and morbidity in many parts of the world, including in these countries. Health professionals and activists argue that restrictive abortion laws force women to seek unsafe procedures, leading to preventable deaths and injuries. This public health perspective advocates for more liberal abortion laws to ensure that women have access to safe and legal abortion services, thereby protecting their health and well-being.

Reform movements within Muslim-majority countries are also driven by broader human rights and women's rights frameworks. International human rights organizations and local advocacy groups emphasize that women's autonomy and reproductive rights are fundamental human rights that should be respected and protected. These movements often call for legal reforms to decriminalize abortion and to ensure that women can make decisions about their own bodies without fear of legal repercussions or social stigma (Shapiro, 2014; Huzaimah et al, 2023).

Muslim countries like Tunisia and Turkey, have taken significant strides towards more liberal abortion policies. Tunisia, for instance, has one of the most progressive abortion laws in the Muslim world, allowing abortion on request up to the end of the first trimester and this policy reflects a commitment to women's rights and public health, providing a model for potential reforms in other Muslim-majority countries. Turkey also permits abortion up to 10 weeks of pregnancy, recognizing the importance of access to safe abortion services as part of comprehensive reproductive healthcare. Conversely, as mentioned, in countries like Saudi Arabia and Iran, abortion laws remain highly restrictive, reflecting conservative interpretations of Islamic teachings and strong religious influence on legal systems (Huzaimah et al, 2023).

The role of religious scholars and leaders is crucial in shaping the discourse on abortion in Muslim-majority countries. Progressive scholars who advocate for more liberal interpretations of Islamic law play a vital role in reform movements. They argue that Islamic teachings should be adapted to contemporary contexts and that the protection of women's health and rights is compatible with Islamic principles.

These scholars often face significant opposition from conservative factions, highlighting the contentious nature of the debate (Shapiro, 2014; Huzaimah et al, 2023).

Grassroots movements and civil society organizations are also pivotal in driving reform and changing public perceptions about abortion. These groups work to raise awareness about the health risks associated with unsafe abortions and advocate for women's reproductive rights. They often engage in public education campaigns, legal advocacy, and support services for women seeking abortions. The work of these organizations is essential in creating a more informed and supportive environment for reproductive health issues (Ansari, 2020).

International influence and the global women's rights movement have also impacted the abortion discourse in Muslim-majority countries. Global initiatives and treaties, such as the Convention on the Elimination of All Forms of Discrimination Against Women (CEDAW), provide frameworks for advocating for women's reproductive rights (Assembly, 1979). These international standards encourage countries to align their laws with global human rights principles, promoting legal reforms that enhance women's autonomy and access to safe abortion services (Ekmekci, 2017)

The economic and social changes in many Muslim-majority countries are also contributing to the evolving discourse on abortion. Urbanization, increased education levels, and greater participation of women in the workforce are shifting societal attitudes towards gender roles and reproductive rights (Shapiro, 2014). These changes create a more conducive environment for discussions about reproductive health and the need for policies that support women's autonomy and well-being (Ekmekci, 2017)

Media and technology have also played a transformative role in shaping the abortion debate. Social media platforms and online forums provide spaces for women to share their experiences and advocate for their rights. These platforms also facilitate the dissemination of information about reproductive health and safe abortion practices, empowering women with knowledge and resources. The increasing accessibility of information through digital channels is helping to break down barriers and challenge traditional stigmas associated with abortion (Shapiro, 2014).

Despite these advancements, significant challenges remain in achieving comprehensive reform in abortion laws and policies in Muslim-majority countries. Cultural stigmas, conservative religious interpretations, and political resistance continue to pose barriers to change (Ekmekci, 2017). Efforts to reform abortion laws often face backlash from conservative groups and political entities that view such reforms as contrary to cultural and religious values. Navigating these challenges requires strategic advocacy, inclusive dialogue, and a nuanced understanding of the socio-political context.

In conclusion, the contemporary debates and reform movements around abortion in Muslim-majority countries highlight the evolving and dynamic nature of this discourse. The interplay of Islamic jurisprudence, public health concerns, human rights frameworks, and socio-economic changes is driving a gradual shift towards more nuanced and liberal approaches to abortion. While significant progress has been made in some countries, the path to comprehensive reform remains complex and multifaceted. The ongoing efforts of scholars, activists, and civil society organizations are crucial in advancing women's reproductive rights and ensuring that policies reflect both religious principles and contemporary realities.

## There is Still Hope

Education and awareness about reproductive health are critical in shaping attitudes toward abortion. In Muslim countries where reproductive health education is limited, misconceptions and lack of knowledge can contribute to negative attitudes and risky practices. Increasing awareness and providing comprehensive education can help address these issues. The role of men and family members is significant in decisions about abortion. In many Muslim societies, family dynamics and patriarchal structures mean that husbands, fathers, and other male relatives often have a significant say in whether a woman can seek an abortion. This can limit women's autonomy and decision-making power regarding their own bodies.

Modernization and changing social dynamics are influencing attitudes toward abortion in some Muslim countries. As societies become more urbanized and women gain greater access to education and employment, there is a gradual shift in perspectives on reproductive rights and women's autonomy. These changes can lead to more progressive views on abortion. Activism and advocacy for women's rights are playing an important role in shaping abortion policies and attitudes (Huzaimah et al, 2023). Women's rights organizations in various Muslim countries are working to promote reproductive health and rights, including safe and legal access to abortion. These efforts are often met with resistance but are crucial for advancing women's health and autonomy (Demirel, 2011)

Media and public discourse also influence attitudes toward abortion. In some Muslim countries, media coverage and public debates about abortion can either perpetuate stigma or promote more open and informed discussions. The portrayal of abortion in media can shape public perceptions and influence policy decisions. International influences and human rights frameworks contribute to the abortion discourse in Muslim countries. Global organizations and treaties advocating for women's rights and health impact national policies and practices (Rahajeng, 2020). However, there is often tension between these international standards and local cultural and religious values but there is still hope!

## Some Proposed Solutions

Addressing abortion-related practices and provisions in Muslim-majority countries requires a balanced approach that respects religious beliefs, addresses public health concerns, and supports women's rights. While solutions must be tailored to the specific cultural, legal, and religious contexts of each country, there are several key areas where reforms and strategies can make abortion practices safer and more equitable.

### Context-Sensitive Legal Reforms

Legal reforms must consider the diverse interpretations of Islamic law while addressing the pressing public health concerns of unsafe abortions. A pragmatic approach could include introducing provisions that permit abortion in cases beyond immediate threats to the mother's life including Cases of foetal anomalies, especially when detected before the 120-day (ensoulment) period recognized in most Islamic jurisprudence. Rape and incest, which could be recognized as legitimate grounds for abortion under compassionate and ethical considerations and allowing abortion not only when the mother's life is at risk but also when her physical or mental health is seriously endangered. Establishing clear medical guidelines can help reduce medical discretion and ensure uniformity in the application of abortion rules.

### Strengthening Public Health Approaches

Many abortions occur in unsafe conditions due to legal restrictions, lack of access to services, or social stigma. Where abortion is permitted, ensuring that healthcare facilities are equipped to provide safe abortion services, including post-abortion care. Training healthcare professionals to perform safe abortions under legal provisions can reduce complications from unsafe procedures. Also expanding access to comprehensive reproductive health services, including family planning, contraception, and sexual education and ensuring access to modern contraceptives, especially in rural and underserved areas, can significantly reduce the demand for abortion. Finally, ensuring that women who undergo unsafe abortions receive nonjudgmental and comprehensive post-abortion care to reduce maternal mortality and complications.

### Islamic Jurisprudence (Fiqh) Dialogue and Religious Engagement

Religious scholars play a key role in shaping public opinion and influencing abortion laws in Muslim-majority countries. Fostering a dialogue between healthcare providers, legal experts, and religious leaders can help create a consensus on abortion-related issues. Encouraging religious scholars (Ulema) to engage in discussions about the health risks associated with unsafe abortions and explore lenient interpretations of Islamic texts. For example, many scholars from the Hanafi school or Shia Islam allow abortion under certain circumstances, which can be highlighted as part of public policy. Educating the public and healthcare providers about the diversity of Islamic opinions on abortion can also be helpful. In many Muslim countries, people are unaware of the more lenient positions in Islamic law regarding abortion, leading to more restrictive practices than the religion may require.

## Addressing Social Stigma

Stigma and societal pressure often prevent women from seeking safe abortions, even when they are legally permitted. Reducing stigma is crucial for improving access to safe abortion care. Launching awareness campaigns to educate communities about the health risks of unsafe abortions and the circumstances under which abortion is legally allowed can highlight real-life stories and experiences to humanize the issue. Establishing confidential counselling services and hotlines where women can access information about reproductive health, legal abortion services, and support for those facing stigma or family pressure can also be useful along with including men and family members in reproductive health education to foster a supportive environment for women facing unplanned pregnancies or health-related abortion decisions.

## Strengthening Reproductive Rights and Women's Empowerment

Governments should frame abortion laws within broader women's rights and health policies. This includes improving access to healthcare, legal support, and protection for women's reproductive autonomy. It may include establishing legal protections for women seeking abortions under permissible circumstances, ensuring they are not criminalized or discriminated against and protecting healthcare providers from legal repercussions when they perform lawful abortions.

## Regional Cooperation and Role of NGOs

Muslim-majority countries with more flexible abortion laws, such as Tunisia and Turkey, can serve as case studies for other countries in the region. Governments and NGOs in countries with restrictive laws can learn from the policies and public health outcomes of countries with more progressive abortion laws in the Muslim world. Tunisia's liberal abortion policies, for example, have contributed to a significantly lower rate of unsafe abortions. NGOs in partnership with local government can organize regional conferences to bring together public health officials, legal experts, and religious scholars to share experiences and discuss best practices in abortion law reform and reproductive health services. Muslim-majority countries can also work with international health organizations such as the World Health Organization (WHO) to improve access to safe abortion services and reduce maternal mortality due to unsafe procedures.

Agencies like the United Nations Population Fund (UNFPA) and the World Health Organization (WHO) work to influence national policies by emphasizing the links between restrictive abortion laws and public health risks, such as maternal mortality from unsafe abortions. They often partner with local governments to create legal frameworks that protect women's health. Similarly, Organizations like the Centre for Reproductive Rights and IPPF (International Planned Parenthood Federation) collaborate with local stakeholders to promote abortion law reform.

International NGOs like Marie Stopes International and IPPF operate clinics in Muslim-majority countries that provide family planning services, contraception, and post-abortion care. While they may face restrictions on providing abortion services directly due to local laws, they often provide essential reproductive health services that help prevent unintended pregnancies, reducing the need for abortions. UNFPA, WHO, and IPPF promote the use of family planning and contraception to prevent unintended pregnancies, thus reducing the need for abortions. They run awareness campaigns that emphasize the importance of reproductive health and educate women and families about available contraceptive methods. These organizations often collaborate with local governments and religious leaders to ensure that educational programs align with local cultural and religious values, making them more acceptable to communities. Likewise, Amnesty International and Human Rights Watch have campaigned to reduce the stigma surrounding abortion in Muslim-majority countries by highlighting the human rights dimensions of access to reproductive healthcare. They produce reports and media campaigns that underscore the harmful effects of criminalizing abortion and the need for women to have access to safe healthcare. For example, in countries like Morocco and Pakistan, research conducted by international organizations has been used to advocate for better healthcare access and more flexible abortion provisions. International organizations and NGOs also provide legal aid and assistance to women who face criminal charges for seeking abortions or who are victims of forced pregnancies due to rape or incest.

A key strength of international agencies and NGOs is their ability to collaborate with local organizations, activists, and governments to address abortion-related issues in a culturally appropriate way. International agencies frequently collaborate with ministries of health and legislators to influence policy changes in ways that align with both international standards and local contexts. For example, UNFPA has worked with governments in countries like Morocco and Tunisia to develop policies that improve access to reproductive health services while respecting religious and cultural sensitivities.

### Comprehensive Sexual Education

Introducing sexual and reproductive health education into school curricula can help reduce the rate of unintended pregnancies, and subsequently, the need for abortions as it can provide comprehensive sexual education that aligns with Islamic values while offering practical information on family planning, contraception, and responsible sexual behaviour. Further, developing youth outreach programs that engage young people in discussions about reproductive health and rights, while addressing the realities of early marriage, contraception, and unwanted pregnancies can also be useful.

### Improve Data Collection and Research

Data on abortion, particularly unsafe abortions, is often scarce in Muslim-majority countries due to legal restrictions and social stigma. To create effective policies, governments should conduct comprehensive studies to assess the prevalence of abortion, maternal mortality, and the factors contributing to unsafe abortions. This will help train healthcare providers to record data on abortion-related health complications and deaths, providing a clearer picture of the public health impact of restrictive laws.

## CONCLUSION (THE FINAL WORD)

The intersection of abortion with other social issues, such as gender equality, poverty, and healthcare access, highlights the complexity of the topic. Addressing abortion in Muslim countries requires a holistic approach that considers these interconnected factors and seeks to promote the overall well-being of women and their families. Ultimately, the discourse on abortion in Muslim countries reflects broader social, cultural, and religious dynamics. It is a topic that encapsulates the tensions between tradition and modernity, individual rights and collective values, and religious beliefs and human rights. Understanding these complexities is essential for developing policies and practices that respect cultural values while promoting women's health and rights. In conclusion, abortion in Muslim countries is shaped by a diverse array of social and cultural values, religious beliefs, and legal frameworks. The interplay of these factors creates a complex and often contentious landscape, where women's experiences and rights are deeply influenced by the broader societal context. As these countries continue to evolve, the discourse on abortion will likely remain a key issue in the ongoing negotiation between tradition and progress.

## REFERENCES


Adamczyk, A. (2022). Religion as a micro and macro property: Investigating the multilevel relationship between religion and abortion attitudes across the globe. *European Sociological Review*, 38(5), 816–831. DOI: 10.1093/esr/jcac017

Al-Bar, M. A. (2021). *Abortion: Shafi'i Perspective. Abortion: Global Positions and Practices*. Religious and Legal Perspectives.

Allotey, P., Ravindran, T. S., & Sathivelu, V. (2021). Trends in abortion policies in low-and middle-income countries. *Annual Review of Public Health*, 42(1), 505–518. DOI: 10.1146/annurev-publhealth-082619-102442 PMID: 33138701

Ansari, M. (2020). A Comparative Study of Reproductive Law: An Analysis of Saudi Arabia, Iraq, and Malaysia. *Dalhousie Journal of Legal Studies*, 29, 11.

Asman, O. (2004). Abortion in Islamic countries-legal and religious aspects. *Med. & L.*, 23, 73. PMID: 15163077

Bagheri, A. (2021). *Abortion: Shi'ite Perspective. Abortion: Global Positions and Practices*. Religious and Legal Perspectives.

Bhalotra, S., Clots-Figueras, I., & Iyer, L. (2021). Religion and abortion: The role of politician identity. *Journal of Development Economics*, 153, 102746. DOI: 10.1016/j.jdeveco.2021.102746

Chang, R. C., Rao, A., Zhong, Q., Wojcieszak, M., & Lerman, K. 2023, June. # RoeOverturned: Twitter Dataset on the Abortion Rights Controversy. In *Proceedings of the International AAAI Conference on Web and Social Media* (Vol. 17, pp. 997-1005). DOI: 10.1609/icwsm.v17i1.22207

Cohen, D. S., Donley, G., & Rebouché, R. (2023). The new abortion battleground. *Colum. L. Rev.*, 123, 1.

Corbin, C. M. (2023). Religious liberty for all? A religious right to abortion. *Wisconsin Law Review*, •••, 475.

Demirel, S. (2011). Abortion from an Islamic ethical point of view. *International Journal of Business and Social Science*, 2(1), 230–237.

Dorff, E. N. 2021. Conservative Judaism on abortion and related issues. *Abortion: Global positions and practices, religious and legal perspectives*, pp.9-22.

Ekmekci, P. E. (2017). Abortion in Islamic ethics, and how it is perceived in Turkey: A secular, Muslim country. *Journal of Religion and Health*, 56(3), 884–895. DOI: 10.1007/s10943-016-0277-9 PMID: 27364347

Eskandar, K. (2024). Advancements in Gynecology: A Comprehensive Review of Emerging Research and Innovations. *J Med Clin Nurs Stud*, 2(1), 1–12.

Fidan, A., Alagoz, R., & Karaman, N. (2021). Liberal sexual morality, religion, and attitudes toward abortion in Turkey. *Journal for the Scientific Study of Religion*, 60(4), 914–933. DOI: 10.1111/jssr.12755

Francome, C. (2024). *Abortion freedom: A worldwide movement*. Taylor & Francis. DOI: 10.4324/9781003478348

Gomez, J. (2022). North Africa and the Middle East. Women and Sexuality: Global Lives in Focus, 93.

Harris, S. (2020). Women's Rights as Human Rights: A Study of Muslim Women's Reproductive Justice in Contemporary Saudi Arabia and Egypt.

Hatun, D., & Yılmaz, M. (2020). Religiosity and public attitudes toward abortion among Turkish adults: From an Islamic perspective. *Sakarya Üniversitesi İlahiyat Fakültesi Dergisi*, 22(42), 433–456.

Huzaimah, A., Abdillah, M., Laila, N. Q., Tamudin, M., & Astuti, T. M. P. (2023). Disregarding the Reproductive Rights of Women in Child Marriage in Indonesia. *Samarah: Jurnal Hukum Keluarga Dan Hukum Islam*, 7(2), 1097–1120. DOI: 10.22373/sjhk.v7i2.17392

Inhorn, M. C. (2020). Two 'quiet'reproductive revolutions: Islam, gender, and (in) fertility. In *The Routledge Handbook of Islam and Gender* (pp. 343–357). Routledge. DOI: 10.4324/9781351256568-23

Lewis, J. (Ed.). (2024). *Women's welfare, women's rights*. Taylor & Francis. DOI: 10.4324/9781003469865

Machalow, D. (2021). Religious Diversity and a Women's Right to Choose: The Religious Right's Mistakenly Assumed Monopoly on Belief and Religious Support for Abortion. *Rutgers JL & Religion*, 22, 476.

Maffi, I., & Tønnessen, L. (2023). Abortion, law, and health in the Arab world. In *Research Handbook on International Abortion Law* (pp. 303–320). Edward Elgar Publishing. DOI: 10.4337/9781839108150.00027

Minkoff, H., Vullikanti, R. U., & Marshall, M. F. (2024). The two front war on reproductive rights—When the right to abortion is banned, can the right to refuse obstetrical interventions be far behind? *The American Journal of Bioethics*, 24(2), 11–20. DOI: 10.1080/15265161.2023.2262960 PMID: 37830758

Ngo, N. V., Pemunta, N. V., Basil, N., Fokunang, E. T., Mbong, S. E., Ezra, K., Che, H. N., & Umbugadu, E. S. (2024). Reproductive health policy Saga: Restrictive abortion laws in low-and middle-income countries (LMICs), unnecessary cause of maternal mortality. *Health Care for Women International*, 45(1), 5–23. DOI: 10.1080/07399332.2021.1994971 PMID: 34726567

Osman, A. (2022). Abortion laws in Muslim countries: Modern reconfiguration of pre-modern logic. *Muslim World Journal of Human Rights*, 19(1), 19–52. DOI: 10.1515/mwjhr-2021-0007

Outka, G. (2021). *Islamic ethics of life: abortion, war, and euthanasia*. Univ of South Carolina Press.

Pagoto, S. L., Palmer, L., & Horwitz-Willis, N. (2023). The next infodemic: Abortion misinformation. *Journal of Medical Internet Research*, 25, e42582. DOI: 10.2196/42582 PMID: 37140975

Petchesky, R. P. (2024). *Abortion and woman's choice: the state, sexuality and reproductive freedom*. Verso Books.

Rahajeng, A. N. (2020). *Abortion in Islamic Law and Its Intersection with Human Rights. Journal of Islamic Law Studies* (Vol. 3). JILS.

Scharp Brilly, N. (2021). The Right to Abortion: A qualitative analysis of NGOs viewpoint on what hinders women's access to abortion in Tunisia.

Schwartzman, M., & Schragger, R. (2022). Religious Freedom and Abortion. *Iowa Law Review*, 108, 2299.

Shapiro, G. K. (2014). Abortion law in Muslim-majority countries: An overview of the Islamic discourse with policy implications. *Health Policy and Planning*, 29(4), 483–494. DOI: 10.1093/heapol/czt040 PMID: 23749735

Sugarman, J., Wenner, D. M., Rid, A., Henry, L. M., Luna, F., Klitzman, R., MacQueen, K. M., Rennie, S., Singh, J. A., & Gostin, L. O. (2023). Ethical research when abortion access is legally restricted. *Science*, 380(6651), 1224–1226. DOI: 10.1126/science.adh3104 PMID: 37347876

Tsai, R. L., & Ziegler, M. (2023). Abortion Politics and the Rise of Movement Jurists. *U.C. Davis Law Review*, 57, 2149.

Women, U. N. (1979). Convention on the elimination of all forms of discrimination against women. diakses melalui: http://www. un. org/womenwatch/daw/cedaw/text/econvention. htm, pada, 12.

Yadav, G. (2022). Abortion (Hinduism). In *Hinduism and Tribal Religions* (pp. 9–12). Springer Netherlands. DOI: 10.1007/978-94-024-1188-1_484

# Chapter 6
# Contours of Choice: Interpreting the Medical Termination of Pregnancy Act 1971 in the Context of Women's Rights

**Syed Mohd Uzair Iqbal**
https://orcid.org/0000-0002-5096-9165
*Symbiosis Law School, Symbiosis International University (Deemed), Pune, India*

**Hritika Jannawar**
*Symbiosis Law School, Symbiosis International University (Deemed), Pune, India*

## ABSTRACT

*There has been a long-running debate between the fetal rights and reproductive rights of women surrounding the topic of abortion. The world is divided into the groups of pro-life and pro-choice. Amid this debate, India, despite having an issue of female infanticide due to its social history and structure, has proactively taken a stand through legislation and adjudication for the 'reproductive rights of women.' The commendable efforts in Indian jurisdiction through the 2021 Amendment to the 'Medical Termination Act, 1971' along with its few limitations and the recent developments by the Supreme Court of India, have been examined in this chapter.*

## INTRODUCTION

The revolution in abortion laws in India came after the passing of The Medical Termination of Pregnancy Act of 1971. The said Act was passed against the backdrop of a large number of illegal and unsafe abortion practices, leading to a high

DOI: 10.4018/979-8-3693-7837-3.ch006

mortality rate among women. Earlier in this Act, the only law governing abortion instead of criminalizing it was the provisions under the Indian Penal Code of 1860 (Bhartiye Nyay Sanhita, 2024). Although the MTP Act was the first step toward the recognition of the reproductive choices of women, it is more towards the doctor-centric approach to providing immunity under the Penal Code (BNS, 2024). The term abortion is not mentioned in any of the legislation in India; at present, what is recognized is the medical termination of Pregnancy. Although the legal foundation of reproductive choice as the right to abortion and reproductive choices has been guaranteed under the fundamental rights of the Indian Constitution by the Hon'ble Apex Court, the termination of the pregnancy still has to be justified on the grounds enumerated in the Act. The recent amendment of 2021 to the Act has brought about few progressive changes, and the liberal interpretation of the provisions and the Hon'ble Supreme Court upholding the right to reproductive choices of women and their right to dignity has made applauding changes in the reproductive choices laws in India, but there are few limitations still present.

The concept of abortion involves a philosophical as to whether women should have control over their bodies. Abortion as a concept has a lot of sociological, legal, and religious implications. The idea of abortion is a debate between the foetal rights and the reproductive choices of the women. The laws relating to Abortion in India at present are liberal and progressive. When identified, the limitations are mitigated by the progressive judicial interpretation of the Act honoring women's reproductive choices. In the present times, when female foeticide or selective abortion of a female fetus is prevalent, the nation still moves forward with liberalized policies recognizing the right to abortions and reproductive choices of women. Albeit the legislation in place for Abortion, there are few practical limitations to this Act, which will be further explored throughout this analysis by tracing the historical evolution of this legislation and Judicial interpretations.

## RESEARCH METHODOLOGY

This research utilizes automated framing analysis and evaluation of textual aspects to triangulate many methodologies to evaluate how the problem of abortion still persists in the 21st century. Primary sources include the Constitutional provisions of India, statutes, Rules, Bills, etc. These foundational documents provide the legal and regulatory context necessary for the research. The authors' framing and textual analysis findings reveal disparities in the women's choice right.

## LITERATURE REVIEW

This work provides a comprehensive analysis of how the denial of reproductive rights promotes gender inequality, subjugating women under the control of men and the state. It explores the idea that the international jurisprudence surrounding the discussion of reproductive rights has emphasized the need for the basing the legal framework for abortion on the grounds of equality and not privacy (Stark, 2011). However, in India at present the basis of these reproductive rights is privacy. This work showcases how courts in India read Article 21 of the Constitution to give the "inner" parts of the right to life—namely, the right to privacy and the freedom to make one's own decisions—more weight and specificity. As state interference in personal decision-making grows and previous ideas about what constitutes a matter of choice are called into doubt, the Supreme On several essential matters court will be asked to decide how much of a citizen's life and liberty are theirs (Kumar, 2016). The discussion in the present paper is essential to continue on the point of reproductive choices. This research also discusses privacy judgment and its relation to the reproductive choice of women (Ghosh & Khaitan, 2017). In the rights discourse, abortion has always been a contentious topic, especially when it is framed as a battle between a woman's right to choose and the life of her unborn child. In addition to immediate health concerns and even death, an unsafe abortion can result in long-term problems that are harmful to a woman's physical and mental health. The present piece provides a thorough analysis of the legislation and practices surrounding abortion in Bangladesh, India, the US, and Russia. Few stringent laws are acceptable for their intended purpose, even though they are frequently broken(Kapoor, 2023). Another paper that is quite pertinent for review because of its way of highlighting the need for the 2021 Amendment to go through the case of a 10-year-old victim of rape who also has become pregnant and has unfortunately been denied permission by the courts because her pregnancy has exceeded 20 weeks limit (Dalvie, 2017). This work dwells on constitutional aspects of reproductive rights and how sexual crime against women hinders their access to rights (Shakantala & Raj, 2022).

Moving further, 'Contrived Confusions' is the work where the dilemma surrounding the rights of the unborn child and the woman's human rights has been briefly discussed (Prasad, 2015). However, these works lacked a precise analysis of the debate of pro-choice and pro-life controversy in the backdrop of the Indian Scenario and its development in the medical sciences. All these works commonly lacked the thorough discussion surrounding the 'Medical Termination Act of 1971', its amendment of 2021, and its implications on the current discourse of reproductive rights in the country and its limitations. The work up until now also lacked the discussion on the pro-choice and pro-life debate surrounding this issue on the backdrop of Indian abortion jurisprudence. The researcher in the current chapter is dwelling on the deep discussion of women's reproductive rights in consonance with the judicial and legislative developments. However, India is one of the most liberal countries in terms of recognition afforded to reproductive rights; the researcher finds it imperative to outline the current Act's limitations and the necessary changes.

## HISTORICAL DEVELOPMENT OF MEDICAL TERMINATION OF PREGNANCY IN INDIA

### Medical Termination Pregnancy and Women's Rights

Earlier, the concept of Abortion was not at all recognized, and what was made punishable was causing voluntary miscarriage of the women under the Indian Penal Code. The punishment for termination of pregnancy was provided under Sections 312 to 316 of the Indian Penal Code (88-92 BNS). Under the purview of this section, all medical practitioners, men and women, were punished. Under the Code, a person inducing an abortion was charged with culpable homicide and can be imprisoned for three or more years.[1] These sections did not differentiate between unwanted and wanted pregnancies.

Later, a lot of cases of increased female mortality were observed due to unsafe and illegal abortions administered, as there was no safe and legal recourse for such women to turn to. The primary reason for the growing concern and rise in mortality rate was because the abortions were performed by unprofessional, ill-equipped, and partially trained or untrained persons (Singh, 2023). The need for balancing the rights of society and the women's right to reproductive choices was felt, and under the recommendations of the Shah Committee, the policy surrounding abortion was liberalized, and 'The Medical Termination of Pregnancy Act of 1971 was passed (hereinafter referred as MTP Act).

In the Landmark decision of the Hon'ble Supreme Court in Suchita Srivastava's case it was held that the .,'right of a woman to reproductive autonomy' is guaranteed as a personal liberty under Article 21 of the Indian Constitution. However, till today, a woman cannot walk into a healthcare facility and demand an abortion without any questions being asked of her. Abortion is permitted at the discretion of the Medical practitioner when such grounds prescribed under the act, such as continuance of the pregnancy, can cause grave mental or physical harm, contraceptive failure, etc.

## The Medical Termination of Pregnancy Act of 1971

The MTP Act, which was considered to be progressive at the time of its passing, was supposed to be more focused on providing immunity to the medical practitioners performing the procedures for abortion rather than ensuring reproductive rights for the women. The objective of the Act is itself indicative of the said fact, which has been mentioned as follows: "An Act to provide for the termination of certain pregnancies by registered medical practitioners." This can also be observed from the start of section 3 of the MTP Act, which is with the Non-obstinate clause to provide immunity to medical practitioners if they terminate any pregnancy, which qualifies the eligibility under the Act to be terminated. The term abortion was not used in the Indian Penal Code (BNS) as well as the MTP Act; what the Act entails is the medical termination of the pregnancy.

The Act is premised on three objectives for terminating the pregnancy medically:

"a. When the pregnant woman's life is in danger, or there is a risk to the physical or mental health of that woman.

b. Humanitarian ground- the pregnant woman is the victim of rape, and the pregnancy is the result of such offense committed against such woman.
c. When there is a risk that the child will be born with diseases or deformities (Gaur, 1986).

Another objective was to bring the population growth under control by providing an option to abort if conceived due to contraceptive failure (Shantanu, 2020).

The Section 3 of the MTP Act provided for the conditions under which the pregnancy can be medically terminated- "*A registered medical practitioner may terminate the pregnancy –*

i. The continuance of the pregnancy would involve a risk to the life of the pregnant woman or of grave injury to physical or mental health; or
ii. there is a substantial risk that if the child were born, it would suffer from such physical or mental abnormalities as to be seriously handicapped.
    a) where the length of the pregnancy does not exceed twelve weeks, the opinion of only one practitioner is required.
    b) When the length of the pregnancy exceeds twelve weeks but does not exceed twenty weeks, the opinion of a minimum of two registered medical practitioners is essential".

Explanations I and II of Sec 3(2) of the Act stated pregnancy alleged to be caused by rape and that unwanted pregnancy due to contraceptive failure is considered to cause grave injury to the mental health of the pregnant woman.

The Act provides to ascertain the fact whether the continuance of the pregnancy of a woman would involve grave injury and risk to the mental and physical health of the woman by taking into account the woman's actual or reasonably foreseeable environment (MTP Act, S.3 (3)).

Furthermore, in regards to the consent to terminate the pregnancy – for lunatics or minors, the guardian's consent is imperative. At the same time, in all the other cases, the pregnant woman's consent alone is necessary.

The conditions of the length of the pregnancy and the opinion of the medical practitioners can be waived in case the termination of such pregnancy in the opinion of the registered medical practitioner is immediately necessary to save the life of the pregnant woman (MTP Act, S.5 (1)).

This legislation was a progressive step toward the modernization of Indian Society and honoring women's reproductive choices. Under this legislative framework, there isn't any difference between the unmarried, married, divorced, or widowed pregnant women except in cases of contraceptive failure, the unmarried and married women are treated differently.

## Evolution of Provisions: Acts and Amendments Overtime

The MTP Act was amended three times; the most significant amendment to date is in 2021, wherein many changes have been introduced to make the legislation more feasible and attempt to promote women's bodily autonomy more rigorously.

### Medical Termination of Pregnancy Amendment Act, 2002

In this Amendment, the responsibility to decide whether private bodies should be allowed to conduct abortions was given to the district committee. The punishment for violating the provision of this Act was made more stringent. Moreover, the term lunatic was replaced by the 'mentally ill person' (Ministry of Health and Family Welfare).

### Medical Termination of Pregnancy Amendment Act, 2003

Under the MTP Act of 1971, section 6 empowers the central government to make rules for making the provisions of the Act effective. In this amendment act, the Central Government exercised this authority. It made regulations relating to abortion certification after 3 hours of terminating the pregnancy by the medical practitioner and other forms and maintenance records (Ministry of Health and Family Welfare).

## Medical Termination of Pregnancy Amendment Act, 2021

India was among the first few countries to legalize abortion on 'threats,' 'eugenic,' and 'humanitarian grounds.' However, with the passage of time and development in medical technology, it was felt by the state that there is scope for the upper gestational limit to be increased for terminating pregnancies through which a wide section of vulnerable women, like survivors of rape, incest, minor girls or differently abled women and pregnancy with substantial fetal abnormalities detected late. The 'fetal anomaly scan' is done at the 20th or 21st week of gestation, and before this amendment, 20 weeks was the upper limit for a medical termination. After the $20^{th}$ week, all these women who wished to terminate the pregnancy were left with no other option than to fight a legal battle, which adds to the stress of already distressed women. Therefore, this amendment was a step towards enhancing the safety and well-being of the women, providing them access to safe abortions.

Also, it is an important initiative of the state to achieve the 'Sustainable Development Goal for India,' aiming to reduce the maternal mortality rate. (Loksabha, third session, 2020/1941, page 284)

The gestational Limit has been increased –

*Table 1. Gestational limits and MTP*

| GESTATIONAL LIMITS | MTP ACT 1971 | MTP AMENDMENT ACT 2021 |
|---|---|---|
| Until 12 Weeks | Advice of one doctor | Advice of one doctor |
| 12 to 20 Weeks | Advice of two doctors | Advice of one doctor |
| 20 to 24 Weeks | Only to save the life of the pregnant woman. | Advice of two doctors if the pregnant woman – survivors of rape, victims of incest, minors, women who experience a change in marital status during pregnancy, including widows and women who are divorced, women with physical disabilities qualifying as a major disability under the Disabilities Act, 2016, a woman suffering from mental illness, foetal malformation and other vulnerable women (MTP, Rule 3B). |
| After 24 Weeks | Only to save the life of the pregnant woman. | Approval of Medical Board, and only if there is substantial foetal "abnormality" |

## Failure of Contraception Extended to Unmarried Woman

This ground for seeking abortion is now available till 20 weeks and has been also extended 'the woman and her partner'(MTP Act, §3 Explanation 1). Under the 1971 Act this ground was only available to married woman and her husband (MTP Act, §3 Explanation 2). This Amendment has led to the recognition of pregnancies outside of the conventional marriage setup and is a step forward for de-stigmatizing the pregnancy of unmarried women. Due to this change in the definition, the consensual pregnancy of an unmarried woman falls under the ambit of the MTP Act for termination (Kaur & Bharadwaj, 2023).

## Establishment of Medical Boards

This Amendment provides for setting up medical boards to grant or deny the medical termination of the pregnancy post-20 weeks of the gestational period. This is the added layer of the facility, a third-party authority to approve or deny the abortion. Before the Amendment, the pregnant woman has to approach the Supreme Court or High Court to request for the formation of a medical Board to hear her plea of termination of pregnancy post the upper gestational limit as prescribed under the Act, which was 20 Weeks before the amendment. But through this amendment, when the law is required to establish a medical board, the pregnant woman does not have to approach the Supreme Court or High Court for its constitution and has been saved a lot of hardship (Kaur & Bharadwaj, 2023).

## Privacy in Cases of Abortion

It has been prescribed that the registered medical practitioner shall not reveal the identity of the pregnant woman whose pregnancy has been terminated except to a person authorized by law. Violation of this provision is punished with one year of imprisonment, a fine, or both.

# LIMITATIONS OF THE ACT

The most welcome amendment to this act was regarding the increase in the gestational period to 20 Weeks, wherein the opinion of only one medical practitioner is required. Furthermore, the termination of pregnancy beyond this limit till 24 weeks is only allowed for the categories of pregnant women prescribed under the Act with the opinion of two medical practitioners (Rule 3b, MTP Act). The reasons like death of the partner and change in the economic status are not covered under the ambit of this Act. Although this seems progressive, this provision should have been extended to all pregnant women and not only restrict itself to the prescribed special categories for it to effectively reduce the number of writ petitions filed before the Supreme Court and various High Courts (Palepu, 2020).

The Act in itself is lacking a rights-based approach for the reproductive choices of the woman. Instead, it prescribes the grounds and procedures for the exemption of the criminal liability to undergo medical termination of the pregnancy. This approach towards the Abortion laws is in contrast to the international standards wherein it is considered that the restrictions imposed by the state infringe on several human rights such as the 'right to life', 'right to privacy', 'freedom from Gender discrimination', 'gender stereotyping', and 'freedom from ill-treatment'(Palepu, 2020). The most recent WHO guideline has recommended the complete decriminalization of abortion and the removal of grounds-based abortion access and gestational limits; it propagates abortion on demand (World Health Organisation, 2022). The present Act is still criticized for limiting the choices of women systematically; it affords the interpretation that the termination of the pregnancy can be accessed if there is a contraceptive failure, and it is upon the opinion of the medical practitioners whether there is ground present to permit the abortion. What if there was no use of contraceptives and the couple still wants to abort the child, but they do not have a choice under the existing framework? (Bhandari, 2023). The current framework under the MTP Act allows the termination of pregnancy only when the individual manages to prove how the pregnancy will be harmful to them mentally or physically (Bhandari, 2023). This is a far cry from the rights-based approach.

Further, per Sec 3 (2) (d) of the MTP Act, the confirmation of at least two medical practitioners is required if the termination of the pregnancy is sought after the 20-week gestational limits. This requirement contributes to lagging the process of seeking medical termination of the pregnancy; the people in rural areas won't have access to such medical facilities, wherein it is difficult to find one medical practitioner who is authorized under this Act to confirm the termination and the act is demanding two. It again adds to the hardship of this woman who has already been under the physical and emotional stress of the pregnancy if we see the categories of the woman eligible to seek the abortion after 20 Weeks of gestational period. This whole framework is lacking in providing the agency of the pregnant woman over their bodies.

Another provision that has been brought under the MTP Act after the 2021 Amendment is the setting up of a medical board in every state and union territory consisting of radiologists, a gynecologist, and a pediatrician to decide over the matters of termination of pregnancy after 24 Weeks of gestational period, but the termination will only be possible there is 'substantial foetal abnormality.' Although it seems ideal on paper, the practicability of the provision of medical boards is questionable. Firstly, because India's health care system is inadequate in its reach and availability of such practitioners; secondly, even if such boards are set up, ensuring its accessibility to the rural regions is an arduous task; and thirdly, involving a third-party agency can also entail risks of delays, personal prejudices, etc.

Furthermore, even though the MTP Act is trying to protect the privacy of the pregnant woman terminating her pregnancy. However, the women who request such termination but their request is denied are left outside the purview of this provision, failing the purpose, which is the protection of privacy.

Another shortcoming of the Act has been highlighted in the parliamentary debate (Loksabha, third session, 2020/194, p.304) is that the gender-neutral term 'person' in place of woman has to be used as the persons belonging to the transgender group are also in need for access to safe abortion. With the recognition of transgender as the third gender and affording them equal rights by the Hon'ble Supreme Court of India (National Legal Services v. Union of India, 2014) and the passing of 'The Transgender Persons (Protection of Rights) Act of 2019', transgender all over the country very well deserve an extension of this right to abortion upholding their bodily autonomy.

## PRO-CHOICE VS PRO-LIFE DEBATE SURROUNDING ABORTION

Two lobbies in the world exist: pro-life and pro-choice lobbies. Pro Pro-life lobbies advocate for fetal rights, and the other advocates for the rights of women. The Ministry of Health and Family Welfare has provided data that is indicative of 5 categories of countries in relation to the restrictions on abortion. The first category is where abortion is prohibited completely (26 countries), the second category is when abortion is allowed to only save the life of the woman (39 countries), third category allows termination to preserve health (5 countries), the fourth categories permits abortion on broad social and economic circumstances (to which India belongs), and the last and fifth category is where the countries permit abortion on request (gestational limits vary; 69 countries) (Loksabha, third session, 2020/194, p.283)

Different jurisdictions have different legal boundaries for different stages of gestation. However, in many, viability—generally believed to be the time at which the fetus might survive outside the uterus with medical assistance—is adopted as the demarcation for acceptable abortion (Glover, 1990). The idea of viability was first created to define the parameters of appropriate care for extremely preterm newborns, which is a very different situation from ending a pregnancy. However, since the middle of the 20th century, viability has emerged as a key component of abortion legislation, serving as a cutoff point beyond which a fetus can no longer be legally terminated or a point at which the list of acceptable reasons for pregnancy termination is severely limited. Viability, in turn, serves as a concept to limit the rights of women seeking abortion over their body; it is at this point that the fetus's life will be given more preference over the reproductive choice of the woman.

However, establishing legislation or expert counsel based only on viability is challenging. The idea is vague, intricate, and challenging to put into reality. It is not a fixed threshold but rather a flexible one based on external and fetus-specific factors. Because it depends on several overlapping fetal variables, including weight and sex, viability is inherently fetus-specific (Halliaday et al., 2023).

Moreover, it is impossible to separate prenatal outcomes from outside factors like geography, frequently associated with resources (Singer, 2011). When used as a standard, viability is determined by applying the "human interpretation of statistical probabilities" to all fetuses collectively, disregarding the individual circumstances that may or may not affect a fetus's chance of survival (Cohen & Sayeed, 2011). Because of this, the idea of viability is ill-suited for laws that decide the extent of criminal culpability, which are rules that affect people's access to healthcare.

Furthermore, since an abortion is a medical procedure in which the fetus is not meant to survive, the application of a medical concept meant to decide whether or not to preserve life in the event of an extremely premature birth to the context of abortion is conceptually illegitimate. These are two completely different circumstances. In particular, the World Health Organization (WHO) advises against "laws and other regulations that prohibit abortion based on gestational age limits" because they increase the risk of unsafe abortion, increase the waiting period for access to abortion services, and increase maternal morbidity and mortality (World Health Organization, 2023). Although gestational age restrictions are inherently ambiguous, rules governing abortion sometimes use viability as a threshold concept.

Consider this: The criterion of viability is commonly defined as "attainment of fetal weight of 1000 grams or fetal age of approximately 28 weeks" (Hellman & Pritchard, 1971, p. 493). In 2015, a study by Rysavy et al. revealed that some preterm babies (mean birth weight of 510 g) might be able to live at 22 weeks gestation if they get intensive neonatal care. Whatever the scientific differences between these two papers, there is no denying that obstetrical care and newborn resuscitation have come a long way in the 4.5 decades since they were published.

However, Williams' concept of viability has had one enduring and unanticipated effect. In the majority ruling of Roe v. Wade in 1973, Justice Blackmun also mentioned this text as a medical source. Blackmun wrote the following in the specifics of that choice, defining viability and citing page 493: The Supreme Court acknowledged in Roe v. Wade that the constitution protects the right to terminate a pregnancy, but that the state's interest in potential life at embryonic viability may limit this freedom. Until a fetus is "potentially able to live outside the mother's womb, albeit with artificial aid," the right to an abortion remains unaffected (Roe v. Wade, 1973). A "trimester framework" was proposed by Blackmun J. to distinguish between the various stages of gestation and show the varying degrees of state intervention that are permissible in each. "The State may go so far as to prohibit abortion during that period unless it is necessary to preserve the mother's life or health if it is interested in protecting fetal life after viability" (Roe v. Wade, n.d.). As a result, the legalization of abortion by the US Supreme Court brought it into conflict with the idea of viability. This gave legislators the authority to restrict American women's reproductive options by utilizing the viability criteria (Leo et al., 2018). Although limiting the reproductive choices of women to a certain viability limit, this ruling of the US Supreme Court in Roe v. Wade provided for the federal protection for women's rights to abortion across all the states. However, in a shocking turn of events in June 2022, the US Supreme Court overturned this landmark ruling, eradicating such federal protection on the issue of abortion and relegating it back to the individual states (Dobbs v. Jackson Women's Health Organization, 2022). Resulting in blanket bans on abortion in a few states or putting a gestational limit of as low as 6 weeks. Resulting in hampering the rights of women altogether.

When the term "viability" is used in a binary manner, it creates the assumption that there is a distinct boundary between viable and unviable fetuses. Obstetricians and pediatricians are aware that this boundary is, at most, hazy and that, in practice, strict black-and-white cutoffs are completely inadequate to inform judgments made during this window of time and do not adequately capture the complexities of viability. According to Rysavy et al. (2015), the overall survival rate of 22-week fetuses in the Rysavy trial who received the most intensive medical therapy available, both before and after delivery, was 23%. Nevertheless, real-world factors are absent from this definition of survival.

While proposing the Amendment to the MTP Act 2021 in Parliament and lifting its gestational limits for enabling women to better exercise their right to reproductive choices, a member of parliament has raised concerns regarding the 'abortus' rights. The member advocated that the proposed 24 weeks (upper limit under MTP) should be lowered to '22 weeks' as the fetus is not viable at that time, and till 24 weeks, it becomes viable. This suggestion came from a medical professional who has been working in this field for over 30 years (Loksabha, third session, 2020/194, p.290). Furthermore, stark opposition was faced by a single member of parliament during these deliberations; his stand was pro-life. He stated, "Abortion is a crime against humanity". He vehemently stated that "a pre-term baby at 24 weeks is one with a good chance of survival, an unborn baby's heart begins to beat 18 to 21 days after the fertilization and brain waves can be detected as early as 40 days after conception. By 24 weeks, a pregnancy completes the second trimester, which means a complete child is born. Permitting termination till that extent virtually implies legislation of murder in violation of Articles 14 and 21 of the Indian Constitution." However, these were not considered in the end while the amendment was passed, which showcases India's pro-choice stand to an extent.

A genuine conversation regarding newborn viability involves not only survival but also an open and sincere exchange of ideas about the kind of life the woman and her family can anticipate. Parents want to know if their child will experience pain or suffering and if they will be able to see, speak, walk, and connect with their family. We define viability and life according to our personal beliefs and preferences (Leo et al., 2018).

It is as wrong to attach the abortion provision to the term viability. As long as medicine treats each patient individually, there will never be a clear definition of viability. More problematic is the more general idea that access to abortion should be correlated with viability. Women make the complicated and unique decision to have an abortion for a variety of reasons. Regardless of the gestational age attained, women who decide to terminate for an abnormality or pregnancy issue do so out of fear for their health or for a fetus that would never reach a binary definition of viability.

Most women who decide to have an abortion do so within the first trimester, well before concerns about viability arise (Jatlaoui, 2017). Rather than being a straightforward case of language being dual, these women's decisions to end pregnancies represent the complexity of actual life. Their financial status, the presence of a spouse, the size of their current family, their readiness to care for a child owing to a job or education, and other factors all play a role in their decision (Finer et al., 2005). Sometimes, the woman does not get to know that they are pregnant until after a few weeks have passed, and what if they is not in a mental, physical, or emotional state to carry on with the pregnancy till the full term? For millions of women, this can mean making reproductive decisions based on an irrelevant concept of fetal outcome.

It is reasonable to predict that advances in medical science will lead to further advancements in managing preterm newborns. You may pretty much always expect to have to erase and redrew any viability lines you drew in the past. However, shifting this perceived boundary may also shift a very real one for women (Leo Han et al., 2018).

If we look at the Historical development of abortion laws in India, it was first to protect medical professionals and women from criminal culpability and then to establish the reproductive rights of the woman. The fetal viability and rights of the fetus as against that of the woman who is impregnated have never been much at the heart of its discussion as, all along, the preference for the rights of the woman was advocated. India, by far, has progressively developed its jurisprudence regarding the termination of pregnancy through legislative interventions as well as judicial ones. This development is in stark contrast to what has been happening in the USA, with the overruling of Roe v. Wade exposing women to unsafe abortions, increased mortality, forced pregnancy, and total disregard for their bodily autonomy. Although India has always been a flag bearer for women's choice in matters of abortion, the Supreme Court of India came across one peculiar case where fetal viability had to be taken into consideration to deny abortion to the woman seeking it, which shall be discussed in detail in the upcoming section.

## SPLIT VERDICT OF SUPREME COURT TO BALANCE THE WOMAN'S RIGHTS AS WELL AS UNBORN CHILD'S RIGHTS

The discussion of fetal viability surrounding the abortion law is considerably new in India. This has been recently brought up before the Bench of the Supreme Court dealing with the case of a 26-week pregnant married woman wishing to terminate her pregnancy medically. The petitioner, in this case, was a twenty-seven-year-married lady (X v. Union of India, 2023). The youngest of her two children is roughly one year old. In order to get the state to allow her to have her ongoing pregnancy terminated medically, she filed a petition under Article 32. The petitioner claimed that because she experienced lactational amenorrhea, she did not become aware of her pregnancy until twenty weeks had passed. Women who are nursing do not menstruate due to lactational amenorrhea. She was unaware that the lack of menstruation was a sign of pregnancy as a result. The petitioner claimed that she felt weak, queasy, lightheaded, and uncomfortable in her abdomen after giving birth to her second child, which is why she made her first appointment with a gynecologist. After undergoing an ultrasound scan, she discovered she was pregnant. At that point, the estimated gestational age of the pregnancy was twenty-four weeks.

A special court consisting of Justice BV Nagarathna and Judge Hima Kohli was convened to decide whether to terminate the 26-week pregnancy. The bench gave the petitioner permission to terminate her pregnancy. The order was issued in the mother's favor due to her emotional, financial, and mental health histories. The woman reportedly suffers from postpartum depression. In a thoughtful ruling, the Bench determined that "mental health" as it is defined under MTP Act Section 3(2) is a broad word that includes all illnesses. It used Section 5 of the Act, which permits a woman to terminate a pregnancy if it has advanced past the 20-week mark and is essential in certain circumstances to protect her life (X v. Union of India, 2023).

In order to protect women's rights, the Indian judiciary has read Section 5 broadly and liberally. Per Rule 3(B) of the MTP Rules, 2023, a pregnancy termination may be allowed if the pregnancy is delayed or if the circumstances alter after 20 weeks. Furthermore, disclosed to the court was the petitioner's usage of Lactational Amenorrhea, a method of contraception, during her nursing of her one-year-old second kid. 'Lactational amenorrhea is the absence of menstruation in lactating mothers, which is a natural method of contraception for six months after childbirth.' Even though the contraception had a 95% success rate, it had failed and led to a third pregnancy. In the expert committee that created the guidelines, conceptions due to failure of lactational amenorrhea were taken into consideration as a category for women who could terminate their pregnancy beyond 20 weeks.

The petitioner's abortion rights were established by the previously mentioned sections of the MTP Act and MTP Rules 2023. Apart from conferring relief upon the petitioner, the court instructed AIIMS, Delhi, to admit the mother for treatment and utilize the incubation procedure if necessary.

A dilemma emerged when the Union of India submitted a recall request for the special bench's ruling. The said Application of the Union of India is based on the email addressed to the 'Solicitor General of India' from the Professor in 'The Obstetrics and Gynecology Department of the AIIMS who was also a member of the medical board who gave a green signal for such termination. The question raised by this professor brought forth the argument of Pro-life and Pro-choice regarding the medical termination of the pregnancy in the present case. The Union of India, through this application, based on the concerns raised by this professor, sought clarification on whether foeticide can be carried out before the termination procedure since the infant was viable; otherwise, the birth would be considered premature and not foeticide. In the latter scenario, the newborn will need care and therapy that will require a lengthy stay in an intensive care unit, significantly jeopardizing the child's quality of life and increasing the likelihood of both short-term and long-term physical and mental damage (X v. Union of India, 2023). To give the kid the best chance of survival, it was also advised to deliver the baby at least eight weeks later.

Justice Hima Kohli was unhappy that the same Professor who was part of the medical board did not specify any such concerns in their report and later came forward after the order had been made. Although the information was brought before the court at a later date, the order in the backdrop of these new concerns did not sit well with Justice Hima Kohli, and she refused to allow the termination of such a pregnancy (Order in MA 2157 of 2023 in WP(C) 1137, 2023 para 4).

In an opposing view, Justice B.V. Nagarathna stated that recall had been discussed previously, even prior to the passing of the allowing termination of the pregnancy. Considering the woman's strong decision not intending to continue her pregnancy, also indicated in the affidavit, having no problem if the government, in case of the baby's survival, takes care of the infant or even gives it in adoption. She believed that the woman's choice ought to be honored. She made it clear that "This is not a case where the question of a viable baby being born or unborn is to be considered when the interest of the petitioner mother of two children and expecting the third in a years' time from giving birth to the second child has to be given preference" (Order in MA 2157 of 2023 in WP(C) 1137, 2023 para 4).

Justice Nagarathna emphasized women's reproductive rights by citing X v. Health & Family Welfare Department. According to her, "unwanted pregnancy resulting from sexual assault or from the failure of a family planning method results in the same consequence, even during the period of lactational amenorrhea as in the instant case." The expectant mother has no desire to carry her pregnancy to term. The viability of the pregnancy or the likelihood of a healthy birth are irrelevant factors in this scenario. The important thing to consider is whether or not the expectant mother plans to give birth. This was held and emphasized by the Hon'ble Supreme Court's three-judge bench and would be binding on the present bench.

Justice Nagarathna accepted the fetus's reliance on its mother, acknowledging that it lacked a distinct personality. The Court determined that the decision to proceed with the pregnancy was against Article 21 and 15(3) of the Indian Constitution, which uphold the right to life and liberty, especially for women, in light of the mother's precarious health. The statement went on to say that women are the only ones who can reproduce; a woman experiences menstruation, pregnancy, childbirth, the postpartum period, and menopause throughout her life (Order in MA 2157 of 2023 in WP(C) 1137, 2023 para 5).

Being a woman's human right, the right to reproductive health includes the right to an abortion. Alternatively, a woman coerced into an unintended pregnancy would suffer physical and psychological harm in addition to having to bear the burden of raising a second child during the postpartum period. As a result, she might miss out on other opportunities in life, such as the ability to work and support her family financially.

The Court further stated that in order for the Courts to exercise their jurisdiction under Article 32 of the Constitution, they must keep in mind the fundamental rights of women and affirm them in light of the prayers that the woman requested in light of her status, position, and unstable mental health, as well as the fact that she made it clear that she would not be able to carry her pregnancy to term.

The Court said that "she cannot be made worse off by this Court by declining to grant her the relief she has sought and thereby forcing her to continue with an unwanted pregnancy," but it was cautious not to open the door for orders of pregnancy termination in similar cases and instead stuck to the facts of the case. Justice Nagarathna affirmed the order to terminate the pregnancy in the present case.

Owing to the split verdict of Justice Hema Kohli and Justice Nagarathna based on pro-life and pro-choice arguments, this matter was further referred to the three-judge bench of the Hon'ble Supreme Court comprising Chief Justice D.Y Chandrachud. The Union's legal representative contended that the pregnancy had gone past the 24-week mark and that, according to the MTP Act, terminations of pregnancy are only permitted in extraordinary circumstances. In this instance, the unborn child was healthy and viable. There was also an argument made that the medical board's ruling, which confirmed the viability and health of the fetus, ought to have precedence in making a decision in this matter. The legal team invoked the concept of "Hobson's choice," which maintains that in the event of a preterm delivery, the fetus would lose its chance of survival because it may be born with significant physical and mental defects after being deemed healthy and viable.The pregnancy had progressed above the maximum gestational limit of 24 weeks, the bench declared after considering the arguments from both parties, and allowing a termination would be against Sections 3 and 5 of the MTP Act.

One concern that was brought up was if the fetus's heart could be halted in order to end the pregnancy in question. The bench stated that it was reluctant to approve the order since it might be interpreted as foeticide. It was decided that the fetus was not suffering from any defects, the mother was not in any "immediate threat" from the pregnancy, and the woman's life was given priority under Indian abortion law. The MTP Act permits a pregnancy to be terminated at any time after 24 weeks of gestation, with the two restrictions indicated above. After assessing the mother's mental, emotional, and physical health, the AIIMS medical board concluded that the petitioner had post-partum depression; nonetheless, the fetus was not negatively impacted by the petitioner's medication (X v. Union of India &Anr., 2023).

When the petitioner's attorney brought up Section 5 of the MTP Act, CJI Chandrachud provided an insightful interpretation of the law. CJI Chandrachud clarified that life cannot be understood in accordance with Article 21 of the Indian Constitution, as defined by Section 5 of the MTP Act (X v. Union of India &Anr., 2023, para 24). If that were the case, Section 3 of the MTP Act would have served no useful purpose. It is not possible to grant an overriding power to end the pregnancy. Sec 5 of the MTP Act uses the term 'life' in a very narrow and specific context, meaning the continuance of pregnancy will directly pose a threat to the life of the pregnant woman, leading to her death. Meanwhile, life under Article 21 has broad connotations revolving around the 'quality of life,' 'dignity,' 'personal liberty', and more. The CJI pointed out that if the broad meaning of 'life ' under Article 21 is applied to Sec 5 of the MTP Act, then it will broadly include the threats to the quality of life and other non-immediate risks, giving almost unlimited power to terminate pregnancies at any stage, which will undermine the regulatory framework established under sec 3 of MTP Act, which generally restricts abortions beyond 20 weeks.

The court strikes a compromise between the right to life of the unborn child and pro-choice in its ruling prohibiting the termination of a 26-week pregnancy. After giving careful thought to every aspect of the situation and reaching a decision that supports the rights of the unborn child, the balance is reached. The legislature, as well as the Judiciary of India, has always been on the side of the pro-choice, but the line for the moral standards of such termination has been drawn through this case. There is no winner in the pro-choice and pro-life debate in this country; balancing the rights of both is what is ultimately sought and starkly reflected through this adjudication.

Although the MTP Act is very liberal legislation protecting the reproductive rights of women, there have been few instances where the judiciary had to step in to protect the object of the Act from being violated in its practical approach. The Indian Judiciary, in the debate of the right of the fetus vs. the rights of women's bodily autonomy, is on the side of the latter except in the cases mentioned above. The Judiciary actively protecting the reproductive choices of women has been a breath of relief in the long-drawn struggle for women's rights.

## CONSTITUTION VIS-A-VIS REPRODUCTIVE RIGHTS

In the Landmark decision of the Hon'ble Supreme Court in Suchita Srivastava's case, it was held that the 'right of women to reproductive autonomy' is guaranteed personal liberty under Article 21 of the Indian Constitution. However, till today, a woman cannot walk into a healthcare facility and demand an abortion without any questions being asked of her. Abortion is permitted at the discretion of the medical practitioner when such grounds prescribed under the act, such as continuance of the pregnancy, can cause grave mental or physical harm, contraceptive failure, etc.

In the landmark judgment of Puttaswamy, also, the Hon'ble Supreme Court reiterated the stand in Suchita Srivastav's case while recognizing the 'right to privacy' under the Ambit of Article 21 of the Indian Constitution. It held that the right to abortion falls within the purview of the 'right to privacy.' Thus, by such an interpretation of the rights of women regarding reproductive choices, a legal foundation has been laid down the foundation to recognize the 'right to abortion' as one of the fundamental rights and liberalization of abortion law such as the MTP Act (Jain & Shah, 2020).

According to Justice Chandrachud, the state has a positive duty to take all necessary steps to protect an individual's privacy in addition to a negative duty (not to infringe) (*Justice K S Puttaswamy v Union of India* 2012: para 3[I]). In addition to the privacy ruling, a 2016 Bombay High Court ruling offers helpful reform guidelines (*High Court on Its Own Motion v State of Maharashtra,* 2016). A woman "should have the right to control her body, fertility and motherhood choices," the high court declared emphatically in a suo motu PIL about the horrible conditions of a female prisoner. The legitimacy of the state's interest in preserving "potential life" was another topic covered by the Supreme Court. It said that an unborn fetus cannot be placed above the rights of a live woman because pregnancy occurs within a woman's body and has a significant impact on her health, mental health, and life.

The Judgement stated that, "A pregnant woman has the extremely valuable right to refuse motherhood according to the MTP Act. Women have the right to become mothers and the freedom to choose not to become mothers, and their wishes must be honored. This right stems from her human right to live in society with dignity and is safeguarded as a fundamental right under Article 21 of the Indian Constitution, subject to the reasonable limitations that the Act considers. A woman has ownership and authority over her body. Deciding to have an abortion is always tough and thoughtful, and a woman should make that decision alone. There is no way to elevate the unborn fetus above the rights of a living woman. (Author's emphasis; Johari and Jadhav 2017).

A 14-year-old rape victim was granted permission by the Supreme Court in April 2016 to terminate her 24-week-old fetus. Noting the fact that the girl would have to live the rest of her life with the social stigma attached to the child, the Court allowed her to have an abortion. In July 2016, the Supreme Court (*Ms X v Union of India*, 2016) once again permitted an abortion at 24 weeks for a pregnancy resulting from sexual assault.

The Hon'ble Court, in its liberal interpretation, went a one-step ahead and held a view that amongst the survivors of the rape and sexual abuse, the married women whose husband performs non-consensual sex and impregnate them can be considered for medical termination of pregnancy till 24 Weeks. Hon'ble CJI Chandrachud (*X v. Principal Secretary, Health and Family Welfare Department, Govt. of NCT of Delhi*, 2022) held that it '*it would be negligent if we failed to acknowledge the reality of intimate relationship abuse and there is the misunderstanding that gender-based violence is primarily or largely the fault of a stranger.*' Hence, by bringing marital rape under its purview, this judgment has led to one positive step towards the rights of bodily autonomy of women.

The Bombay High Court and the Supreme Court have so placed a strong focus on women's autonomy to make decisions about their own bodies, fertility, and reproduction based on information. The MTP Act has long been criticized for failing to take a rights-based stance toward women and for providing the doctor with complete decision-making authority. These rulings makes it clear that the ruling might be read to suggest that women have the right to an abortion and that the doctor's primary duty is to make sure the established guidelines perform the procedure

## CONSENT

Under the MTP Act, the consent of women is only considered for the termination of the pregnancy and in one such Appeal of a husband against the wife and her family for terminating the pregnancy without his consent and without any medical need and seeking damages of 30 lakhs to the Hon'ble Supreme Court in the year 2017 upheld the judgment of the High Court of Punjab and Haryana. Wherein the Court held that there is no requirement of consent of the husband of a pregnant woman under section 3(4)(b), Only the consent of the pregnant women undergoing the termination is required (*Anil Kumar Malhotra v. Ajay Pasricha*, 2017).

The Court further held that a woman consenting to sexual intercourse with her husband does not mean she ipso facto consents to conceive and bear the child in her womb till the term. The Court remarked, "*Woman is not a machine in which raw material put and the finished product comes out. She should be mentally prepared to conceive, continue the same, and give birth to the child. Only a woman is the best judge as to whether or not to continue with the pregnancy, and the husband has no right to sue his wife if she terminates pregnancy.*"

Although, on the face of it, this is a progressive judgment furthering the cause reproductive choices of the women, it is detrimental to the institution of marriage.

### Rights of Married vs. Rights of Unmarried Women

Recently, in 2022, the Hon'ble Supreme Court in X v. Principal, Secretary, Health and Family Welfare Department, Govt. The NCT of Delhi declared that 'unmarried women are completely entitled *to seek abortion of a pregnancy resulting from consensual relationship after the 20 weeks of Gestational period is passed.*" Herein, the Delhi High Court had provided a literal interpretation of the Medical Termination of Pregnancy Rules, 2003, under which Rule 3(b) refers to 'change in the marital status of women' such as 'divorce or widowhood.' But in the recent amendment of 2021, the legislature replaced the word 'husband' with partner in Explanation I of Section 3. Therefore, if we read the MTP Act in its entirety along with its supplementary rules, it would defeat the object of the Act by excluding unmarried women from the right to terminate their pregnancy after 20 Weeks when married women have the right to do so. This case has arisen from a 25-year-old unmarried woman who terminated her pregnancy after 23 Weeks and 5 days of the Gestational period had passed, and her partner refused to marry her. Looking at the facts of the cases, it can be easily understood that if the Hon'ble Supreme Court does not afford such an interpretation of the provisions of the Act, it shall defeat the purpose of the Act and would cause unjust discrimination against the unmarried women in violation of her fundamental right to equality (Article 14); leaving with her no option other than to carry the pregnancy to full term and face the social stigma of the pre-marital birth with no financial and emotional help also by the partner. The Hon'ble Court concluded that '*the fetus's survival depends on the mother's body and the choice to end the pregnancy is solidly grounded in their right to bodily autonomy and the women's dignity will be violated if the state compels her to carry an unintended pregnancy to term"* (X v. Principal, Secretary, Health and Family Welfare Department, Govt. The NCT of Delhi, 2022).

## GLOBAL TRENDS IN RELATION TO RIGHTS REGARDING ABORTION

Considering the global level, only 22 countries have a complete ban on Abortion. (Council on Foreign Relations, 2023). On a global scale, abortion laws in time have successfully moved towards liberalization. Most industrialized countries allow abortion without any restrictions in New Zealand. Women have the liberty to choose abortion for 20 weeks without any restrictions other than this gestational limit as the abortion there is just treated as a health issue, but there are many countries that have some restrictions. They permit abortion in specific situations, including socio-economic reasons, risks to the mental and physical health of the woman, or the presence of foetal anomalies. India is one of the countries on this list. The trend globally is actively moving towards the liberalization of abortion laws. Over the period of the last 30 years, 60 countries have liberalized their policies concerning abortion rights. Recently, Argentina and Thailand 2020 legalized abortions subject to gestational limits. Columbia has made its abortions legal for up to 24 weeks of pregnancy. Only four countries have rolled back the legality of abortion within their territory, which are the USA, EL Salvador, Nicaragua, and Poland. Where the global trends are evidently moving towards liberalization, the United States, once a liberal country, has taken a step back and tightened its grip over abortion legislation—restricting the freedom of women's reproductive rights.

If we look at the U.S.A., the June 2022 judgment in Dobbs v. Jackson overturning Roe v. Wade after almost 50 years has shaken the reproductive rights of women throughout the country. The elimination of the constitutional right for abortion has led to a total ban in almost 13 of the states, where in some states, abortion is not available, even in the case of rape and incest. Another 8 states have abortion available for a limited gestational period of 6 – 18 weeks or till the fetus turns viable (CNN, 2024). The complete Ban or limited access to abortion does not deter women from seeking abortion. It only turns them towards unsafe and unregulated ways to carry them out, leading to an increase in female mortality and compromising overall health. (CNN, 2024). The end result is only whether the abortion shall take place in a safe environment or unsafe. Human Rights bodies have been advocating for the decriminalization of abortion and access to safe abortion for decades.

*Table 2. Abortion Policies and categories*

| | |
|---|---|
| **On Request (Gestational Limit may vary)**<br>Category I: All have gestational Limits of 12 weeks with few exceptions<br>77 Countries | Albania, Argentina, Armenia, Austria, Australia, Azerbaijan, Belarus, Belgium, Benin, Bosnia & Herzegovina, Bulgaria, Cambodia, Canada, Cape Verde, China, Colombia, Croatia, Cuba, Cyprus, Czech Rep., Dem, People's Rep. of Korea, Denmark, Equatorial Guinea, Estonia, Finland, France, French Guiana, Georgia, Germany, Greece, Guinea Bissau, Guyana, Hungary, Iceland, Ireland, Italy, Kazakhstan, Kosovo, Kyrgyzstan, Latvia, Lithuania, Luxembourg, Maldives, Moldova, Mongolia, Montenegro, Mozambique, Nepal, Netherlands, New Caledonia, New Zealand, Northern Ireland, Norway, Portugal, Republic of Korea, Romania, Russian Fed. San Marino, Sao Tome & Principe, Serbia, Singapore, Slovak Rep, Slovenia, South Africa, Spain, Sweden, Switzerland, Tajikistan, Thailand, Tunisia, Türkiye, Turkmenistan, Ukraine, Uruguay, Uzbekistan, Vietnam |
| **Broad Social or Economic Grounds**<br>Category II: 12 Countries | Barbados, Belize, Ethiopia, Fiji, Great Britain, Hong Kong, India, Japan, Rwanda, Saint Vincent & Grenadines, Taiwan, Zambia |
| **To Preserve Health**<br>Category III: 47 countries | Algeria, Angola, Bahamas, Bolivia, Botswana, Burkina Faso, Cameron, Central African Rep. Chad, Comoros, Dem. Rep. of Congo, Djibouti, Ecuador, Eritrea, Eswatini, Ghana, Guinea, Israel, Jordon, Kenya, Kuwait, Lesotho, Liberia, Liechtenstein, Malaysia, Mauritius, Monaco, Morocco, Namibia, Nauru, Niger, Pakistan, Peru, Poland, Puerto Rico, Qatar, Saint Lucia, Samoa Saudi Arabia, Seychelles, Togo, Trinidad & Tobago, Vanuatu, Zimbabwe |
| **To save a pregnant person's Life**<br>Category IV: 43 countries | Afghanistan, Antigua & Barbuda, Bahrain, Bangladesh, Bhutan, Brazil, Brunei Darussalam, Chile, Cote d'Ivoire, Dominica, Gabon, Gambia, Guatemala, Indonesia, Iran, Kiribati, Lebanon, Libya, Malawi, Mali, Marshall lands, Micronesia, Myanmar, Nigeria, Oman, Palestine, Panama, Papua New Guinea, Paraguay, Saint Kitts & Nevis, Solomon Islands, Somalia, South Sudan, Sri Lanka, Sudan, Syria, Tanzania, Timor-Leste, Tavula, Uganda, UAE, Venezuela, Yemen |
| **Prohibited Altogether**<br>Category v: 22 countries | Andora, Aruba, Congo, Curacao, Dominican Republic, Egypt, El Salvador, Haiti, Hondarus, Iraq, Jamaica, Laos, Madagascar, Malta, Mauritania. Nicaragua, Palau, Philippines, Sengal, Sierra Leone, Suriname, Tonga |
| **Varies at the State Level**<br>2 Countries | Legal status in the various states of USA and Mexico varies ranging from Category I to Category IV |

Source: Centre for Reproductive Rights

The Centre of Reproductive Rights has divided the countries on the basis of the abortion policies they follow in five categories. The majority of the countries make abortion available on request, but there are also alrming number of countries where the policy is very restrictive, making abortion available only to preserve the health of the pregnant woman or to save her life. India Lies in the Category II countries where the abortion policy is based. If we look at the Abortion policies in India, although abortion is not available on request, the current policy is not moving opposite to the trend; India has been actively making efforts to guarantee the reproductive rights and choices of the woman and one which are left beyond the statutory purview are taken care by the Judiciary.

## CONCLUSION

After giving the issue its fair weight, Indian laws do pass the balancing test for determining the extent of abortion rights. Occasionally, courts are presented with situations in which competing interests are evaluated, and the outcome is determined by whether the party is more persuasive under the particular conditions. A similar situation presented itself to the court when an unmarried lady wanted to end her pregnancy at 24 weeks. Because the MTP Rules only allowed a married woman to abort, they artificially distinguished between married and single women, which is why the court granted her request. Due to the unconstitutionality of such discriminatory laws, the court extended the right to an abortion beyond 24 weeks to include unmarried women. This demonstrates the Indian judiciary's substantively proactive involvement in securing women's access to safe abortion. Furthermore, the denial of a 26-week pregnancy by the Hon'ble Supreme Court virtually seems to be a step backward in the movement for the reproductive rights of women, but in reality, it is not. The higher judiciary is compassionate enough for both women and the unborn child, but in such circumstances when the termination may result in pre-term birth, how can the flag bearers of fundamental rights and human rights allow for human life to be compromised in such a way? The Hon'ble Court, although denied permission for abortion, extended assistance to the pregnant woman for giving up the child in adoption, which is the most human route one can manage to take in such situations. However, we can see that if not for the threat of pre-term birth, the judiciary would have been in favor of permitting abortion and upholding the reproductive rights of women. In all, through the legislative intent as well as the proactive steps by the judiciary, it is blatantly evident where India stands in the pro-choice and pro-life debate surrounding Abortion.

For furthering the cause of women's empowerment and their rights to their bodily autonomy till the period of 12 weeks is that the right to terminate medically should be available on request of the women. The biggest issue with the framing of the MTP Act at present is its doctor-centric language. We can decipher from both the parliamentary debate of 1971 and 2021 regarding the legislation of the MTP Act, 1971 and the deliberations for its amendment that the MTP Act can be construed that the said act is to establish rights of the women over their bodies, enabling a reproductive choice. However, in actual framing, the Act places the onus on the registered medical practitioners to determine the legitimacy of a woman's request to terminate her pregnancy. A woman can nowhere outrightly request an abortion, and it is administered with no questions asked. However, the authors herein understand what implications such liberal laws can bring forward, so to avoid those, a gestational limit of 12 weeks does not harm anyone.

What is essential for the successful implementation of the safe abortion initiative of the state is generating awareness about the Reproductive rights of women. In many of the rural areas of India, to date, women are not aware of their rights regarding their bodily autonomy. Making women aware is half the battle won; complete victory shall be attained when the men are educated and sensitized regarding bodily autonomy, reproductive choices, maternal health, family planning, etc. Only giving rights never solves the issues; its implementation at the grassroots level is the key to development.

## REFERENCES


Anil Kumar Malhotra v. Ajay Pasricha Civ. Appeal 4704 of 2013

Bhandari, A. (2022). Navigating the Sociological and Legal Aspects of Abortion in India in the Context of the MTP Amendment Act 2021. *Jus Corpus LJ*, 3, 258.

Bhatia, G. (2016): "The Bombay High Court's Abortion Judgment: Some Unan-sweredQuestions," *Live Law*, 22 September, http://www.livelaw.in/bombay-high -courts-abortion-judgmentunanswered- questions/

Center For Reproductive Rights. Who's New Abortion Guideline: Highlights Of Its Law And Policy Recommendations (2022) available at https://reproductiverights .org/wpcontent/uploads/2022/03/CRR-Fact-sheet-on-WHO-Guidelines.pdf

Center for Reproductive Rights. (2024). *The world's abortion laws*. https:// reproductiverights.org/maps/worlds-abortion-laws/

CNN. (2024, September 30). *Abortion access restrictions and bans in the U.S.* CNN. https://edition.cnn.com/us/abortion-access-restrictions-bans-us-dg/index.html

IG Cohen and S Sayeed, 'Fetal Pain, Abortion, Viability and the Constitution' (2011) 39 Journal of Law, Medicine & Ethics 235, 237.

Council on Foreign Relations. (2023, April 28). *Abortion law: Global comparisons*. Council on Foreign Relations.https://www.cfr.org/article/abortion-law-global -comparisons

Dalvie, S. (2017). Right to Safe Abortion, 52 (33). *Economic and Political Weekly*, 30–32.

Dobbs v. Jackson Women's Health Organization, 597 U.S. 215 (2022)

Finer, L. B., Frohwirth, L. F., Dauphinee, L. A., Singh, S., & Moore, A. M. (2005). Reasons U.S. women have abortions: Quantitative and qualitative perspectives. *Perspectives on Sexual and Reproductive Health*, 37(3), 110–118. DOI: 10.1363/3711005 PMID: 16150658

Gaur, K. D. (1986). Abortion and the law in India. *Journal of the Indian Law Institute*, 28(3), 348–363.

Ghosh, A., & Khaitan, N. (2017). A womb of one's own: Privacy and reproductive rights. *Economic and Political Weekly*, 52(42-43).

Hallidya, E. R., de Proost, L., & Verweij, E. (2023). The (mis)use of fetal viability as the determinant of non-criminal abortion in the Netherlands and England and Wales. *Medical Law Review*, 31(4), 538–563. DOI: 10.1093/medlaw/fwad015 PMID: 37253391

Han, L., Rodriguez, M. I., & Caughey, A. B. (2018). Blurred lines: Disentangling the concept of fetal viability from abortion law. *Women's Health Issues*, 28(4), 287–288.

Hellman, L. M., & Pritchard, J. A. (1971). *Williams obstetrics* (14th ed.).

High Court on Its Own Motion v The State of Maharashtra, Suo Motu Public Interest Litigation (2016): No 1 of 2016, Judgment dated 20 September 2016.

Indian Penal Code, No.45 of 1860.

Jain, D., & Shah, P. K. (2020). Reimagining reproductive rights jurisprudence in India: Reflections on the recent decisions on privacy and gender equality from the supreme court of India. *Colum. J. Gender & L.*, 39, 1.

Jatlaoui, T. C., Shah, J., Mandel, M. G., Krashin, J. W., Suchdev, D. B., Jamieson, D. J., & Pazol, K. (2017). Abortion surveillance d United States, 2014. *MMWR. Surveillance Summaries*, 66(24), 1–48. DOI: 10.15585/mmwr.ss6624a1 PMID: 29166366

Johari, V., & Jadhav, U. (2017): "Abortion Rights Judgment: A Ray of Hope!" *Indian Journal of Medical Ethics*, 28 February 2017, http://ijme. in/wp-content/ uploads/2017/02/20170228_ abortion_rights_judgment.pd

Kapoor, P., & Laws, E. A. (2023). A Case Study of Bangladesh, India, Russia, and the United States, 53 (29). *Economic and Political Weekly*, 59–63.

Kaur, J., & Bhardwaj, C. (2023). Right to Abortion in India: A Critical Appraisal of Legislative and Judicial Initiatives., No. 1 Int'l JL Mgmt. &. *Human.*, 6, 2223.

Kumar, A. P. (2016). 'Right to Choose'as a Fundamental Right. *Economic and Political Weekly*, 10–11.

Loksabha debates, 17th March, 2020 available at https://eparlib.nic.in/bitstream/ 123456789/794800/1/lsd_17_03_17-03-2020.pdf

Medical Termination of Pregnancy Act, Act No. 34 of 1971

Ministry of Health and Family Welfare. https://main.mohfw.gov.in/?q=acts-rules -and-standards-health-sector/acts/mtp-act-amendment-2002

National Legal Services v. Union of India, (2014) 5 SCC 438.

Palepu, J. (2020, September) *Will the Medical Termination of Pregnancy Amendment Bill reduce abortion cases before Indian High Courts?* THE LEAFLET, https://www.theleaflet.in/will-the-medical-termination-ofpregnancy- amendment-bill-reduce-abortion-cases-before-indian-high-courts/#

Prasad, V., & Confusions, C. (2015). 50 (10). *Economic and Political Weekly.*

Raj, O. (2022). Constitutional and criminal perspectives of women's reproductive rights. *Indian Journal of Integrated Research in Law*, 2(5), 1–10.

Roe v. Wade, U.S. 113 (1973).

Rysavy, M. A., Li, L., Bell, E. F., Das, A., Hintz, S. R., Stoll, B. J., & Higgins, R. D. (2015). Between-hospital variation in treatment and outcomes in extremely preterm infants. *The New England Journal of Medicine*, 372(19), 1801–1811. DOI: 10.1056/NEJMoa1410689 PMID: 25946279

Stark, B. (2011). The women's convention, reproductive rights, and the reproduction of gender. *Duke Journal of Gender Law & Policy*, 18(2), 261–304.

Suchita Srivastava v. Chandigarh Administration (2009) 9 SCC 1

Suchita Srivastava v. Chandigarh Administration (2009) 9 SCC 1

Supreme Court of India. (2023). *Order in MA 2157 of 2023 in WP(C) 1137 of 2023.* Retrieved from https://www.livelaw.in/pdf_upload/ma-2157-of-2023-in-wpc-1137-of-2023-1-1-498107.pdf

The Medical Termination of Pregnancy (Amendment) Rules, 2021, Rule 3B.

World Health Organization. 'Abortion Care Guideline' https://www.who.int/publications/i/item/9789240039483 28.

X v. Union of India &Anr., INSC 919, 2023

## ENDNOTES

1 Indian Penal Code, No.45 of 1860, §312 - Whoever voluntarily causes a woman with child to miscarry, shall, if such miscarriage be not caused in good faith for the purpose of saving the life of the woman, be punished with imprisonment of either description for a term which may extend to three years, or with fine, or with both; and, if the woman be quick with child, shall be punished with

imprisonment of either description for a term which may extend to seven years, and shall also be liable to fine.

# Chapter 7
# Right-Based Approach to Reproductive Autonomy: A Comparative Study Between Indian and US Judiciaries

**Jipson Joseph**
https://orcid.org/0009-0005-1795-5051
*Christ University, India*

**Ananya Pandey**
https://orcid.org/0000-0002-2419-6314
*Christ University, India*

## ABSTRACT

*Discussion on reproductive health became prominent in the second half of the 20th century. The Declaration of the universality of human rights energized a right-based approach to reproductive health. Many women realized that without reproductive rights the questions on their dignity, equality, liberty, and life would become meaningless. This right-based approach got momentum in USA and extended to other countries, including India. But both these countries did not consider right to abortion as an absolute right. In India, the enactment of Medical Termination of Pregnancy Act, 1971 considered it as a limited right. The US judiciary in its Roe judgment in 1973 considered it under right to privacy in the ambit of right to liberty but only as a limited right. However, this judgment was overruled by the Dobbs judgment in 2022. In this context, this chapter attempts to compare the perspectives of both USA and India on reproductive health.*

DOI: 10.4018/979-8-3693-7837-3.ch007

## INTRODUCTION

Women were discriminated against their culturally imposed gender throughout history (Beniwal, 2013). Patriarchal society denied meaningful existence to women. Their independence and decision-making capacity were not respected and treated them as mere possessions of men. Questioning their self-autonomy, the patriarchy even denied their basic rights (Millett, 1970). However, the constitutional provisions of equality and non-discrimination challenged patriarchal hegemony. But still, the societal stigma fails to accept the decision-making roles of women (Kapoor, 2023). This is explicit both in USA and India in varying scales. It is most evident about reproductive rights as well. The core of woman's personality is attached to reproductive rights. These are foundational rights of women as it helps to make free choice with regard to their sexuality and pregnancy.

While framing the Constitution of India, the Constitutional Fathers were highly influenced by the oldest democratic Constitution of USA. Many parts of the Indian constitution owe its origin to the American constitution. This is mainly evident in its Part III that speaks about the fundamental rights. These countries also concentrate their discussions on reproductive rights in the ambit of fundamental rights. Both of them also focus on abortion rights among the plethora of reproductive rights in their heated legislative and judicial discussions. However, the discussions on reproductive rights in USA started with the growing awareness of human rights and women rights. Whereas, in India it started with the question of decriminalization of abortion. When Indian legal system defends women's reproductive by making laws and regulations, the American legal system enlarged its ambit from the perspective of rights. Accordingly, a comparative study on these two countries' understanding of reproductive rights will be helpful in exploring the depth of women's reproductive autonomy.

Contemporary discussions on reproductive rights in India and USA state that while there is a significant progress in the scope of reproductive rights in India, its scope in USA is being restricted. Indian legal system gradually moved towards a more progressive approach, whereas the American legal system became more conservative. This chapter thus aims to make a comparative study of these two judicial systems in view of their approach towards reproductive rights. It analyzes how the US approach influenced the Indian understanding of reproductive rights, the legislative and judicial initiatives of both the countries on reproductive health decisions, and the impact of the latest American judicial decision on the Indian understanding of reproductive rights.

## HISTORICAL BACKGROUND OF REPRODUCTIVE RIGHTS IN INDIA AND USA

Reproductive rights originated in the second half of the 19th century and became prominent in the second half of the 20th century. The declaration of the human rights by the United Nations (UN) in 1948 was the immediate background for this progressive vision. But an overview of the evolution of rights shows that the reproductive rights as such were not a major concern till the 20th century. The post-World War II scenario redefined women's role in the society. Both feminists' and equal rights' movements emphasized the essentiality of women rights. The main thrust of these movements was to uphold women's reproductive rights as they thought that it would establish their uniqueness and individuality.

### International Framework

With the formation of UN, the history of human rights took a decisive turn. It affirmed that human rights should be respected universally without any differentiation based on sex (UN Charter, art. 55). A peaceful and harmonious relationship is impossible without due respect towards human dignity and inalienable rights (UDHR, Preamble). Undue interference into the privacy of an individual is considered as an infringement of one's rights (UDHR, art. 12). States have the responsibility to ensure physical and mental well-being of their citizens (ICESCR, art. 12). It indirectly states that if a pregnancy causes physical and mental issues to the woman, then the State should protect the interests of women (Cook, 2020). States also should give proper and timely care to pregnant women during and after pregnancy (ICESCR, art. 10). This was in view of reducing the maternal mortality-rate. In this context, the right to reproductive health is affirmed as a human right (CRPD, art. 23). The UN further stated that the size of the family should be decided by the individual family even though the State can formulate policies in the ambit of population control. Decisions with regard to various aspects of reproductive health are the prerogatives of each family (UN General Assembly, 1966, res. 2211). The first International Conference on Human Rights considered reproductive decisions as the parents' choice (Momtaz, 2009). Later on, the Convention on the Elimination of All Forms of Discrimination Against Women (CEDAW) affirmed the rights of women to decide the number and spacing of pregnancy (art. 16(e)). But it did not consider it as a particular right of women. A committee constituted under CEDAW instructed the government of Peru to legalize abortion of rape victims (Fine et al., 2017). The International Conference on Population and Development convened in Cairo in 1994 strongly upheld the couple's right to make reproductive choices. It considered reproductive rights as essential human rights (Reichenbach & Roseman,

2009). But the Beijing Proclamation of 1995 took a paradigm shift and stated that women should have control over reproductive decisions (nos. 95-96). All these above-mentioned international frameworks laid a general foundation for the growth of reproductive rights. It shows that the international community took almost 50 years to consider reproductive rights as a prerogative of women.

## Development of Right-Based Approach in USA

The 1776 Declaration of Independence states that all men are created equal. Though it can be argued that the term "men" is used in general, consisting of both man and woman, still the usage is discriminatory. However, the 1791 Bill of Rights used a gender-neutral term 'person.' The change in the usage of terms also underlines the changed perspective. Reproductive rights will be unrealizable without due respect towards the basic equality of men and women. US history of reproductive rights has both ups and downs. The first initiative towards reproductive rights can be traced back to the last quarter of the 19th century, when feminists demanded "voluntary motherhood." The second stage began with the Margaret Sanger's promotion of the idea of "birth control" in 1915, and the third stage arose in the aftermath of the First World War with the "professionalization of birth control" (Presser, 1978). In the second half of the 20th century, various women movements, who fought for the rights of women, took up the lead for the protection of women's claims in reproductive health related matters (McBride & Mazur, 2008). Reproductive rights movements originated during this same period. However, towards the end of the 20th century a reproductive justice movement evolved that stood for economic, social, cultural, and political empowerment of women, enabling them to make decisions regarding their body, sexuality, and reproduction (Joachim, 2007; Kluchin, 2011; Ross, 2020). They argued that women should have access to abortion without any undue interference from external agents (Price, 2010). Right to abortion becomes implemented only when there is access to safe and hygiene abortion procedures.

## Development of Reproductive Rights in India

Evolution of reproductive rights in India started with the incorporation of fundamental rights in the Constitution of India. Its article 14 affirms equality before law to any person without any differentiation on the basis of sex. This equality clause is the rationale behind adult women's right to make reproductive decision even without the consent of her husband or other family members. Based on its Article 15, the State cannot make discriminating laws against women's reproductive choices. Article 21 is the guardian of reproductive rights. It implies that a woman should have the freedom if she wants to terminate her pregnancy. It also warns against undue influence or coercion against women's reproductive choices. The Directive Principles of State Policy, enlisted in Part IV of the Constitution, also gives certain guidelines. Article 39(e) states that the State should consider *inter alia* the health and strength of working women, which cannot be separated from their reproductive health matters. It also affirms women's rights in reproductive matters. Article 42 speaks about maternity relief, which was the cornerstone of the Maternity Act of 1961. This provision affirms India's respect and concern towards maternity.

Compared to many other countries, women rights movements had a late origin in India. It originated in the 1980s as a small group in which women discussed many topics including menstruation, use of contraceptive methods, abortive techniques, women empowerment programs, and importance of education and employment in their private and informal gatherings. These private discussions slowly extended to positive and progressive dialogues and discussions in colleges, housing colonies, and working sites. Gradually their voice and needs became noticed in the legislative bodies either through women or men representatives, who had a progressive vision. Such women movements and feminist advocates also raised their voice against the discrimination of women in reproductive matters. They also demanded safe and effective contraceptive and abortive methods for reducing maternal mortality-rate (Saheli, 2000).

## REPRODUCTIVE RIGHTS: AN OVERVIEW

Many people equate reproductive rights with right to abortion as it is the most controversial topic in the umbrella of reproductive rights. But reproductive rights include a group of rights connected with reproductive health. These rights are essential to women's autonomy and dignity as they are closely related to their life, sexuality, and pregnancy. Some people oppose these arguments claiming that men also should be credited crucial role in reproductive matters. But compared to men, women's body and mind are more allied to pregnancy (Berer, 2000). Reproductive rights are essential for the personal, educational, professional, and familial well-being of women. Denying reproductive rights to women endangers their very dignity. In the past, women's subordination to the male family members was considered as a virtue. But the present-day women are far superior to their counterparts in many fields and they strive to establish their unique position in the society. This necessitates women's active role in reproductive health decisions as well. Reproductive rights are the self-determination of woman with regard to her body and sexuality (Petchesky, 1980). Its scope is in the ambit of right and freedom that are essential for the full realization of her personality and equality in the society (Moen, 1981).

## Right to Life

The Constitutions of US and India guarantee right to life to every citizen irrespective of sexual differences. Right to life and maternal health is closely associated as many women lose their lives due to complications in pregnancy and childbirth in the absence of appropriate healthcare facilities. Right to life is the most violated reproductive right throughout the world. For a good period of time, the society did not give required attention to pregnant woman's right to life. Both human rights and women rights movements propagated against the increasing maternal mortality-rate. Some suggested to increase the spacing between childbirths to respect woman's health and life (Cook, 2020). Right to life cannot be realized without proper medical care. States should take precaution against unsafe clinics and unqualified medical practitioners in order to protect the lives of pregnant women (Shalev, 2000).

## Right to Marriage and Family

Right to marriage and family is a basic right of both men and women for sustainable future. Men exercised free choice with regard to marriage from time immemorial. But women were denied of this right as their family members took decision on their behalf. Freedom to choose in relation to marriage is an essential right for ensuring one's personality and dignity. In order to have this right woman should have the freedom to decide her marriage. Consent for marriage should come from within, without any coercion or undue influence. Both man and woman are the choice-makers, and their families have only supporting-roles. Their choice-making role should not be replaced by the family. Compared to developed countries, the family's involvement is more evident in developing countries. Without real consent, marriage becomes problematic. Right to marriage and family includes factors like right to decide marriageable age, right to choose the person for marriage, and right to decide the spacing and number of childbirths. Right to family includes her right to say yes or no throughout the marital life. She can even deny sexual relationship with her husband, if she is not interested on a particular day (Cook, 2020).

## Right to Contraceptives

Neo-Malthusians were the prime advocates of population control. Only a very few countries adopted population control strategies in the beginning but the number increased with the involvement of feminist and women rights movements. Both voluntary and involuntary models of birth control mechanisms can be seen in the history of reproductive health (Connelly, 2003). China is a model of involuntary approach. India too had undergone through a dark age in its history of reproductive rights, where the State mechanisms used coercion and force for contraception during the time of national emergency. Obligation to use contraceptives is not a right. States can suggest to control the rapid population growth through the use of contraceptives but the choice should be made by individuals (Pillay & Wang, 1999). Even the government advertisements that propagate family planning programs is an unfair influence as many of women feel ashamed when they become pregnant for the third or fourth time. Conscientization of contraceptives is essential but it should not lead to undue influence. They should have complete freedom to make their own choices (Cook, 2020).

## Right to Abortion

Right to abortion is the pregnant woman's right to terminate pregnancy at her will (Berer, 2002). Absolute right to abortion is not guaranteed by either US or Indian legal systems. World religions always criticized abortion arguing that it is against the divine design. They equate it with culpable homicide claiming that the unborn from the very first moment of its origin is a person. They advocate the tube to tomb theory arguing that the life starts from the fallopian tube, where the sperm interrelates with the egg, and ends at the tomb. The life of any person is sacred and inviolable throughout this life-span. To add quality to pregnant woman's life, an innocent's sacred life cannot be destroyed (Chamakala, 2009). However, in the second half of the 20th century, international conventions and women rights movements argued for women's right to make decision with regard to the continuance of pregnancy. Many abortive methods can be seen throughout the centuries; most of them were unsafe. Even when the Hippocrates Oath forbade the doctors to practice such things, it was practiced (Prokopijević, 1994). The society should protect women's right to abortion by providing safe and effective methods for affirming their dignity and equality of status. Affirmation of their right to abortion also leads to the recognition of their control over their own body, sexuality, and life (Berer, 2002). It helps them to be free from unintended pregnancy and make choice in the areas of educational and professional demands. They can prioritize their interests in life. However, such a decision is very complex as it also involves physical, psychological, and emotional aspects (Visaria & Ramachandran, 2007).

## Right to Privacy

Right to privacy is a vital component of reproductive rights. Reproductive health service providers should keep the privacy of their clients. Disclosing the client's personal identity and other personal facts is against the parameters of medical ethics (Shalev, 2000). Right to privacy refers to one's absolute freedom to make a choice in reproductive matters. Any interference into the decision-making role of woman would lead to an encroachment into her privacy. The European Court on Human Rights stated that the pregnant woman's right to privacy to abort her pregnancy is far beyond the choice of the child's biological father or the State. Not even a consultation with the father of the child is required (Cook, 2020). However, in India, the ultimate deciding person is the Registered Medical Practitioner (RMP). Termination of pregnancy cannot be done without the pregnant woman's consent but she cannot decide by herself. In Justice Puttaswamy's case, the Supreme Court of India affirmed right to abortion as a matter of right to privacy on the basis of three essential attributes of privacy: liberty, autonomy, and dignity. But the law prioritizes the decision of the RMP (Magill, 2020).

## LEGISLATIVE FRAMEWORK: A COMPARISON

Enforcement of reproductive rights becomes easy in view of a specific legislative framework. All the campaigns and movements for reproductive rights will be ineffective in the absence of proper legislation. Legalization of abortion can elucidate most of the doubts and apprehensions in this area. While the USA focused on approaching reproductive health matters, particularly the right to abortion, in line with judicial interventions, India enacted a proper legislation and cleared confusions on this intricate question. In this section, an analysis is done on the legislative frameworks of both India and USA in the ambit of reproductive health with a specific focus on right to abortion.

### Abortion: Indian Legislative Framework

The basic legislation that shaped the termination of pregnancy in India is the Medical Termination of Pregnancy (MTP) Act of 1971, which was amended in 2002 and 2021 respectively. Based on the parent Act, the Medical Termination of Pregnancy Rules, 1975 were formulated, which was amended in 2003 and 2021. The MTP Act was enacted due to the necessity of decriminalization of abortion.

#### The Indian Penal Code, 1860

Abortion was illegal in India and if any person voluntarily causes miscarriage, it would lead to an imprisonment of three years and fine (IPC, 1860, §312). The punishment will be prolonged to seven years together with fine, if the woman already had the feeling of fetus' movement. But this provision also could criminalize the action of RMP if the abortion is done without any medical necessity just because of the pregnant woman's demand. It also caused liability to woman as well, if she herself caused miscarriage. Legal abortion was possible only in extreme necessities to save the mother's life. No other reason was accepted as justifiable (Shah et al., 1967). This provision of the IPC strictly followed the spirit of both Victorian morality and the English Christian tradition. The Indian Hindu tradition that gave high respect and sacredness towards the mother and the child is also visible.

Any person causing miscarriage to a woman without her consent, regardless of the feeling of fetus' movement, shall be punished for life imprisonment or for a period of up to ten years besides being imposed of certain amount of fine (IPC, 1860, §313). IPC thus differentiates between causing miscarriage with and without the consent of woman. There is an exception in §312 if it is done to save the woman's life. In such case, it will not amount to crime. But in §313 there is no exception as it is always considered a crime. If the woman dies in the process of miscarriage, which is done with the consent of woman, then who causes miscarriage shall be punished up to a period of ten years together with fine; and if it is done without her consent then the offender shall be punished with life imprisonment (IPC, 1860, §314). Besides, severe punishment will be given in cases where a child is not permitted to be born alive or causing it to die soon after its birth if it is not done for saving the mother's life (IPC, 1860, §315). Under the IPC framework, women had no freedom to terminate pregnancy except when it was a serious threat to their life. RMPs also had to risk their life if the abortion is done without any medical emergency.

## Shanti Lal Shah Committee Report

The impracticality of unnecessary restrictions on abortion caused an increase in unsafe abortion practices and clinics that led to enormous increase in maternal mortality rate. Faced with this dilemma, the then Central government constituted a committee under Dr. Shanti Lal Shah in 1964 to study the possibilities of legalization of abortion. Its immediate reason was the anxiety expressed by the 1964 Central Family Planning Board meeting about the increase in illegal abortions performed by untrained persons in unhygienic places that cause severe health issues and deaths to women. Shanti Lal Shah committee consisted of nine members including the chairman and then two more members were added (Jalnawalla, 1974). The committee studied the medical, social, moral, and legal questions on the legalization of abortion. It underlined the increase in maternal mortality rate in connection with illegal abortions. The committee thus strongly recommended for the liberalization of abortion laws and noted that it could also reduce the uncontrollable population growth (Shah et al., 1967)

## Medical Termination of Pregnancy (MTP) Act

The MTP Act was enacted in 1971 to provide an option to legally abort certain pregnancies that cause physical or mental issues to the pregnant woman. Its basic intention was to save the RMP from the legal liability of abortion. The Act preferred 'medical termination of pregnancy' over abortion to tackle the protest from the socio-religious groups against the abortive methods. They preferred medical termination of pregnancy thinking that it would give a feeling that it is done out of some medical necessity. Its 'notwithstanding' clause overrides the IPC provisions with regard to miscarriage (§3). It does not legalize abortion but liberates the RMP from the culpability of miscarriage by widening the scope of IPC provisions. The only possibility of abortion under IPC was to save the mother's life, but the MTP Act enlarged it with the provisions of physical and mental health of the mother and physical and mental health issues of the unborn (§3(1)).

The RMP can terminate pregnancy at the pregnant woman's demand and consent if the pregnancy is within the limit of 12 weeks. If it is beyond twelve weeks but not above twenty weeks then the RMP can terminate pregnancy only in consultation with another RMP (§3(2)). The decision to terminate pregnancy must be based on the reasons provided in §3(1). Physical and mental health of the pregnant woman is very wide in scope and so, the RMP can find a reason in support of pregnant woman's choice to terminate pregnancy. The decision of the RMP is final in terminating pregnancy but it is depended on the pregnant woman's choice and desire. The explanations of §3(2) address the pregnancies of rape victims and the persons with failed contraceptive methods. Both rape and failure of contraceptives cause severe physical and mental issues to pregnant women and if they desire the RMP can decide in their favor. The maximum possible span for terminating a pregnancy was 20 weeks under the Act but it will not be applicable in cases where it becomes a medical emergency to save the mother's life (§5(1)). However, in any case a pregnancy should not be terminated without pregnant woman's consent (§3(4)(b)). Neither husband nor parents of an adult woman of sound mind can substitute her consent. It should epitomize the choice of her free will and full consent. But the Act says that if the pregnant woman is a lunatic or a minor, then the RMP cannot make decision without the written consent of her guardian (§3(4)(a)). The Act also specifies that a pregnancy can be terminated either in a government owned and run hospital or in a place approved by the government (§4). It was to forbid illegal and unsafe abortions that can cause health risks to women.

In 1975, the government of India formulated the rules and regulations for the better functioning and implementation of the Act. These rules had the objective to regulate unexpert procedures in unsafe places. It specified appropriate training and experience for the RMP to terminate pregnancy. It also specified the required quality and hygiene of the places where such procedures should be undertaken.

In 2002, the principal Act was amended. It substituted the term 'lunatic' with 'mentally ill person' (§2(i)). It arranged an option for District Level Committee (DLC) to permit places for terminating pregnancy, after due inspection. It provided punishment with rigorous imprisonment for a period of two years extendable to seven years if any person other than the RMP terminates pregnancy (§5(2)). In order to ensure hygiene place for the procedure, the Act stated punishment with rigorous imprisonment for a term of two years extendable to seven years for any person terminating pregnancy in a place not specified by the Act (§5(3)). The owner or the administrative head of such places also will have the same punishment (§5(4)). The amendment was in view of establishing expert persons and safe places for the procedure so that the health and life of women can be protected. Based on the amendment Act, the MTP Rules were codified in 2003. It mainly spoke about the composition of DLC, the required experience and training of the RMPs, and the approval of places for abortion. The DLC should approve a place only by inspecting that particular place. It should verify the hygiene and safety of the place (§6).

In 2021, the MTP Act was further amended. Termination of pregnancy is defined as a procedure to terminate pregnancy either by surgical or medical method (§2(ii)). It also extended the 12 weeks period of the principal Act to 20 weeks wherein the RMP could decide by himself with the consent of pregnant woman and the 20 weeks period to 24 weeks wherein the decision should be taken in consultation with another RMP (§3). The amendment provided the option for abortion up to the completion of first two trimesters (six months) of pregnancy. Most interestingly, the amendment does not differentiate women into married or unmarried. It uses 'partner' instead of 'husband'. It gives high respect towards the privacy of woman (§4(i)). It also added a new provision, the medical board (§2(i)). Based on the amendment of the Act, the MTP Rules were also amended in 2021. It specified the functions of the medical board. Its main function is with regard to the termination of pregnancy beyond the 24 weeks period (§3). It also enlisted the categories of women, who can terminate their pregnancy (§3B).

From 1971 to 2021, the MTP Act underwent changes and modifications in favor of women. The Act, its amendments, and the Rules provided legal framework for safe termination of pregnancy in hygiene place by expert RMPs. However, it does not give absolute right to women as the decision-making role is bestowed on the RMP if the pregnancy is within the prescribed life-span.

## Abortion: US Legislations

Unlike India, there is no federal legislation in US in the ambit of termination of pregnancy. The US Supreme Cout in Roe v. Wade had given a judicial protection to abortion but it was overruled in Dobbs v. Jackson Mental Health Organization. Currently, abortion is illegal in 12 states and many other states plan to pass such laws due to the absence of judicial protection (CRR, 2023). The conflict of interest between the Democrats and Republicans is the main obstacle for the legalization of abortion. Though there is no specific legislation that permit abortion, there is a kind of legislative framework with regard to reproductive health and that will be analyzed in this section.

### The Freedom of Access to Clinic Entrances Act, 1994 (FACE Act, 1994)

The Congress enacted the FACE Act to amend Chapter 13 of Title 18 of the US Code, which discusses civil rights. The amendment added new sections to ensure freedom of access to reproductive health services. Its objective was to protect and promote health and safety of people, who approach the reproductive services, against the injuring, intimidating, and interfering activities of certain others (§2). The Act provided free access to reproductive health centers and those who violate this provision will be punished either with imprisonment for one year or fine or with both (§3(b)). The Act had no intention to legalize abortion as it was done by the Roe judgment. Its main concern was to protect reproductive health service providers and their clients against those who act against their interests.

### Women's Health Act: Proposed Legislation

The bill of Women's Health Protection Act (WHP Act) was introduced in 2013 but did not even get the assent of the committee. It was reintroduced in 2015, 2017, 2019, and 2022. The House of Representatives passed it but the Senate defeated it by 2 votes in February 2022 and again in May 2022. Its objective is to legalize abortion by giving decision-making capacity to the individual and freedom to the healthcare sector to provide abortion services. It wants to empower individuals with decisional autonomy in the areas of pregnancy, family, and life (§2(a)(1)). It states that individuals are the ultimate authority in this choice, and not the State. Affirming reproductive justice, it echoes individual's self-determination capacity (§2(a)(4)). Restrictions on abortion deny bodily autonomy and dignity to women (§2(a)(7)). It defines women in a wider ambit including all those persons having the capacity of pregnancy (§2(a)(8)). It criticizes that the hospitals do not provide abortion facilities but only clinics and, in many counties, there are no clinics forcing people to travel a long distance for having access to abortion clinics (§2(13)). It also states that in the absence of a federal legislation, each State has its own legislation and that in many instances cause burden to women (§2(27)). Basically, the Act's main objective is to protect women's right to abortion if the fetus has not achieved the period of viability. It shows that this proposed legislation also does not want to make it as an absolute right.

## Analysis of the Executive Order of 2022

The US Supreme Court's overturning of Roe judgment caused a convoluted situation and thus the President of USA, Joseph R. Biden, on 03 August 2022 issued an executive order that provided certain possibilities for reproductive health services. It was to clarify the confusions of the reproductive healthcare providers whether they should provide emergency healthcare facilities to pregnant women that necessitates termination of pregnancy. The situation is more complex in the States where there are strict anti-abortion laws. RMPs even deny necessary medical care to pregnant women fearing legal liability. But this may adversely affect their pregnancy and life. Pharmacies also deny prescribed medication to pregnant women fearing legal liability as the prescribed medication may risk their pregnancy. Some clinics and hospitals in the anti-abortion law States deny contraceptive services to their clients. In this background, the President had to give an executive order to ensure access to reproductive healthcare services (§1), which were defined as all those medical and surgical services including counselling in the area of pregnancy and its termination (§2). It also affirmed that all healthcare providers, who receive financial support from the federal government, have the responsibility to provide such services (§4). However, the Order does not give any entitlement of rights against the State (§6(ii)(c)).

# JUDICIAL DECISIONS AND REPRODUCTIVE RIGHTS: A COMPARATIVE STUDY

The judicial framework was more predominant in US with regard to reproductive health. Indian judiciary has been actively involved in reproductive health matters only since the last decade of the 20th century. Indian judicial system mostly inspired by its US counterpart. Both these judiciaries had to interfere when women or RMPs challenged the legal barriers in reproductive health. Various women empowerment groups also filed petitions regarding women's bodily autonomy and reproductive health. Judiciary preferred to consider reproductive health matters under the ambit of human rights widening its scope.

## Judicial Pronouncements in USA

The US Supreme Court has given plenty of decisions with regard to reproductive health. It would not be possible to analyze all those judgments, and hence, an attempt is made to examine the important judgments for exploring the growth of its right-based-approach towards reproductive health and its influence on other judicial systems.

### Griswold v. Connecticut

This case of 1965 is a historic judgment in the ambit of reproductive health. It was with regard to the use of contraceptives. The Connecticut laws forbade the use of contraceptive medicine or device. But the Planned Parenthood League of Connecticut and its RMP provided contraceptive information to married persons helping them to prevent conception They were convicted of violating the above-mentioned law of Connecticut. They approached the Federal Supreme Court, arguing that such a law was against the Constitution's Fourteenth Amendment. The judiciary affirmed its role in interpreting and widening the ambit of rights to protect individual claims. Though two judges stated that it is a constitutionally valid enactment, five judges unanimously declared that the Connecticut law intruded into the married persons' right to privacy, which is against the 'due process' clause of $14^{th}$ amendment. They said that married persons have the right to privacy and in that private sphere they can make decisions about contraceptives. They also noted right to privacy as an integral part of right to liberty. However, this was applicable only to married persons. This case introduced a right-based approach in reproductive health matters.

### Eisenstadt v. Baird

This case of 1972 was against the Massachusetts law, which forbade the use of contraceptives by unmarried persons and prescribed contraceptives to unmarried persons by the RMPs. Baird was a prominent proponent of contraceptives, who at the end of one his lectures to students on its use and advantages gave a contraceptive foam to an unmarried woman. He was convicted, and an appeal arose against the State law arguing that it challenges his fundamental rights. This case was a connecting link between Griswold and Roe. Basing on the Griswold judgment the court said that if the prescription, distribution, and use of contraceptives is legal for married, it should be equally applicable to unmarried persons. Among the eight judges, five judges concurred to the decision, one judge dissented and two others did not participate in the proceedings. The court stated that all contraceptives are unhealthy but if they can be used by the married then the unmarried also should have the right to use them (Appleton, 2016). The court also noted that it does not want to entertain the questions of morality and premarital sex as it is intimately related to one's personal choice. It thus liberalized sex from the control of ethical codes.

## Roe v. Wade

The US Supreme Court had recognized marital and familial rights as part of right to privacy read under the right to liberty clause of the fourteenth amendment. According to them, it included the right to marry (Meyer v. Nebraska; Loving v. Virginia), to procreate (Skinner v. Oklahoma), and to use contraceptives (Eisenstadt v. Baird). But it never considered right to abortion as part of right to privacy (Keynes & Miller, 1989). However, this 1973 case became historic due to its progressive vision towards right to abortion.

Jane Roe (pseudonym) was a single pregnant woman but when the case reached at the supreme court there had already taken place a natural miscarriage, but the court continued with her petition. She had challenged the abortion laws of Texas that prohibited abortion except to save the life of the mother (Kranz, 2002). The court said that there can have many influencing factors like conservative or progressive mentality and population growth on one's opinion about abortion. Such parameters will not be considered over the constitutional provisions. The court opined that the anti-abortion laws are not age-old as they originated only in the second half of the $19^{th}$ century. There can have three reasons for the evolution of these laws like the influence of Victorian morality, the State's interest to protect pregnant women from unsafe abortion practices, and the State's interest to protect the unborn. The court noted that pregnancy can cause both physical and mental health issues to women. The court thus recognized right to abortion as part of right to privacy but as a qualified right (Ehrlich, 2006).

Since the court did not recognize it as an absolute right, it pointed to a "compelling" point for the State's intervention. It prescribed the end of the first trimester as the compelling point. It was in connection with the viability of the fetus. It affirmed that during the first trimester the RMP can terminate pregnancy with the consent of the pregnant woman without the State's interference. In the second trimester, the State can make reasonable restrictions on the right to abortion. But it cannot deny their right to abortion. In the third trimester, the abortion can be done only in extreme cases to save the mother's life. The State can regulate and prohibit abortion during this stage (Keynes & Miller, 1989).

## Planned Parenthood v. Casey

This case of 1992 was an appeal against the stringent provisions of the Pennsylvania Abortion Control Act of 1982. The Act insisted for the pregnant women's informed consent. Besides, married women had to give an affidavit stating that she had notified her husband about the procedure and the minor woman had to present the informed consent of one of her parents. The court affirmed its responsibility to be faithful to the *stare decisis* of the Roe judgment. The court however said that women have only "some freedom" to terminate pregnancy and that ends with the viability of the fetus. It denied the rigid trimester formula of Roe and said that the State can interfere by giving information on life and adoption possibilities. It tried to protect the State's interests rather than women's rights. The restrictions that were placed on State intervention were taken away. The court favored the State's insistence on informed consent of the pregnant woman and the informed consent of one of the parents of the minor pregnant woman. But it invalidated the clause that required the notification to the husband.

## Dobbs v. Jackson Women's Health Organization

This 2022 judgment might be the most unexpected, undesired, unsupported, and unethical one in the history of US Supreme Court. This case was in the context of the Mississippi law that forbade abortion after the completion of 15 weeks except for saving the mother's life and due to fetal abnormalities. The petitioners argued that this law is constitutionally invalid and stated that the judgments of Roe and Casey are not reasonably framed. They thus argued to overrule those decisions. Overruling those landmark judgments, the court denied constitutional protection to abortion. It claimed that such a decision is not vested on the court but on the people and their elected representatives. The court noted that more than half of the States approached it to overrule both Roe and Casey judgments and to give back the law-making power to the States. It criticized the Roe reasoning stating that it has no basis in American and Common Laws. It further criticized the trimester line for the State intervention, which is drawn by the Roe judges, as irrational. They said that there is no such right in the constitution or in its broader interpretation. It added that right to abortion is not part of American culture and tradition. It also denied to apply 'due process' clause claiming that it is an entirely different idea. Overruling both Roe and Casey the court empowered the States to make laws either in favor or against of abortion.

## Judicial Decisions in India

The cultural, religious, and ethical code of India always upheld the dignity of pregnant women as children were considered a blessing. Terminating pregnancy was unthinkable except to save the pregnant woman's life. This cultural background was the rationale behind the criminalization of abortion. However, the MTP Act, based on its specific provisions, protected those who wanted to terminate their pregnancy. Hence, there were only few judicial interventions in the Indian scenario compared to the USA. But in the 21st century there are a good number of cases in which judiciary stepped in to protect the reproductive health matters.

### Suchita Srivastava v. Chandigarh Administration

The Punjab and Haryana High Court's division bench at the demand of a government-run hostel authorities where she was an inmate, granted abortion to a mentally retarded woman, who was a rape victim. The expert committee constituted by the division bench noted that the woman likes to continue her pregnancy. But even then, the High Court permitted to terminate pregnancy. Against this order an appeal was raised in the division bench of Supreme Court. The Supreme Court stated that as per the provision of the MTP Act, the consent of the woman has paramount importance. The woman has absolute power to make the choice. Her consenting power cannot be substituted with any other person. The Supreme Court thus over-ruled the judgment of the high court.

### Laxmi Mandal v. Deen Dayal Harinagar Hospital

This case addressed the poor people's lack of safe and hygiene facilities to realize their reproductive rights. This writ petition was filed on behalf Shanti Devi who was denied reproductive healthcare by the public and private health sectors and the central and Haryana State governments (Kaur, 2012). In the absence of public and private affordable healthcare services, people approach unqualified medical practitioners that lead to health risks. The procedure in government hospitals is lengthy and requires many documents causing troubles to patients. The court thus instructed that no poor pregnant woman should be sent out of a public health center due to the absence of necessary documents for proving her BPL status.

## Sandesh Bansal v. Union of India

The petitioner, a social activist, was seriously concerned of the increasing maternal mortality rate in Madhya Pradesh. This was mainly due to the failure of public healthcare service sector as it does not reach to the rural poor people. Due to lack of transport facilities, rural people fail to bring pregnant women with complications to the hospital promptly, which finally cause their life. The court affirmed women's fundamental right to survive pregnancy and childbirth under Article 21 of the Constitution. If any woman fails to survive pregnancy and childbirth in India, it is a violation of her basic right to life. The State has high responsibility to protect the pregnant woman's life as guaranteed by the Constitution. The court gave an action plan for the Madhya Pradesh government to address the maternal mortality issue in its rural areas. The court also said that the government and its officials would be accountable for any violation in the ambit of reproductive rights of women (Kaur, 2012).

## Devika Biswas v. Union of India

This case was a public interest litigation and the petitioner was a social worker in many North Indian States. She argued that the sterilization procedures in India are not following any norms or regulations. The immediate background for the petition was the unsafe and unhygienic conducting of a sterilization camp in Bihar in which 53 women were sterilized on a single day without giving them proper counselling or awareness. There was only one surgeon, who did not even change his glove after each procedure. After the procedure, many women underwent through physical and mental health issues, and thus complaints were registered in the nearby police station. Such kind of camps that cause health hazards to women were conducted in many other States also. Though sterilization procedure is not complicated, it causes many lives in India. Poor people of rural areas are the main victims of this unsafe procedure. The petitioner thus pleaded the court to interfere and give justice to many innocent people. The Court stated that though family planning is a concurrent list entry, the Central government should ensure safe and effective sterilization procedures. Both central and state governments should collaborate with each other to protect the lives of the citizens. Right to reproductive health is a facet of right to life and personal liberty. No person should undergo the sterilization procedure without giving an informed consent, which is an expression of her personal choice. Informed consent implies that the person must be given all vital information with regard to the effects and drawbacks of the procedure.

## X v. Principal secretary, Health and Family Welfare Department, Delhi

An unmarried woman living in Delhi became pregnant from a consensual relationship and she wanted to terminate pregnancy before the completion of the 24$^{th}$ week as the partner left her. She approached the Delhi high court pleading three things: permit to terminate her pregnancy before the 24$^{th}$ week, no criminal proceedings should be initiated against her and the RMP, and to give direction to include unmarried women also into the ambit of rule 3B of the MTP Rules of 2003. She argued that as her partner refused to marry her, she is worried of the social stigma and harassment if she gives birth to the child. She also claimed that she has no source of living and not mentally healthy to accept the child. The High court observed that being an unmarried pregnant woman, her plea does not come under the ambit of MTP Rules 2003. She appealed to the Supreme Court arguing that the judgment of the High Court is a violation of Article 14. The Supreme Court stated that the law must be interpreted on the basis of the purpose of the enactment. The MTP Act is primarily a beneficial legislation as it intends to provide access to women to safe and hygiene pregnancy termination procedures. Interpretation of law should be in view of the changing needs of times and circumstances. Now, both pre-marital sex and live-in relationships are not viewed through the lens of criminality. The very purpose of the legislation is to include both married and unmarried women into the ambit of the MTP Act. The artificial distinction between married and unmarried women in terminating pregnancy is not constitutionally sustainable. The choice with regard to reproductive health is equally applicable to all women under Articles 14 and 21 of the Constitution. Accordingly, the Supreme Court granted her plea.

## POSSIBLE IMPACT OF DOBBS JUDGMENT ON INDIAN JUDICIARY

Indian judiciary considered many US Supreme Court decisions as important sources. Indian Judges like justice Krishna Iyer frequently referred to US Supreme Court decisions in their judgments. The US judiciary always had a right-based approach. Its promotion of human rights always inspired Indian judiciary. The right-based approach towards reproductive health originated in US as well. From the mid of the 20$^{th}$ century, the US judiciary approached reproductive health matters through the lens of rights. The Roe judgment even fortified this approach as US judiciary connected right to abortion with right to privacy under the ambit of right to liberty. Such progressive approach became visible in Indian judicial decisions in the 21$^{st}$ century while dealing with reproductive matters. However, the US Supreme

Court's 2022 Dobbs judgment overruled the Roe judgment by which it denied right-based approach to reproductive health. In such a context, what would be the impact of this latest judgment on the Indian judicial system? In line with the US judiciary, Indian judiciary also considered reproductive rights under the ambit of right to liberty (Suchita Srivastava v. Chandigarh Administration). Making a direct reference to Roe judgment, it considered reproductive health matters under right to privacy in the ambit of Article 21 of the Constitution (Justice K. S. Puttaswamy v. Union of India). However, it did not solely depend on the US judicial reasonings as it had to uphold India's legislative framework. The MTP Act was even prior to Roe judgment. Indian judiciary thus tried to relate law with rights and explained reproductive rights only as limited rights under the ambit of the MTP Act.

Reproductive rights consist of a plethora of rights. The confusion arises only with regard to right to abortion. Both US and Indian legislatures and judiciaries value all other reproductive rights. But with regard to right to abortion, the US judiciary through Roe judgment considered it as a limited right and the Indian judiciary also considered it as a limited right under the MTP Act provisions. However, when the US Supreme Court overruled Roe judgment and denied constitutional protection to abortion (Dobbs v. Jackson Women's Health Organization), the Indian Supreme Court gave purposive interpretation to the MTP Act and stated that the unmarried women can also make choice with regard to the termination of pregnancy (X v. Principal Secretary).

The change in US judiciary's approach is due to many factors. *Firstly*, the judges are appointed by the executive for a lifetime. The President of USA appoints the judges on the basis of their political ideology. The conservative or democratic background of the judges influence their decisions. If the majority of the judges are conservatives, then the Supreme Court's judgment also will be conservative (von Hagel & Mansbach, 2016). This is not the case in India. *Secondly*, reproductive rights are a campaign issue for the election of President in USA (Pacelle, 2003). But in India there is a clear legislative framework and the court can make purposive interpretation. Indian politicians are not interested to involve in reproductive health matters. *Thirdly*, there is no federal legislation in US on abortion and hence, many States according to their political ideology make laws. This leads to many litigations. But in India there is a specific central legislation. *Fourthly*, while the US judges stand for their political ideology, Indian judges proclaim a progressive vision of life.

In India, abortion was already de-criminalized by the central legislation of 1971. Thereafter, its various amendments enlarged the provisions of the MTP Act giving more liberal approaches. Indian judiciary mainly focused on the other areas of reproductive health rather than limiting itself to right to abortion as there had a well-established legislation. Whenever questions on the scope of termination of pregnancy were raised, the court addressed them by giving a purposive interpretation to the legislation. Neither India nor US consider right to abortion as a constitutional right. But Indian judiciary considered women's right for informed consent to terminate pregnancy as a constitutional right under Article 21.

In sum, the latest Dobbs judgment of the US Supreme Court will not have any impact on the reproductive decisions of Indian judiciary.

## CONCLUSION

Reproductive health is an important area of concern for humanity's sustainable future. It is equally applicable to both men and women. But compared to men, women are the main protagonists of reproductive matters as their bodies, minds, and emotions are closely associated with the reproductive procedure. For a good period of time, women had no voice in reproductive health matters. The power-politics of the patriarchy subjugated women even by making reproductive choices and decisions on their behalf. In the second half of the 20th century, many changes happened in the global scenario due to the influence of various human rights and women rights movements that favored women's rights and decision-making role in reproductive matters. A right-based approach to reproductive health emerged in the US, which influenced many other countries including India.

However, with regard to right to abortion there was no consensus among the judiciaries. Most of them considered it as a limited right. India enacted a legislation in 1971 providing the option of termination of pregnancy depending on the choice of woman. But in US, the Supreme Court in its Roe judgment favored a right-based approach to abortion considering it under the ambit of right to privacy. However, neither Indian legislature nor US judiciary considered it as an absolute right of women as it will lead to many problems. If it is considered as their absolute right then women may demand it at any stage of pregnancy, which may risk their own life if it is done at a later stage of pregnancy. It may also infringe the rights of unborn. Questions with regard to the rights of the father are also a serious concern.

Equating reproductive rights with right to abortion is not justifiable. Reproductive rights include a plethora of rights. Except right to abortion, all other rights are highly appreciated and respected by both US and Indian legal systems. They consider these rights as absolute rights of women under the right to liberty of the Constitution. But right to abortion is considered only as a limited right. Overruling Roe's judgment, the US Supreme Court in its latest judgment (Dobbs v. Jackson Women's Health Organization) denied right-based approach to abortion claiming that it is a prerogative of the legislature. But Indian legal system considers it as a limited right under the ambit of MTP Act 1971.

## REFERENCES


Appleton, S. F. (2016). The Forgotten Family Law of Eisenstadt v Baird. *Yale Journal of Law and Feminism*, 28(1), 1–9.

Beniwal, A. (2013). Gender Discrimination and Empowerment of Women in India: A View. *Indian Journal of Poultry Science*, 74(1), 27–38.

Berer, M. (2000). Reproductive Rights, Advocacy and Changing the Law. *Reproductive Health Matters*, 8(16), 6–9. DOI: 10.1016/S0968-8080(00)90182-4 PMID: 11424251

Berer, M. (2002). Making Abortion a Woman's Right Worldwide. *Reproductive Health Matters*, 10(19), 1–8. DOI: 10.1016/S0968-8080(02)00010-1 PMID: 12369311

Biden, J. R.Jr. (2022). *Executive Order on Securing Access to Reproductive and Other Healthcare Services*. The White House.

Chamakala, L. (2009). *Quality of Life Versus Sanctity of Life*. Dharmaram Publications.

Connelly, M. (2003). Population Control is History: New Perspectives on the International Campaign to Limit Population Growth. *Comparative Studies in Society and History*, 45(1), 122–147. DOI: 10.1017/S0010417503000069

Cook, R. J. (2020). International Human Rights and Women's Reproductive Health. In Sherwin, S., & Parish, B. (Eds.), *Women, Medicine, Ethics and the Law* (pp. 37–50). Routledge. DOI: 10.4324/9781003073789-3

CRR (Centre for Reproductive Rights). (2023). Women's Health Protection Act (WHPA). https://reproductiverights.org/the-womens-health-protection-act-federal-legislation-to-protect-the-right-to-access-abortion-care/

Devika Biswas v. Union of India (2016) 10 SCC 726.

Dobbs v. Jackson Women's Health Organization (2022) 19-1392 U.S. 597.

Ehrlich, J. S. (2006). *Who Decides? The Abortion Rights of Teens*. Praeger. DOI: 10.5040/9798216035404

Eisenstadt v. Baird (1972) 405 U.S. 438.

Fine, J. B., Mayall, K., & Sepùlveda, L. (2017). The Role of International Human Rights Norms in the Liberalization of Abortion Laws Globally. *Health and Human Rights*, 19(1), 69–79. PMID: 28630542

Griswold v. Connecticut (1965) 381 U.S. 479.

Jalnawalla, S. F. (1974). Medical Termination of Pregnancy Act: A Preliminary Report of the First Twenty Months of Implementation. *Journal of Obstetrics and Gynecology of India*, •••, 588–592. PMID: 1228023

Joachim, J. M. (2007). *Agenda Setting, The UN, and NGOs*. Georgetown University Press.

Justice K S Puttaswamy v. Union of India (2017) 10 SCC 1.

Kapoor, P. (2023). Exploring Abortion Laws. *Economic and Political Weekly*, 58(29), 59–63.

Kaur, J. (2012). The Role of Litigation in Ensuring Women's Reproductive Rights: An Analysis of the Shanti Devi Judgment in India. *Reproductive Health Matters*, 20(39), 21–30. DOI: 10.1016/S0968-8080(12)39604-3 PMID: 22789079

Keynes, E., & Miller, R. K. (1989). *The Court v. Congress*. Duke University Press.

Kluchin, R. M. (2011). *Fit to be Tied: Sterilization and Reproductive Rights in America, 1950-1980*. Rutgers University Press.

Kranz, R. (2002). *Reproductive Rights and Technology*. Facts on File.

Laxmi Mandal v. Deen Dayal Harinagar Hospital 2010 (172) DLT 9.

Loving v. Virginia (1967) 388 U.S. 1.

Magill, S. (2020). The Right to Privacy and Access to Abortion in a Post Puttaswamy World. *University of Oxford Human Rights Hub Journal*, 3(2), 160–194.

McBride, D. E., & Mazur, A. G. (2008). *Women's Movements, Feminism, and Feminist Movements*. Cambridge University Press.

Meyer v. Nebraska (1923) 262 U.S. 390.

Millett, K. (1970). *Sexual Politics*. University of Illinois Press.

Moen, E. (1981). Women's Rights and Reproductive Freedom. *Human Rights Quarterly*, 3(2), 53–60. DOI: 10.2307/761857

Pacelle, R. L. (2003). *Between Law and Politics*. A & M University Press.

Petchesky, R. P. (1980). Reproductive Freedom: Beyond "a Woman's Right to Choose.". *Signs (Chicago, Ill.)*, 5(4), 661–685. DOI: 10.1086/493757

Pillay, V., & Wang, G. (1999). Social Structural Model of Women's Reproductive Rights: A Cross-National Study of Developing Countries. *Canadian Journal of Sociology*, 24(2), 255–281. DOI: 10.2307/3341731

Planned Parenthood v. Casey (1992) 505 U.S. 833.

Presser, H. B., Gordon, L., Rich, A., & Norton, W. W. (1978). Review: Birth Control and the Control of Motherhood. *Family Planning Perspectives*, 10(6), 374–376. DOI: 10.2307/2134425

Price, K. (2010). What is Reproductive Justice? How Women of Color Activists are Redefining the Pro-Choice Paradigm? *Meridians (Middletown, Conn.)*, 10(2), 42–65. DOI: 10.2979/meridians.2010.10.2.42

Prokopijević, M. (1994). In Defense of Abortion. *Archives for Philosophy of Law and Social Philosophy*, 80(3), 363–382.

Reichenbach, L., & Roseman, M. J. (2009). *Reproductive Health and Human Rights: The Way Forward*. University of Pennsylvania Press. DOI: 10.9783/9780812206104

Roe v. Wade (1973) 410 U.S. 113.

Ross, L. (2021). Understanding Reproductive Justice. In McCann, C., Kim, S.-k., & Ergun, E. (Eds.), *Feminist Theory Reader: Global and Local Perspectives* (pp. 77–82). Routledge.

Saheli. (2000). Reproductive Rights in the Indian Context. Saheli Women's Resource Centre. https://sites.google.com/site/saheliorgsite/health/reproductive-rights-in-the-indian-context

Sandesh Bansal v. Union of India (PIL) W. P. No. 9061/2008.

Shah, S. L., Mathai, A., & Wadis, A. P.. (1967). *Report of the Committee to Study the Question of Legalization of Abortion*. Ministry of Health and Family Planning.

Shalev, C. (2000). Rights to Sexual and Reproductive Health: The ICPD and the Convention on the Elimination of all Forms of Discrimination against Women. *Health and Human Rights*, 4(2), 38–66. DOI: 10.2307/4065196 PMID: 10796970

Skinner v. Oklahoma (1942) 361 U.S. 535.

Suchita Srivastava v. Chandigarh Administration (2009) 9 SCC 1.

Th Medical Termination of Pregnancy Act, 1971, No. 34, Acts of Parliament, 1971 (India).

Visaria, L., & Ramachandran, V. (2007). *Abortion in India: Ground Realities*. Routledge.

von Hagel, A., & Mansbach, D. (2016). *Reproductive Rights in the Age of Human Rights*. Macmillan. DOI: 10.1057/978-1-137-53952-6

# Chapter 8
# Legal Frameworks Governing Reproductive Rights and Policies

**Hemendra Singh**
https://orcid.org/0000-0003-1160-8284
*O.P. Jindal Global University, Sonipat, India*

## ABSTRACT

*This chapter provides a comprehensive analysis of the legal frameworks governing reproductive rights and policies, covering their historical evolution, international and regional contexts and national implementations. It examines key international treaties including CEDAW, ICESCR and the Sustainable Development Goals, and their influence on global reproductive health policies. It also explores regional legal frameworks in Europe, Africa and the Americas, and their impact on national laws. A comparative analysis of national approaches highlights variations in legal traditions and effectiveness in safeguarding reproductive rights. The chapter also addresses key issues in reproductive health like contraception, maternal health, abortion laws and assisted reproductive technologies (ART), assessing legal status, barriers and successful interventions. The chapter underscores the critical role of legal frameworks in ensuring access to reproductive health services and protecting individual rights.*

## INTRODUCTION

Reproductive rights are a fundamental component of human rights, encompassing a wide range of entitlements that ensure individuals can make autonomous decisions about their reproductive health and lives. Guzman Alejandro (2020) dis-

DOI: 10.4018/979-8-3693-7837-3.ch008

cusses reproductive rights in detail, he states that these rights affirm the ability of every person, regardless of gender, age, ethnicity, or socio-economic status, to make informed and voluntary choices about whether, when, and how to have children. Central to reproductive rights is the principle of bodily autonomy, which recognizes that decisions about one's reproductive life are deeply personal and must be made free from coercion, discrimination, and violence (Williams, 2018).

The scope of reproductive rights is expansive and multifaceted. It includes the right to access comprehensive reproductive health services, such as contraception, safe abortion, prenatal and postnatal care, and infertility treatments (Cook, Dickens, & Fathalla, 2011). Ensuring access to these services is essential for individuals to maintain control over their reproductive lives, allowing them to prevent unintended pregnancies, manage pregnancies safely and receive the necessary care throughout their reproductive journey. Additionally, reproductive rights encompass the right to make informed decisions about reproductive health (Dakic, 2015). This involves access to accurate, unbiased information that enables individuals to understand their options and make choices that align with their health, circumstances and values. As per Wen (2003), the right to informed consent is a critical aspect of this which ensures that individuals are fully aware of the potential risks, benefits and alternatives to any medical procedure or treatment related to their reproductive health.

Education and access to information are also key elements of reproductive rights. Comprehensive sexuality education provides individuals with the knowledge they need to make informed decisions about their sexual and reproductive health, covering topics such as contraception, sexually transmitted infections, sexual orientation and gender identity, as Fayokun (2015) discusses in relation to reproductive rights and female education in Nigeria. Accurate and inclusive information is vital for individuals to understand their bodies, protect their health, and exercise their reproductive rights fully (Mehlman, 2015). Reproductive rights are intrinsically linked to the right to privacy and bodily autonomy, which asserts that decisions about one's reproductive health should be made free from external interference, whether from the state, medical professionals or family members. This principle recognizes that individuals have the ultimate authority over their bodies and reproductive choices.

Moreover, reproductive rights are closely tied to the broader principles of non-discrimination and equality. All individuals, regardless of their background, have the right to access reproductive health services and make reproductive decisions without facing discrimination. Upholding these rights is essential for achieving gender equality as it empowers women and marginalized groups to exercise control over their reproductive lives, which is crucial for their overall well-being and empowerment, as Colker (1994) emphasizes in her discussion of equality theory and reproductive freedom. Finally, reproductive rights include the right to live in environments that support and facilitate the exercise of these rights. This involves legal protections against violations such as forced sterilization and coerced abortion, as well as the availability of supportive services like counseling and legal assistance (Iemelianenko, Gornostay, & Ivantsova, 2019).

In essence, reproductive rights are about ensuring that every individual has the freedom and capacity to make decisions about their reproductive health in a safe, informed and autonomous manner. These rights are crucial not only for individual health and well-being but also for the broader pursuit of social justice, gender equality, and human dignity. By upholding reproductive rights, societies can ensure that all individuals have the opportunity to lead healthy, empowered, and fulfilling lives.

## HISTORICAL DEVELOPMENT AND EVOLUTION

Initially, reproductive health was largely confined to matters of maternal health and family planning, with a focus on controlling population growth rather than empowering individuals with the right to make informed choices about their reproductive lives. The early 20th century saw limited recognition of reproductive health as a distinct issue, often viewed through the lens of public health and morality, with little regard for individual autonomy or gender equality.

The mid-20th century marked a significant turning point in the evolution of reproductive rights, driven by the broader movement for women's rights and the push for gender equality. The post-World War II era, characterized by rapid social change and the emergence of human rights as a global concern, provided fertile ground for the advancement of reproductive rights. The introduction of the birth control pill in the 1960s, for example, revolutionized reproductive autonomy, giving women unprecedented control over their fertility and contributing to the broader feminist movement. This period also saw the emergence of advocacy for legal abortion, with landmark cases such as Roe v. Wade in the United States establishing the legal right to abortion as a critical component of reproductive rights (Myers, 2014).

The recognition of reproductive rights as human rights gained further momentum during the late 20th century, particularly through international conferences and agreements. The 1994 International Conference on Population and Development (ICPD) in Cairo and the 1995 Fourth World Conference on Women in Beijing were pivotal in reframing reproductive health as a matter of human rights and gender equality. These conferences emphasized the importance of reproductive autonomy, informed choice, and access to a full range of reproductive health services which shifted the focus from population control to individual rights and empowerment. The ICPD's Programme of Action, in particular, was groundbreaking in its recognition of reproductive rights as central to sustainable development and the well-being of individuals and communities.

In the decades following these conferences, the global understanding of reproductive rights continued to expand, incorporating issues such as access to contraception, safe abortion, maternal health care, and the rights of marginalized groups. The adoption of various international treaties and conventions, such as the Convention on the Elimination of All Forms of Discrimination Against Women (CEDAW) and the International Covenant on Economic, Social, and Cultural Rights (ICESCR), further solidified the legal framework for protecting and promoting reproductive rights. These instruments explicitly recognized reproductive rights as fundamental human rights, calling on states to ensure that all individuals have access to the services, information, and education necessary to exercise these rights fully (Cook, 1992).

Despite these significant advancements, the evolution of reproductive rights has not been uniform across all regions and societies. Cultural, religious, and political factors have played a significant role in shaping the implementation and acceptance of reproductive rights in different contexts. In some regions, reproductive rights remain contested, with restrictive laws and policies limiting access to essential services and perpetuating gender inequality. Nonetheless, the ongoing efforts of activists, policymakers, and international organizations continue to push for the full realization of reproductive rights as an integral part of human rights.

## Importance of Legal Frameworks in Ensuring Reproductive Rights

Legal frameworks play a crucial role in the protection and promotion of reproductive rights, serving as the foundation upon which these rights are recognized, enforced and upheld within societies. The existence of robust legal frameworks ensures that reproductive rights are not merely aspirational but are codified as enforceable rights, accessible to all individuals. By embedding reproductive rights within national constitutions, statutes and international agreements, legal frameworks provide a clear mandate for governments and institutions to protect these rights, establish accountability, and create mechanisms for redress when violations occur.

One of the key functions of legal frameworks is to safeguard individuals from coercive practices, discrimination and violations of their reproductive autonomy. Laws that protect access to contraception, safe abortion and maternal healthcare are essential for ensuring that individuals can exercise control over their reproductive lives without facing barriers imposed by the state, healthcare providers or societal norms (Babor, 1999). Furthermore, legal frameworks that explicitly prohibit practices such as forced sterilization, gender-based violence and discrimination in reproductive healthcare are vital in protecting the most vulnerable populations, including women, marginalized communities, and individuals with disabilities.

Legal frameworks also play a critical role in advancing gender equality by addressing the structural inequalities that often underlie reproductive rights violations. By ensuring that reproductive rights are recognized as fundamental human rights, legal frameworks help to challenge and dismantle discriminatory laws, policies, and practices that perpetuate gender inequality (Baruah, 2022). For example, laws that mandate comprehensive sexuality education or guarantee access to reproductive health services for all individuals, regardless of their socio-economic status, contribute to levelling the playing field and empowering individuals to make informed choices about their reproductive lives.

Moreover, legal frameworks provide a basis for advocacy and social change, offering tools for activists, civil society organizations and international bodies to hold governments accountable for their obligations to protect and promote reproductive rights. Through litigation, policy advocacy and public education, legal frameworks can be leveraged to challenge restrictive laws, expand access to reproductive healthcare, and ensure that reproductive rights are respected and fulfilled in practice. They also serve as a benchmark for measuring progress, enabling the international community to monitor compliance with human rights standards and push for reforms where necessary.

## INTERNATIONAL LEGAL FRAMEWORKS

This section examines the international legal frameworks and organizations that shape the protection and promotion of reproductive rights. Key documents, including the Universal Declaration of Human Rights (UDHR), the International Covenant on Economic, Social and Cultural Rights, and the Convention on the Elimination of All Forms of Discrimination Against Women, provide foundational standards for reproductive rights. The roles of the WHO and UNFPA in setting standards and advocating for these rights globally are also discussed.

### Key International Legal Instruments

The protection and promotion of reproductive rights on a global scale are grounded in several key international legal instruments that recognize these rights as fundamental to human dignity and well-being. These instruments provide a legal foundation for the recognition of reproductive rights, establishing standards and obligations that member states are expected to uphold and implement within their domestic legal systems.

One of the most foundational documents in this regard is the Universal Declaration of Human Rights, adopted by the United Nations General Assembly in 1948. Although the UDHR does not explicitly mention reproductive rights, its broad articulation of human rights lays the groundwork for their protection (Guzman Alejandro, 2020). Articles such as Article 1, which states that "all human beings are born free and equal in dignity and rights," and Article 3, which affirms the right to life, liberty, and security of person, have been interpreted to encompass the right to make decisions about one's body and reproductive life. The UDHR's emphasis on non-discrimination, particularly in Articles 2 and 7, further supports the argument that reproductive rights must be protected equally for all individuals, regardless of gender or other status.

Building on the principles of the UDHR, the International Covenant on Economic, Social and Cultural Rights adopted in 1966, explicitly recognizes the right to health, which is a crucial aspect of reproductive rights. Article 12 of the ICESCR obligates state parties to recognize "the right of everyone to the enjoyment of the highest attainable standard of physical and mental health." This includes the right to access reproductive health services, such as maternal care, contraception, and family planning. General Comment No. 22 on the right to sexual and reproductive health, issued by the Committee on Economic, Social and Cultural Rights, further clarifies that reproductive health is an integral part of the right to health, and that states must ensure access to services without discrimination, coercion, or violence.

Another significant instrument is the Convention on the Elimination of All Forms of Discrimination Against Women adopted in 1979. Often referred to as the "women's bill of rights," CEDAW explicitly addresses reproductive rights in several provisions. Article 12 requires states to "ensure to women appropriate services in connection with pregnancy, confinement, and the post-natal period," as well as adequate nutrition during pregnancy and lactation. Article 16 further emphasizes the rights of women to make decisions freely and responsibly regarding the number and spacing of their children. CEDAW's General Recommendation No. 24 on women and health elaborates on these rights, emphasizing the importance of access to family planning services, safe abortion, and comprehensive reproductive healthcare as essential to women's health and equality.

In addition to these core human rights treaties, other international instruments and declarations also play a pivotal role in shaping the global legal landscape for reproductive rights. For instance, the Programme of Action adopted at the 1994 International Conference on Population and Development (ICPD) in Cairo marked a significant shift in the global approach to reproductive rights (Fine, Mayall, & Sepúlveda, 2017). It reframed population policies to focus on the rights and needs of individuals, rather than demographic targets, emphasizing that reproductive health and rights are central to human development. The ICPD's Programme of Action affirmed the right of individuals to make decisions about reproduction free of discrimination, coercion, and violence, and called for universal access to reproductive health services by 2015, a goal that has since been integrated into the Sustainable Development Goals.

The Beijing Declaration and Platform for Action, adopted at the Fourth World Conference on Women in 1995, reinforced these commitments, calling on governments to "take all appropriate measures to eliminate discrimination against women in the field of health care" and to ensure access to reproductive health services. The Platform for Action recognized that the ability of women to control their own fertility is fundamental to their empowerment and equality and called for comprehensive strategies to improve women's health, including access to safe abortion where not against the law, family planning, and maternal health care. Together these international legal instruments establish a robust framework for the protection and promotion of reproductive rights worldwide. They provide a legal and normative basis for states to develop and implement policies and laws that ensure access to reproductive health services, protect reproductive autonomy, and promote gender equality. While the implementation of these instruments varies across different national contexts, their collective influence has been instrumental in advancing reproductive rights as an essential component of human rights and social justice globally.

## Sustainable Development Goals (SDGs)

The Sustainable Development Goals (SDGs), adopted by the United Nations in 2015, represent a global blueprint for achieving a more equitable, sustainable, and prosperous world by 2030. Within this framework, reproductive rights are integral to several of the 17 goals, underscoring their importance in promoting overall health, gender equality, and social development. The SDGs explicitly recognize that access to reproductive health services and the protection of reproductive rights are not only essential for individual well-being but also critical for broader societal progress (Albertyn, 2019).

**Goal 3: Good Health and Well-Being** directly addresses reproductive health by aiming to ensure healthy lives and promote well-being for all at all ages. This goal includes specific targets related to reproductive health, such as reducing the global maternal mortality ratio, ensuring universal access to sexual and reproductive health care services, including family planning, and integrating reproductive health into national strategies and programs. By focusing on these targets, the SDGs highlight the critical role of reproductive health in achieving broader health outcomes, reducing inequalities, and improving the quality of life for women and girls worldwide.

**Goal 5: Gender Equality** is another key area where reproductive rights are prominently featured. This goal aims to achieve gender equality and empower all women and girls, recognizing that gender equality cannot be realized without ensuring access to reproductive health services and the protection of reproductive rights (Kunchit, 2023). Targets under this goal include eliminating all harmful practices, such as child, early, and forced marriage, and ensuring universal access to sexual and reproductive health and reproductive rights as agreed in accordance with the Programme of Action of the International Conference on Population and Development and the Beijing Platform for Action. By linking reproductive rights to gender equality, the SDGs emphasize that empowering women and girls requires safeguarding their reproductive autonomy and providing them with the resources and support needed to make informed decisions about their bodies and futures.

**Goal 1: No Poverty** and **Goal 10: Reduced Inequalities** also intersect with reproductive rights as access to reproductive health services is critical for breaking the cycle of poverty and addressing the socio-economic disparities that disproportionately affect women and marginalized communities. By ensuring that all individuals, regardless of their socio-economic status, have access to essential reproductive health services, the SDGs aim to reduce inequalities and create more inclusive and just societies. Access to reproductive health services, including family planning, enables women to make choices about their reproductive lives that are in line with their economic circumstances, thereby contributing to poverty reduction and social mobility.

The SDGs recognize that reproductive rights are not isolated issues but are interconnected with broader development goals. Achieving sustainable development requires a comprehensive approach that includes the protection and promotion of reproductive rights as a fundamental component of human rights. The inclusion of reproductive health and rights within the SDGs underscores their importance in creating a world where all individuals can live healthy, empowered, and dignified lives. As nations work towards the 2030 Agenda, the SDGs serve as a critical framework for ensuring that reproductive rights are upheld and that all individuals have the opportunity to exercise their rights fully and without discrimination.

## Role of International Organizations in Reproductive Rights

International organizations play a pivotal role in the promotion, protection, and advancement of reproductive rights globally. These organizations, including the World Health Organization (WHO) and the United Nations Population Fund (UNFPA), are instrumental in shaping global standards, providing guidance to national governments, and advocating for the integration of reproductive rights into broader human rights frameworks. Their efforts have been crucial in ensuring that reproductive rights are recognized as fundamental human rights, and they continue to drive progress in areas where reproductive rights are threatened or underdeveloped.

The World Health Organization is a leading authority on global health and has been at the forefront of efforts to promote reproductive rights. Through its research, policy guidance, and technical assistance, WHO plays a critical role in setting international standards for reproductive health services. WHO's guidelines on topics such as safe abortion, maternal health, and contraception are widely recognized as benchmarks for best practices in reproductive health care. Additionally, WHO works closely with governments to implement these guidelines, ensuring that health systems are equipped to provide comprehensive and equitable reproductive health services. WHO also monitors global progress on reproductive health indicators, providing valuable data that informs policy decisions and advocacy efforts.

The United Nations Population Fund (UNFPA) is another key player in the field of reproductive rights, with a specific mandate to ensure universal access to reproductive health services, promote gender equality, and support population and development strategies (Prakash & Asthana, 2019). UNFPA's work is centered on the belief that reproductive rights are essential to achieving sustainable development and human dignity. The organization provides financial and technical support to countries to strengthen their health systems, improve access to reproductive health services, and address inequalities in reproductive health outcomes. UNFPA also plays a critical role in advocating for the rights of women and girls, particularly in contexts where these rights are most at risk, such as in conflict zones or areas with high rates of gender-based violence.

Both WHO and UNFPA are deeply involved in global initiatives and partnerships aimed at advancing reproductive rights. They collaborate with other international organizations, governments, civil society, and the private sector to mobilize resources, share best practices, and drive coordinated action on reproductive health issues. For instance, their involvement in the implementation of the Sustainable Development Goals (SDGs) has been pivotal in ensuring that reproductive rights are recognized as a key component of global development efforts. Specifically, SDG 3 (Good Health and Well-being) and SDG 5 (Gender Equality) emphasize the importance of universal access to reproductive health services, and both WHO and UNFPA are leading efforts to achieve these goals by 2030.

In addition to their direct work in promoting reproductive health services, international organizations like WHO and UNFPA also play an advocacy role, raising awareness of reproductive rights as human rights and pushing for legal and policy reforms at the national and international levels. Their advocacy efforts have been crucial in challenging restrictive laws and practices, promoting gender equality, and ensuring that reproductive rights are integrated into broader human rights agendas. International organizations such as WHO and UNFPA are indispensable in the global effort to promote and protect reproductive rights (Isfahan Merali, 2000). Through their leadership, technical expertise, and advocacy, these organizations help set global standards, support national health systems, and drive progress towards the realization of reproductive rights for all. Their work is vital in ensuring that reproductive rights are recognized, respected, and fulfilled worldwide, contributing to broader goals of health, gender equality, and human rights.

## REGIONAL LEGAL FRAMEWORKS

This section explores the regional legal frameworks governing reproductive rights across Europe, Africa and the Americas. It highlights the distinct approaches and challenges faced by each region, focusing on pivotal legal instruments and landmark judicial rulings. By examining key legal instruments and landmark judicial rulings within each region, we will explore how these frameworks influence reproductive health policies and practices. Understanding these regional contexts highlights the diverse approaches to reproductive rights and the ongoing efforts to address challenges and promote human rights in reproductive health.

### European Legal Framework

The European legal framework on reproductive rights is shaped by several key instruments and institutions, particularly the European Convention on Human Rights (ECHR) and the European Court of Human Rights (ECtHR). Although the ECHR does not explicitly mention reproductive rights, its provisions have been interpreted to encompass aspects of reproductive health, autonomy, and freedom. These interpretations have significantly influenced national laws and policies across European countries, compelling them to align with the evolving standards set by the ECtHR's jurisprudence.

## 1. The European Convention on Human Rights (ECHR)

The ECHR, adopted in 1950, is a foundational document that guarantees a range of civil and political rights to individuals within its jurisdiction. While the Convention does not specifically address reproductive rights, several articles have been interpreted by the ECtHR to protect aspects of reproductive autonomy and access to reproductive healthcare:

**Article 2 (Right to Life):** This article primarily safeguards the right to life, but it has been invoked in cases involving abortion, where there is a need to balance the rights of the mother against the potential rights of the fetus. The ECtHR has consistently emphasized that states must respect and protect women's health and life, particularly in circumstances where restrictive abortion laws are in place. The Court has also highlighted that the right to life does not impose an absolute prohibition on abortion but requires a careful consideration of the competing interests involved.

**Article 3 (Prohibition of Torture and Inhuman or Degrading Treatment):** Article 3 has been applied in situations where denial of reproductive healthcare, such as access to safe abortion services or essential maternal health interventions, has resulted in severe physical or psychological suffering. The ECtHR has ruled that subjecting women to such suffering by denying them access to necessary reproductive healthcare can constitute inhuman or degrading treatment, thus violating Article 3. This interpretation underscores the importance of state obligations to ensure access to reproductive healthcare to prevent harm and suffering.

**Article 8 (Right to Respect for Private and Family Life):** Article 8 has been the most instrumental in shaping reproductive rights in Europe. The ECtHR has interpreted this provision to encompass the right to make decisions about one's own body and reproductive choices, which includes access to contraception, fertility treatments, and abortion services under certain conditions. The Court has repeatedly affirmed that the right to respect for private life includes the ability to make decisions regarding one's reproductive health free from arbitrary interference by the state. This broad interpretation of Article 8 has established a robust framework for protecting reproductive autonomy within the context of privacy rights.

**Article 14 (Prohibition of Discrimination):** This article has been crucial in challenging discriminatory practices in the provision of reproductive health services. The ECtHR has used Article 14 to ensure that reproductive rights are accessible to all individuals without discrimination based on gender, socioeconomic status, disability, or other factors. This has led to a more inclusive understanding of reproductive rights as fundamental human rights that must be upheld equally for all.

## 2. Key Rulings by the European Court of Human Rights (ECtHR)

The ECtHR has played a pivotal role in interpreting the ECHR to include protections for reproductive rights. Through its rulings, the Court has clarified the scope and limits of these rights, influencing national policies and practices:

**Tysiąc v. Poland (2007):** This case involved a Polish woman who was denied a therapeutic abortion despite the severe risk to her eyesight posed by continuing the pregnancy. The ECtHR found that Poland violated Article 8 by failing to provide an effective mechanism for accessing lawful abortion. The Court emphasized the importance of procedural safeguards to protect women's rights, including the need for a clear legal framework that allows women to challenge decisions denying them access to reproductive healthcare. This case underscored the necessity of effective legal and administrative processes to ensure that reproductive rights are more than theoretical but practically accessible (Komanovics, 2009).

**A, B, and C v. Ireland (2010):** In this landmark case, three women challenged Ireland's restrictive abortion laws, arguing that the inability to access abortion services in Ireland violated their rights under the ECHR. The ECtHR ruled that while the Convention does not guarantee a right to abortion on demand, Ireland's failure to provide a clear and accessible legal framework for determining when abortion is permitted under Irish law violated the applicants' rights under Article 8. The Court's decision highlighted the importance of clarity and accessibility in national abortion laws, reinforcing that restrictive laws must still provide practical and effective means for women to exercise their rights in cases where abortion is legally permissible (Staunton, 2011).

**P. and S. v. Poland (2012):** This case concerned a 14-year-old girl who became pregnant as a result of rape and faced numerous obstacles in accessing a legal abortion in Poland. The ECtHR found multiple violations of the ECHR, including Articles 3, 5 (right to liberty and security), and 8. The Court ruled that the Polish authorities had failed to ensure the applicant's access to a lawful abortion, subjecting her to inhuman and degrading treatment. The decision underscored the state's obligation to ensure that vulnerable individuals, particularly minors, can access reproductive healthcare services without undue hardship or delay.

**K.L. v. Latvia (2020):** In this case, the ECtHR addressed the right to access comprehensive information about prenatal testing. The Court ruled that withholding or providing inadequate information regarding prenatal health violated the applicant's right to private life under Article 8. This decision reinforced the principle that informed choice is a critical component of reproductive rights and that states have a duty to provide accurate and complete information to enable individuals to make informed decisions about their reproductive health.

## 3. Impact on National Laws and Policies

The rulings of the ECtHR have had a profound impact on national laws and policies related to reproductive rights across Europe. Member states of the Council of Europe are required to implement the Court's judgments, which often necessitates reforms to align domestic laws with the standards set by the Court. For example, following the Tysiąc and A, B, and C cases, Poland and Ireland were compelled to amend their abortion laws and practices to comply with the ECHR's requirements for clarity, accessibility, and effective legal recourse.

In addition, the ECtHR's emphasis on the right to privacy and the prohibition of inhuman treatment has led to broader reforms in reproductive healthcare. Several countries have revised their policies to ensure that reproductive health services are accessible and non-discriminatory, reflecting a commitment to uphold reproductive rights as integral to human rights. These changes have been particularly evident in the areas of abortion law reform, access to contraception, and the rights of individuals undergoing assisted reproductive technologies (ART).

Furthermore, the Court's jurisprudence has encouraged European states to adopt a human rights-based approach to reproductive health, recognizing that access to reproductive services is essential for achieving gender equality and protecting individual autonomy. This perspective has influenced a range of policies, from comprehensive sex education to the regulation of ART, ensuring that reproductive rights are protected and promoted as fundamental human rights across Europe.

Overall, the ECtHR's interpretations and rulings have significantly advanced the protection of reproductive rights in Europe. By requiring states to comply with its judgments, the Court has helped to create a more consistent and rights-based approach to reproductive healthcare across the continent, ensuring that individuals have the autonomy and freedom to make informed decisions about their reproductive health in a manner that is respectful of their rights and dignity.

## African Legal Framework

The African continent presents a unique landscape for reproductive rights, shaped by diverse legal traditions, cultural practices, and socio-economic conditions. This section explores the key regional legal frameworks governing reproductive rights in Africa, focusing on the African Charter on Human and Peoples' Rights and the Maputo Protocol. It examines the provisions related to reproductive health, the challenges in implementing these frameworks, and the successes achieved in advancing reproductive rights across the continent.

## 1. The African Charter on Human and Peoples' Rights

Adopted in 1981 and coming into force in 1986, the African Charter on Human and Peoples' Rights (often referred to as the "Banjul Charter") is a foundational document that enshrines a wide range of civil, political, economic, social, and cultural rights. While the Charter does not explicitly mention reproductive rights, it provides a broad framework for the protection of health and the rights of women, which are essential for advancing reproductive rights (Ngwena, Brookman-Amissah, & Skuster, 2015).

Key Provisions Relevant to Reproductive Rights:

**Right to Health (Article 16):** The Charter guarantees the right of every individual to enjoy the best attainable state of physical and mental health. This provision has been interpreted to include access to reproductive health services, including family planning, maternal health care, and safe abortion where permitted by law.

**Rights of Women (Article 18):** It calls on member states to ensure the elimination of discrimination against women and to protect their rights, taking into consideration their specific needs. This has implications for reproductive rights, as it encompasses the protection of women's autonomy in making decisions about their reproductive health.

## 2. The Maputo Protocol: A Landmark for Women's Reproductive Rights

The Protocol to the African Charter on Human and Peoples' Rights on the Rights of Women in Africa, commonly known as the Maputo Protocol, was adopted in 2003 and entered into force in 2005. This Protocol is one of the most comprehensive legal instruments globally regarding women's rights, explicitly addressing reproductive rights and setting out obligations for member states to protect these rights.

Key Provisions of the Maputo Protocol:

**Article 14: Health and Reproductive Rights:** This article is pivotal as it explicitly recognizes women's rights to control their fertility, decide freely and responsibly on the number and spacing of their children, and have access to family planning education and services. It also mandates the protection of reproductive rights by authorizing medical abortion in specific cases, such as sexual assault, rape, incest, and when the continued pregnancy endangers the mental and physical health of the mother or the life of the mother or the fetus.

**Article 13: Economic and Social Welfare Rights:** This includes the right to food security and adequate housing, which are intrinsically linked to reproductive health. Ensuring economic rights helps create a supportive environment for women to exercise their reproductive rights fully.

## 3. Challenges in Implementing Reproductive Rights in Africa

Despite the progressive nature of the Maputo Protocol and the provisions of the African Charter, the implementation of reproductive rights across African countries faces several challenges. One significant challenge is the legal and policy gaps that exist in many African nations. Several countries have not fully aligned their national laws and policies with the provisions of the Maputo Protocol, resulting in limited access to safe abortion services, contraceptives, and comprehensive reproductive health care (Ebeku, 2004). This misalignment creates inconsistencies in the protection and promotion of reproductive rights across the continent.

Cultural and religious barriers also play a crucial role in hindering the realization of reproductive rights in Africa. Deep-seated cultural beliefs and religious doctrines in many African societies often conflict with the concept of reproductive autonomy, especially concerning contraception, family planning, and abortion. These barriers can lead to restrictive laws and policies that prevent women from exercising their reproductive rights freely. Additionally, there is a lack of access to healthcare services, particularly in rural areas where healthcare infrastructure is limited, and funding for reproductive health services is often inadequate. As a result, women in many African countries face significant obstacles in accessing quality reproductive health care, including maternal health services, safe delivery, and post-abortion care.

Gender inequality and discrimination against women further exacerbate the challenges to achieving full reproductive rights in Africa. Persistent gender disparities limit women's access to education and economic opportunities, which in turn restricts their ability to make informed decisions about their reproductive health. Addressing these barriers is crucial for advancing reproductive rights and ensuring that all women can exercise their rights to health, autonomy, and bodily integrity.

## 4. Successes and Best Practices in Advancing Reproductive Rights

Despite these challenges, several African countries have made notable progress in advancing reproductive rights. Legal reforms and policy advances in countries like South Africa and Mozambique have been significant. These countries have reformed their laws to align more closely with international and regional standards, allowing greater access to reproductive health services, including safe abortion and contraception. Such legal reforms demonstrate a commitment to upholding reproductive rights and ensuring women have the autonomy to make decisions about their reproductive health.

In addition to legal reforms, innovative health programs have been implemented in countries like Rwanda and Ethiopia. These nations have developed successful community-based health programs that improve access to family planning services and maternal health care, significantly reducing maternal mortality rates. By focusing on community involvement and education, these programs have effectively addressed some of the barriers to reproductive health services and have set a model for other countries to follow.

Civil society advocacy and education have also played a critical role in advancing reproductive rights across the continent. Strong advocacy efforts by civil society organizations have helped educate communities, challenge discriminatory practices, and hold governments accountable for their obligations under regional and international legal frameworks. These organizations have been instrumental in promoting awareness of reproductive rights and pushing for legal and policy changes that enhance women's access to reproductive health services.

## American Legal Framework

The American context for reproductive rights is primarily shaped by the Inter-American System for the Protection of Human Rights, which includes the Inter-American Commission on Human Rights (IACHR) and the Inter-American Court of Human Rights (IACtHR). This system plays a crucial role in setting legal standards and interpreting reproductive rights across the Americas.

### 1. The Inter-American Convention on Human Rights and Reproductive Rights

The Inter-American Convention on Human Rights (often referred to as the American Convention on Human Rights, or ACHR) establishes a comprehensive framework for the protection of human rights, including those related to reproductive health and autonomy. Although the convention does not explicitly mention reproductive rights, several of its provisions, such as the rights to life (Article 4), personal integrity (Article 5), privacy (Article 11), and non-discrimination (Article 24), have been interpreted to encompass aspects of reproductive rights.

Key Provisions and Interpretations:

**Right to Life (Article 4)**: The right to life has been a contentious issue in the context of abortion laws. The interpretation of when life begins has varied among member states, leading to diverse legal landscapes. The IACtHR has taken a nuanced approach, recognizing both the protection of prenatal life and the rights of women to access reproductive health services.

**Right to Privacy (Article 11)**: This article has been interpreted to protect individuals' autonomy over their reproductive choices, including the right to make decisions about one's own body without interference.

**Non-Discrimination (Article 24)**: The IACtHR has emphasized the need to ensure equal access to reproductive health services for all individuals, regardless of gender, economic status, or other factors, recognizing that discrimination in this area exacerbates social inequalities.

## 2. Jurisprudence of the Inter-American Court of Human Rights

The IACtHR has addressed several cases related to reproductive rights, shaping the interpretation of the ACHR and setting precedents for member states. Some landmark cases include:

**Artavia Murillo et al. ("In Vitro Fertilization") v. Costa Rica (2012)**: This landmark ruling addressed the ban on in vitro fertilization (IVF) in Costa Rica, which the Court found violated the rights to privacy, family, and to have a family. The Court ruled that the absolute ban on IVF was disproportionate and constituted discrimination against those with fertility issues. This decision underscored the importance of access to reproductive technologies as a fundamental right under the ACHR.

**Manuela et al. v. El Salvador (2021)**: This case involved the criminal prosecution of a woman who suffered an obstetric emergency and was subsequently convicted of aggravated homicide. The IACtHR found that El Salvador violated Manuela's rights to life, personal integrity, and judicial protection. The decision highlighted the severe implications of restrictive abortion laws and underscored the need for member states to ensure that their reproductive health laws align with international human rights standards, particularly concerning women's health and autonomy.

**Gonzales Lluy et al. v. Ecuador (2015)**: Although not directly related to abortion or contraception, this case involved issues of medical negligence and discrimination affecting reproductive health. The Court emphasized states' obligations to ensure access to health care services without discrimination, which can be extended to reproductive health services.

## 3. Impact on National Laws and Policies

The rulings of the Inter-American Court of Human Rights (IACtHR) have had profound implications for national laws and policies across the Americas, particularly in advancing reproductive rights and setting crucial legal precedents. Landmark decisions, such as those in the cases of Artavia Murillo v. Costa Rica and Manuela v. El Salvador, have forced several countries to reassess and, in some instances, reform their reproductive health laws to align with the human rights standards established by the Court. In Artavia Murillo, the IACtHR ruled that Costa Rica's ban on in vitro fertilization (IVF) violated the right to personal integrity and reproductive autonomy, as protected under the American Convention on Human Rights. This decision compelled Costa Rica to lift its IVF ban, enabling access to assisted reproductive technologies (ART) and setting a significant precedent for reproductive rights in the region (Hevia & Vacaflor, 2013). The ruling not only provided a legal foundation for ART access in Costa Rica but also influenced debates and policy reforms throughout Latin America, reinforcing the importance of reproductive autonomy within the broader human rights framework.

Similarly, the Manuela case has become a pivotal moment in the ongoing struggle to reform El Salvador's draconian abortion laws, which are among the most restrictive in the world. The case involved a woman who was convicted of aggravated homicide after suffering an obstetric emergency, highlighting the extreme consequences of El Salvador's absolute ban on abortion. The IACtHR's ruling found that the state's actions violated Manuela's rights to health, dignity, and due process, and called for the government to take immediate measures to prevent further human rights violations related to reproductive health (Morgan, 2021). The ruling has since sparked broader debates over the country's restrictive abortion policies, prompting increased advocacy for legal reform. It also brought attention to the systemic violations of women's reproductive rights in El Salvador and similar contexts, emphasizing the role of the IACtHR in pushing states to harmonize their domestic laws with international human rights obligations.

These cases illustrate the IACtHR's critical role in shaping national reproductive health policies across the Americas, as its rulings encourage states to modernize legal frameworks that uphold reproductive autonomy and dignity. By holding governments accountable to international human rights standards, the Court plays a transformative role in promoting legal changes that enhance the protection of reproductive rights, setting essential legal benchmarks for the entire region.

## 4. Challenges and Future Directions

Despite the progress facilitated by the Inter-American System, significant challenges remain in ensuring the comprehensive protection of reproductive rights across the Americas. Cultural, religious, and political factors continue to shape national policies and impede the full realization of reproductive rights. Many countries in the region, including El Salvador, Honduras, and the Dominican Republic, maintain highly restrictive abortion laws that severely limit access to safe and legal abortion services. Additionally, inequities in access to reproductive health services persist, particularly in rural and marginalized communities, where discriminatory practices and inadequate healthcare infrastructure exacerbate these disparities. Strong cultural and religious beliefs also pose substantial barriers to advancing reproductive rights, especially in more conservative societies resistant to changing long-standing norms.

To address these challenges, continued advocacy and legal reform are essential. Strategic litigation and public awareness campaigns can drive the legal reforms needed to align national laws with international human rights standards. Moreover, increased regional collaboration among countries in the Americas could strengthen efforts to harmonize laws and policies with the American Convention on Human Rights and IACtHR jurisprudence, fostering a more unified approach to reproductive rights. Strengthening mechanisms for monitoring compliance with IACtHR rulings and holding states accountable for violations of reproductive rights is also crucial for ensuring lasting change.

In essence, the American context presents a complex landscape for reproductive rights, shaped by a combination of progressive jurisprudence from the Inter-American Court and ongoing challenges at the national level. As countries navigate these dynamics, there is a critical need for continued advocacy, legal reform, and regional cooperation to uphold and advance reproductive rights across the Americas.

## COMPARATIVE ANALYSIS OF NATIONAL APPROACHES

Reproductive rights are approached differently across the globe, shaped by each country's unique cultural, religious, political, and historical context. The variety in legal frameworks reveals a complex global landscape where progressive, moderate, and restrictive approaches coexist. These differences have significant implications for the accessibility and quality of reproductive health services, as well as the overall protection of reproductive rights.

### Progressive Legal Frameworks

Countries with progressive legal frameworks prioritize the protection and promotion of reproductive rights, viewing them as integral to individual autonomy, gender equality, and public health. These nations often have comprehensive policies that ensure broad access to reproductive health services, supported by robust legal protections.

**Sweden** is a prime example of a country with a highly progressive approach to reproductive rights. Swedish law guarantees access to contraception, abortion, and comprehensive sexual education. Abortion is legal up to the 18th week of pregnancy without restriction and later if there are specific medical reasons. The government provides extensive support for maternal health, ensuring that women have access to high-quality healthcare services. Sweden's approach is underpinned by its broader commitment to gender equality, public health, and human rights, resulting in low rates of unintended pregnancies and excellent maternal health outcomes.

**South Africa** represents another example of progressive reproductive rights legislation, particularly in the context of a developing country. The Choice on Termination of Pregnancy Act of 1996 is one of the most liberal abortion laws in Africa, allowing abortion on demand up to 12 weeks of pregnancy, and under broader conditions up to 20 weeks. The law is a reflection of post-apartheid South Africa's commitment to human rights, including the right to bodily autonomy. Despite challenges in implementation, especially in rural areas, the legal framework provides a strong foundation for advancing women's reproductive rights and has led to significant improvements in women's health outcomes (Shozi, 2020).

## Moderate Legal Frameworks

Some countries adopt a moderate approach, balancing legal restrictions with provisions that protect certain aspects of reproductive rights. These nations may allow access to reproductive health services like contraception and abortion but impose certain conditions or limitations.

**India** presents a mixed approach to reproductive rights, combining progressive elements with significant challenges in implementation. The Medical Termination of Pregnancy Act of 1971 allows abortion under broad conditions, including risks to the woman's physical or mental health, fetal abnormalities, and contraceptive failure. However, access to abortion services is often limited by social stigma, lack of awareness, and inadequate healthcare infrastructure, particularly in rural areas (Combellick-Bidney, 2017). Additionally, while contraception is widely available, there are still substantial barriers to access, including cultural resistance and gender-based discrimination. Despite these challenges, India's legal framework has enabled significant advancements in reproductive health, particularly in urban areas.

**Mexico** offers another example of a moderate approach, where reproductive rights are protected in certain states but heavily restricted in others. Mexico City, the capital, has one of the most liberal abortion laws in Latin America, allowing abortion on demand up to 12 weeks of pregnancy. However, other states in Mexico maintain strict abortion laws, allowing the procedure only under limited circumstances, such as rape or threat to the woman's life. This disparity within the same country highlights the impact of regional differences on reproductive rights and underscores the challenges of ensuring uniform access to reproductive health services in a federal system.

## Restrictive Legal Frameworks

At the other end of the spectrum, some countries maintain highly restrictive legal frameworks that severely limit access to reproductive health services. These restrictions are often rooted in conservative cultural norms, religious beliefs, or political ideologies, and can lead to significant human rights concerns.

**El Salvador** is one of the most restrictive countries globally concerning reproductive rights. The country has a total ban on abortion, criminalizing the procedure under all circumstances, including cases of rape, incest, or threats to the mother's life. Women who undergo abortions, as well as those who assist them, can face long prison sentences. This strict legal framework is deeply influenced by the country's strong Catholic traditions and has led to severe consequences for women's health, including high rates of maternal mortality and unsafe abortions.

**The Philippines** also enforces restrictive laws on reproductive rights, largely influenced by the Catholic Church's significant role in society. Abortion is illegal under all circumstances, and access to contraception is limited, particularly in rural areas. The Responsible Parenthood and Reproductive Health Act of 2012 aimed to improve access to contraception and maternal care, but its implementation has faced strong opposition from religious groups. As a result, the law's impact has been uneven, with many women still lacking access to essential reproductive health services (Smith, 2014).

The comparative analysis of national approaches to reproductive rights reveals a world deeply divided in how these rights are understood, protected, and implemented. Progressive countries prioritize access to reproductive health services and protect individual autonomy, while restrictive nations impose significant barriers that often lead to adverse health outcomes and human rights violations. As global dynamics continue to evolve, the landscape of reproductive rights remains in flux, requiring ongoing advocacy and international cooperation to ensure that these fundamental rights are universally recognized and upheld.

## Case Studies in National Legal Frameworks

Examining specific case studies of national legal frameworks reveals how legal structures influence reproductive rights in different countries. By analyzing key court rulings and landmark cases, we can understand the dynamic relationship between law, policy, and reproductive rights, as well as the broader implications for individuals and society.

## Ireland: Savita Halappanavar and the Repeal of the Eighth Amendment

Ireland's restrictive abortion laws, rooted in the Eighth Amendment to the Constitution, were challenged by the tragic case of Savita Halappanavar in 2012. Savita, a pregnant woman, was denied an abortion despite severe complications that eventually led to her death from sepsis. The Eighth Amendment, enacted in 1983, equated the life of the mother with that of the unborn, resulting in a near-total ban on abortion.

Savita's death sparked national and international outrage, leading to widespread protests and calls for legal reform. The case became a symbol of the dangers posed by restrictive abortion laws. In 2018, following years of advocacy, a national referendum was held, resulting in the repeal of the Eighth Amendment. This historic decision led to the legalization of abortion in Ireland up to 12 weeks of pregnancy, with provisions for later-term abortions under specific circumstances. The Savita Halappanavar case underscores the critical impact of restrictive laws on women's health and highlights the role of public advocacy in driving significant legal change.

## United States: Roe v. Wade and Dobbs v. Jackson Women's Health Organization

The United States has been at the forefront of the global debate on reproductive rights, with the landmark Supreme Court case Roe v. Wade (1973) serving as a foundational moment. In Roe v. Wade, the Supreme Court ruled that the Constitution protects a woman's right to choose to have an abortion, effectively legalizing the procedure nationwide. This decision was based on the right to privacy under the Due Process Clause of the 14th Amendment and established a framework for regulating abortion based on the trimesters of pregnancy.

However, the legal landscape changed dramatically with the 2022 Supreme Court decision in Dobbs v. Jackson Women's Health Organization, which overturned Roe v. Wade. The Dobbs ruling returned the authority to regulate abortion to the states, leading to a highly fragmented legal environment where some states have imposed strict abortion bans, while others have expanded protections. The aftermath of Dobbs has highlighted the vulnerability of reproductive rights to shifts in the political and judicial landscape, resulting in significant disparities in access to reproductive healthcare across the United States (Machaj, 2023).

## Argentina: Law 27.610 and the Legalization of Abortion

Argentina's journey toward the legalization of abortion culminated in the passing of Law 27.610 in December 2020, a landmark achievement for reproductive rights in Latin America. Prior to this law, abortion in Argentina was only permitted in cases of rape or when the mother's life was at risk, leading to widespread unsafe abortions and significant health risks for women.

The legalization of abortion up to 14 weeks of pregnancy was the result of years of activism led by the feminist movement "Ni Una Menos" and other women's rights organizations. The movement galvanized public support, leading to massive demonstrations and a shift in public opinion. Law 27.610 represents a significant victory in a region traditionally characterized by restrictive abortion laws. This case study illustrates the power of grassroots advocacy and the importance of legislative change in advancing reproductive rights.

## India: X v. Principal Secretary, Health & Family Welfare Department and Marital Rape

India's approach to reproductive rights is complex, involving a mix of progressive laws and significant socio-cultural challenges. One significant case is X v. Principal Secretary, Health & Family Welfare Department (2022), where the Supreme Court of India expanded the scope of the Medical Termination of Pregnancy (MTP) Act to include all women, regardless of marital status, and acknowledged marital rape as a factor for seeking an abortion.

The case arose when a woman challenged the restrictive interpretation of the MTP Act, which initially limited access to abortion based on marital status. The Supreme Court ruled that unmarried women could not be denied the right to a safe abortion and recognized the impact of marital rape, a significant step forward in a country where marital rape is not criminalized. This ruling reflects the evolving nature of reproductive rights in India, where judicial interpretations are playing a crucial role in expanding access to reproductive health services.

## El Salvador: Manuela v. El Salvador and the Consequences of a Total Abortion Ban

El Salvador's total ban on abortion has led to extreme cases of human rights violations, exemplified by the case of Manuela v. El Salvador (2021), which was heard by the Inter-American Court of Human Rights. Manuela, a young woman, was imprisoned for homicide after suffering a miscarriage. She was sentenced to 30 years in prison, where she died from untreated cancer.

The case brought international attention to the severe consequences of El Salvador's strict abortion laws, which criminalize abortion under all circumstances, including cases where the mother's life is at risk. In its ruling, the Inter-American Court condemned El Salvador for violating Manuela's rights, highlighting the inhumane treatment of women under the country's abortion laws. This case underscores the devastating impact of restrictive legal frameworks on women's lives and health and emphasizes the need for international human rights mechanisms to challenge such laws.

These case studies from Ireland, the United States, Argentina, India, and El Salvador illustrate the varied approaches to reproductive rights across the world. They highlight how legal frameworks can either protect or severely restrict these rights, with profound implications for women's health, autonomy, and dignity. Each case reflects the complex interplay between law, society, and politics, and underscores the ongoing need for vigilance, advocacy, and reform to ensure that reproductive rights are protected and upheld globally.

## REPRODUCTIVE HEALTH AND RIGHTS

Reproductive health and rights are central to individual autonomy and well-being, encompassing access to contraception and family planning, protection of maternal health, regulation of abortion, and the governance of assisted reproductive technologies (ART). Legal frameworks at the national and international levels play a crucial role in safeguarding these rights, ensuring access, and addressing ethical considerations. This section examines the legal perspectives on these aspects of reproductive health, focusing on how laws shape, protect, and sometimes limit reproductive rights.

### Contraception and Family Planning: Legal Status and Availability

Contraception and family planning are vital components of reproductive rights, and their legal status is pivotal in ensuring that individuals can make informed decisions about their reproductive lives. In many countries, laws explicitly protect access to contraception as part of the broader right to health. For instance, in France and the United Kingdom, national healthcare systems are legally required to provide free or subsidized contraceptive services, ensuring widespread access. These laws are often rooted in broader commitments to public health and gender equality, recognizing the importance of family planning in empowering individuals, particularly women, to control their reproductive lives (Kurland, 2006).

Conversely, some countries impose legal restrictions that limit access to contraception. In several Middle Eastern and African nations, cultural and religious considerations are deeply embedded in the legal system, resulting in laws that restrict the availability of contraceptives, particularly to unmarried individuals. In countries like Iran and Nigeria, legal barriers are reinforced by social norms that stigmatize the use of contraception, especially for women, leading to limited access and widespread misinformation.

Legal barriers to contraception often stem from restrictive laws or policies that either limit who can access contraceptives or place unnecessary burdens on their availability. For example, in the United States, certain states have implemented "conscience clauses" that allow healthcare providers to refuse to prescribe or dispense contraceptives based on religious or moral beliefs. These legal provisions create significant obstacles for individuals seeking contraception, particularly in rural or underserved areas.

Despite these barriers, legal interventions have been successful in expanding access to contraception. In Kenya, the Reproductive Health Care Bill seeks to remove legal and policy barriers to contraceptive access by ensuring that reproductive health services, including contraception, are provided without discrimination and that they are available to all, regardless of marital status or age. Such legal frameworks are crucial for overcoming both legal and social barriers, ensuring that family planning services are accessible to those who need them most.

## Maternal Health: National and International Legal Obligations

Maternal health is a critical aspect of reproductive rights, protected under various international legal instruments. The Convention on the Elimination of All Forms of Discrimination Against Women (CEDAW) and the International Covenant on Economic, Social and Cultural Rights (ICESCR) obligate states to ensure that women have access to adequate healthcare services, including those related to pregnancy and childbirth. These international treaties emphasize the state's duty to protect women's health and rights, mandating that national laws provide for safe and accessible maternal health services.

Additionally, the Sustainable Development Goals (SDGs), particularly Goal 3.1, aim to reduce the global maternal mortality ratio. This goal reinforces international legal commitments, pushing countries to enact laws that protect maternal health and improve healthcare infrastructure. For example, countries are legally required to ensure that maternal health services are accessible, affordable, and of high quality, with specific focus on vulnerable populations.

At the national level, countries have adopted various legal measures to protect maternal health. In South Africa, the National Health Act mandates the provision of free maternal health services, reflecting the country's commitment to reducing maternal mortality and improving health outcomes. This law ensures that all women, regardless of socio-economic status, have access to essential maternal healthcare services, including prenatal care, skilled birth attendance, and emergency obstetric services (Ikeatu, 2020).

However, in many countries, legal protections for maternal health are insufficient or poorly implemented. In Nigeria, despite existing laws that aim to improve maternal health, the lack of effective enforcement and healthcare infrastructure has led to persistently high maternal mortality rates. Legal frameworks must therefore be supported by adequate funding, training of healthcare personnel, and public health campaigns to be effective.

## Abortion Laws: Comparative Legal Approaches

Abortion laws vary widely across the world, with significant differences in how countries regulate the procedure. In liberal legal regimes, such as those in Canada and most of Western Europe, abortion is permitted on broad grounds, often up to a certain point in pregnancy. These legal frameworks are grounded in the principles of autonomy and privacy, recognizing the right of individuals to make decisions about their own bodies without undue interference from the state. In Canada, for example, abortion was decriminalized in 1988 following the R. v. Morgentaler decision, which struck down the existing abortion law as unconstitutional. This decision established a legal framework where abortion is treated as a healthcare issue rather than a criminal one.

In contrast, many countries maintain highly restrictive abortion laws, often rooted in religious or cultural values. In El Salvador, for instance, abortion is completely banned under all circumstances, with no exceptions even for cases of rape or when the woman's life is at risk. This legal framework criminalizes both women who seek abortions and healthcare providers who perform them, leading to severe penalties. The restrictive nature of such laws often forces women to seek unsafe, illegal abortions, with significant risks to their health and lives.

The impact of abortion laws on reproductive health is profound. In countries with liberal abortion laws, women generally have better access to safe and legal abortion services, leading to lower rates of maternal mortality and morbidity. Conversely, in countries with restrictive abortion laws, women are more likely to resort to unsafe abortion methods, contributing to higher maternal mortality rates and serious health complications. International human rights organizations, such as the United Nations Human Rights Committee, have consistently advocated for the decriminalization of abortion, arguing that restrictive abortion laws violate the rights to life, health, and non-discrimination.

### Assisted Reproductive Technologies (ART)

Assisted Reproductive Technologies, including in vitro fertilization (IVF) and surrogacy, are subject to complex legal regulations that vary significantly by country. In many Western nations, ART is regulated through comprehensive legal frameworks that establish standards for the ethical and safe practice of reproductive technologies. For instance, the United Kingdom's Human Fertilisation and Embryology Act 1990 regulates all aspects of ART, from the licensing of clinics to the legal status of embryos and the rights of donors, surrogates, and intended parents. This act ensures that ART is practiced in a manner that protects the rights and well-being of all parties involved, while also addressing ethical concerns such as the welfare of children born through ART (Adamson, 2002).

In other countries, the regulation of ART is less clear, leading to legal ambiguities and potential ethical issues. In India, before the Surrogacy (Regulation) Act 2021, the surrogacy industry was largely unregulated, leading to concerns about the exploitation of poor women who served as surrogates. The new law, while imposing important restrictions such as banning commercial surrogacy, also raised issues about access to ART services for unmarried and LGBTQ+ individuals, reflecting the ongoing tension between regulation and reproductive rights.

The legal frameworks governing reproductive health and rights are crucial in determining access to essential services such as contraception, maternal healthcare, abortion, and assisted reproductive technologies. These laws not only protect individual rights but also reflect broader societal values and commitments to public health and gender equality. However, the effectiveness of these legal protections varies widely, depending on the strength of the legal framework, its implementation, and the socio-political context. As reproductive technologies and societal attitudes continue to evolve, legal frameworks must adapt to ensure that reproductive rights are fully protected and accessible to all.

## CONCLUSION AND FINAL REFLECTIONS

The legal frameworks governing reproductive health and rights are foundational to shaping individual autonomy and access to essential services worldwide. This chapter has explored how various legal instruments and policies significantly impact key areas, including contraception, maternal health, abortion, and assisted reproductive technologies (ART). Each of these areas reflects a complex interplay among legal provisions, societal values, cultural norms, and international human rights standards, underscoring the necessity for ongoing reform and advocacy.

Legal frameworks are vital in determining access to contraception and family planning services. Countries that have established comprehensive laws—such as France and the United Kingdom—illustrate a commitment to reproductive health and gender equality by ensuring widespread access to contraceptive services, often at no cost or subsidized rates. These policies empower individuals to make informed choices about their reproductive lives and contribute to broader societal health outcomes. However, legal restrictions in certain regions, heavily influenced by cultural and religious norms, present significant barriers to contraception access. Such barriers often manifest in laws that impose requirements like spousal consent or limit access based on marital status. These issues highlight the urgent need for legal reforms to dismantle obstacles and ensure equitable access to reproductive healthcare.

Maternal health is another critical domain shaped by legal frameworks. International treaties such as the Convention on the Elimination of All Forms of Discrimination Against Women (CEDAW) and the Sustainable Development Goals (SDGs) establish clear obligations for states to ensure safe and accessible maternal health services. While many countries have enacted laws mandating the provision of maternal healthcare, disparities in implementation and enforcement remain significant. Effective maternal health policies are essential for reducing mortality and morbidity rates, especially in underserved areas. For instance, South Africa's National Health Act reflects a commitment to improving maternal health outcomes, yet challenges persist where legal protections are weak or poorly enforced. Strengthening these frameworks and ensuring robust enforcement mechanisms are critical to safeguarding the health of mothers and infants alike.

Abortion laws exhibit a wide spectrum of legal approaches, from liberal frameworks that uphold reproductive autonomy to highly restrictive regimes. In countries with liberal abortion laws, such as Canada and much of Western Europe, access to abortion is legally protected and is associated with positive health outcomes and social equity. Conversely, restrictive abortion laws in countries like El Salvador and the Philippines criminalize the procedure under nearly all circumstances, leading to significant health risks and exacerbating human rights concerns. The impact of these legal frameworks on women's health and rights underscores the need for reform, pushing for legal alignment with international human rights standards to protect women's health and autonomy.

The regulation of Assisted Reproductive Technologies (ART) presents a complex legal landscape, influenced by diverse ethical considerations and societal attitudes. Countries with established regulatory frameworks, such as the United Kingdom and Israel, provide comprehensive guidelines that ensure ethical practices and protect the rights of all parties involved, including patients, donors, and resulting children. However, the lack of a unified international approach complicates cross-border reproductive care, where individuals seek ART services in different jurisdictions. As ART technologies evolve, it is imperative to develop clear and balanced legal frameworks that effectively address ethical dilemmas while safeguarding reproductive rights and ensuring informed consent.

As reproductive technologies advance and societal attitudes shift, emerging trends will continue to shape the future of reproductive health and rights. Advances in medical technology, changing cultural norms regarding gender and sexuality, and increasing advocacy for gender equality will all drive changes in legal frameworks and policies. Future research and policy development should prioritize addressing existing gaps in laws, exploring innovative solutions to emerging challenges, and ensuring the protection of reproductive rights in a rapidly evolving global landscape.

In conclusion, the legal frameworks governing reproductive health and rights are crucial in determining access, quality, and respect for reproductive freedoms. While significant progress has been made, persistent challenges remain that necessitate a sustained commitment to strengthening legal protections, addressing ethical considerations, and improving access to services. Ensuring that all individuals can exercise their reproductive freedoms with dignity, respect, and autonomy must remain at the forefront of legal and policy agendas. By advocating for reforms that prioritize reproductive health as a fundamental human right, we can create a more equitable and just society where reproductive rights are universally recognized and protected.

## REFERENCES


Adamson, D. (2002). Regulation of assisted reproductive technologies in the United States. *Fertility and Sterility*, 78(5), 932–942. DOI: 10.1016/S0015-0282(02)04199-7 PMID: 12413975

Albertyn, C. (2019). Abortion, reproductive rights and the possibilities of reproductive justice in South African courts. *University of Oxford Human Rights Hub Journal*, 2019, 87–119.

Babor, D. D. M. (1999). Population growth and reproductive rights in international human rights law. *Connecticut Journal of International Law*, 14(1), 83–122.

Baruah, M. (2022). International and national legal framework on Sustainable Development Goal (Gender equality). *Indian Journal of Law and Legal Research*, 4, 1–20.

Colker, R. (1994). Equality theory and reproductive freedom. *Texas Journal of Women and the Law*, 3(1), 99–122. PMID: 12645608

Combellick-Bidney, S. (2017). Reproductive rights as human rights: Stories from advocates in Brazil, India and South Africa. *International Journal of Human Rights*, 21(7), 800–822. DOI: 10.1080/13642987.2016.1276446

Cook, R. J. (1992). International protection of women's reproductive rights. *New York University Journal of International Law & Politics. New York University. International Law Society*, 24(2), 645–728. PMID: 11656212

Cook, R. J., Dickens, B. M., & Fathalla, M. F. (2011). Reproductive health and human rights: Integrating medicine, ethics, and law (Oxford, 2003; online edn, Oxford Academic). Oxford University Press. https://doi.org/DOI: 10.1093/acprof:oso/9780199241323.001.0001

Dakic, D. (2015). Requirements of informed consent in the reproductive sphere under the European Convention on Human Rights. Ave Maria International Law Journal, 4, 72-105.

Ebeku, K. S. A. (2004). New dawn for African women: Prospects of Africa's Protocol on women's rights. *Sri Lanka Journal of International Law*, 16, 83–138.

Fayokun, K. O. (2015). Reproductive rights and female education in Nigeria. *US-China Law Review*, 12(11), 906–921.

Fine, J. B., Mayall, K., & Sepúlveda, L. (2017). The role of international human rights norms in the liberalization of abortion laws globally. *Health and Human Rights*, 19(1), 69–80. DOI: 10.1111/1467-9280.00006 PMID: 28630542

Guzman Alejandro, P. A. (2020). Reproductive rights. *Revista Juridica de la Universidad de Puerto Rico*, 89(1), 249–298.

Hevia, M., & Vacaflor, C. H. (2013). The legal status of in vitro fertilization in Latin America and the American Convention on Human Rights. *Suffolk Transnational Law Review*, 36(1), 51–88.

Iemelianenko, V., Gornostay, A., & Ivantsova, A. (2019). Reproductive rights violations: Forced sterilization and restriction of voluntary sterilization. *Wiadomosci Lekarskie (Warsaw, Poland: 1960), 72*, 2536-2540.

Ikeatu, E. G. (2020). Violations of women's reproductive rights in Nigeria. *Nnamdi Azikiwe University Journal of International Law and Jurisprudence*, 11(2), 157–174.

Komanovics, A. (2009). Effective enforcement of human rights: The Tysiac v. Poland case. Studia Iuridica Auctoritate Universitatis Pecs Publicata, 143, 186-225.

Kunchit. (2023). Women's Health and Reproductive Rights. Issue 4 Int'l JL Mgmt. & Human., 6, 1008.

Kurland, A. S. (2006). Access to contraception. *The Georgetown Journal of Gender and the Law*, 7(3), 1129–1142.

Machaj, Ł. (2023). Dobbs v. Jackson Women's Health Organization: The epitaph for Roe v. Wade. Bialostockie Studia Prawnicze, 28(3), 259-278.

Mehlman, M. J. (2015). Reproductive information and reproductive decision-making. *The Journal of Law, Medicine & Ethics*, 43(2), 241–244. PMID: 26242944

Merali, I. (2000). Advancing women's reproductive and sexual health rights: Using the international human rights system. *Development in Practice*, 10(5), 609–624. https://www.jstor.org/stable/4029536. DOI: 10.1080/09614520020008797

Morgan, L. M. (2021). Costa Rica's oversized role in Latin American sexual and reproductive rights lawfare. *Revista Direito GV*, 17(3), 1–31. DOI: 10.1590/2317-6172202137

Myers, R. S. (2014). Re-reading Roe v. Wade. *Washington and Lee Law Review*, 71(2), 1025–1046.

Prakash, S., & Asthana, N. (2019). Reproductive rights of women: Constitutional and global perspective. *Supremo Amicus*, 10, 294–303.

Shozi, B. (2020). Something old, something new: Applying reproductive rights to new reproductive technologies in South Africa. *South African Journal on Human Rights*, 36(1), 1–24. DOI: 10.1080/02587203.2020.1776632

Smith, E. S. (2014). Reproductive justice begins with contraceptive access in the Philippines. *Pacific Rim Law & Policy Journal*, 23(1), 203–250.

Staunton, C. (2011). As easy as A, and C: Will A, and v. Ireland be Ireland's wake-up call for abortion rights. *European Journal of Health Law*, 18(2), 205–220. DOI: 10.1163/157180911X564589 PMID: 21644438

Wen, C. (2003). Informed choice in rural Anhui. *Human Rights (Chicago, Ill.)*, 2(4), 22–23.

Williams, A. (2018). State regulatory efforts in protecting surrogate's bodily autonomy. *Seton Hall Law Review*, 49(1), 205–232. PMID: 30557923

## KEY TERMS AND DEFINITIONS

**Reproductive Rights:** It refers to the legal and human rights related to individuals' ability to make autonomous decisions about reproduction, including access to contraception, abortion, maternal health services, and assisted reproductive technologies.

**Contraception:** It refers to methods or devices used to prevent pregnancy by inhibiting fertilization or implantation, including hormonal, barrier, and permanent solutions.

**Maternal Health:** It refers to the health and well-being of women during pregnancy, childbirth, and the postpartum period, including access to essential healthcare services and protection against maternal mortality.

**Abortion:** It refers to the medical procedure that terminates a pregnancy, with legal frameworks ranging from unrestricted access to severe restrictions, impacting women's ability to safely and legally end a pregnancy.

**Assisted Reproductive Technologies (ART):** It encompasses medical procedures, such as in vitro fertilization and surrogacy, designed to aid individuals in conceiving and carrying a pregnancy to term, governed by legal regulations addressing ethical, medical, and social concerns.

**Sustainable Development Goals (SDGs):** These are a set of 17 global goals established by the United Nations to address a range of issues, including reproductive health and rights, aiming to end poverty, protect the environment, and ensure prosperity for all by 2030.

**Reproductive Autonomy:** It refers to the right of individuals to make independent and informed decisions about their reproductive lives, free from coercion, discrimination, or undue influence from others.

# Chapter 9 Reproductive Challenges and Rights of Surrogates: A Mixed Methods Study From Indian Urban Inhabitants

**Sushmita Das**
https://orcid.org/0009-0002-5002-2702
*Amity University, Gwalior, India*

**Shubhang Gomasta**
https://orcid.org/0009-0000-7834-2084
*Amity University, Gwalior, India*

**Sanjum Bedi**
https://orcid.org/0009-0008-8601-4257
*Amity University, Gwalior, India*

## ABSTRACT

*"The more law the less justice."- Marcus Tullius Cicero The reproductive challenges are very common now a days in a modern world particularly in the urban inhabitants of an Indian society and almost in every western cultures globally and due to stereotype society adult humans aren't aware of their reproductive rights and duties and they have to knock the doors of the courts despite of numerous legislations and reproductive case precedents of abortion, Assisted Reproductive technology, Surrogacy challenges in their respective legislations. The reproductive challenges are mainly due to infertility issues, unsafe abortion, lack of awareness in STD's (sexually transmitted diseases), HIV, forced pregnancies etc. The authors in this chapter will explore about surrogacy and abortion laws as a solution to the reproductive challenges and proposes an effective remedy for the dispute's settle-*

DOI: 10.4018/979-8-3693-7837-3.ch009

*ment mechanism.*

## INTRODUCTION

The authors cite a famous quote by Sir Walter Scott, "Bloods is thicker than the water," which conveys the idea that only blood can establish a strong bond with one's own relatives in terms of loyalty. This is particularly relevant in urban and rural communities where the belief in raising biological children is still prevalent. Numerous religions and communities in India recognise that close relatives and cousins are entitled to marry in adulthood, but they prohibit adoption, surrogacy, and IVF (in-vitro fertilisation). However, in a few communities where adoption, surrogacy, and other Assisted Reproductive technologies are permitted, individuals face numerous obstacles in gaining acceptance from society and the court. This is due to the absence of comprehensive legislations that provide a unified solution for addressing such matters. The reproductive difficulties faced by urban residents can be attributed to the adopted lifestyle of urban women, which is characterised by a hectic working culture. In the past, there was a patriarchal society where men were the primary earners and women were responsible for managing the household. However, in contemporary times, it is clear that urban women are now employed and have predominantly relocated to major cities in India such as Delhi, Mumbai, Bengaluru, Chennai, Gurgaon, Pune, and others. The authors emphasises that the urban working structure disproportionately affects the reproductive health of women, leading married couples to resort to procedures such as IVF (in-vitro fertilisation), abortion, surrogacy, and assisted reproductive technology. Furthermore, the researcher investigated that in certain urban areas of India, couples in live-in relationships are permitted to reside in rented homes and hotels. However, they are also required to engage in legal disputes over abortion, surrogacy, and in-vitro-fertilization (IVF). The urban lifestyle in India exhibits notable disparities in terms of working culture and lifestyle, which therefore give rise to reproductive difficulties among women. In the year 1944, Professor John Rock Miriam Menkin Lab technician of Harvard University for the first time experimented with fertilizing egg outside human body which was a man-made process of creating a natural offspring same like the process of divine but later this magical process of human made technique turned out as a business. Louise Brown was the first "test-tube baby", was born in United Kingdom, the product of the first successful IVF *(in vitro fertilization)* procedure in the year 1978 (The Independent, 2018 Jul 25). The concept of surrogacy was experimented scientifically but there is still on-going legal battle for surrogacy tracing back to the historical times of mid 80's in United States where there was legal battle between the surrogate mother and biological mother who refused to hand over the child

(Johnson v. Calvert) where the New Jersey court gave the custody to the intended couple. Similarly, in California (1990) another case which 1st time declare "gestational surrogacy" by the Supreme court of California on 20th May 1993.

The reproductive legislation such as Surrogacy, Abortion, Assisted Reproductive Technologies (ART), etc. are consistently top stories in the media, regardless of their legality. In ancient India, the patriarchal society has consistently associated the birth of biological male children with inheritance, property ownership, economic contributions, religious and ritual obligations, and the prohibition of social evils. This led to the enactment of the PCPNDT Act (Pre-conception and Pre-natal Diagnostic Techniques Act) 1994. The purpose of this act is to prohibit and prevent the misuse of techniques used for determining sex. Even in modern times, educated and literate women are still unable to advocate for their own reproductive rights. The Medical Termination of Pregnancy Act 1971 in India is a legislation that grants women the reproductive rights to deliberately end a pregnancy under specific circumstances. Surrogacy presents a formidable obstacle for women who must advocate for their reproductive rights. It serves as the final resort to achieving a biological child, particularly when couples are unable to conceive naturally. In such cases, they resort to IVF treatments, in vitro fertilisation, or Assisted Reproductive Technology (ART), which is also regulated by the Assisted Reproductive Technology Act 2021 in India. Although there are provisions in place, the issue at hand is the level of acceptance among Indian families towards biological children conceived through surrogacy. The comprehensive prohibition of commercial surrogacy fails to address the concerns pertaining to the reproductive rights of women. With the increasing number of infertility cases, India is poised to become the epicentre of infertility, posing a concerning threat to future generations. Medical professionals report that both men and women, as well as couples, are experiencing infertility as a result of contemporary lifestyle issues such as smoking and mental stress in urban residents of India.

## LITERATURE REVIEW

The researchers conducted a comprehensive doctrinal analysis of surrogacy laws in Ukraine, which is considered a leading global destination for surrogacy. Ukraine has established itself as a prominent hub for international intended parents due to its well-regulated system. However, recent political unrest and conflicts have hindered Ukraine's ability to provide global surrogacy services. Due to the country's favourable legal system, economic conditions, and the presence of highly skilled medical professionals, it is a popular choice for individuals seeking to produce children through surrogacy. The progression of reproductive technologies, first regulated by the government, has transitioned towards the commercialisation of surrogacy (Oksana Kashyntseva 2022). The Ukraine was considered to be the best destination for gestational surrogacy (Jacobson, H., König, A., & Majumdar, A. (2024) and India currently being following the gestational surrogacy although for the Indian intending parents. The lawmakers are constantly concerns for the protection of children and women in a surrogacy arrangement in Ukraine which is discussed in the Hague Conference. (Emma Lamberton 2020). In Georgia, gestational model of surrogacy is adopted which lack of regulation as discussed, the best bet and regulations which is worth reviewing (Madeline Mae Neel 2019).

As the authors are concerned about the reproductive rights and challenges of the parties to the surrogates and in countries like Russia and Ukraine it is considered like a work (Veronika Siegl 2023) whereas in India currently altruistic model of surrogacy is followed. The ART and commercial surrogacy are growing fashion which lack in ethical and legalisation in this industry (Sylvie Armstrong 2022). The surrogacy is not only having a legal issue as also has emotional (Tehran, H. A. et., al 2014), Psychosocial (Olga B.A. van den Akker 2007) and ethical (Dr Herjeet Marway 2018) aspects to deal with as explored. There are no global surrogacy laws but it is advisable to forbid at a global level as threatening to human dignity (Hannah Rahim 2024). There should be legislative uniformity in the global surrogacy law and collective international effort. (Paola Frati et,,al 2021). The authors (Susanna Marinelli et., al 2024) well looked into some pragmatic cases dealt with European Courts of Human Rights with related to Surrogacy.

The fashion of alternative dispute started a way back but the citizens in most of the state are relied on the courts, the authors (Prasad, M. et., al 2014) in the research has discussed about transnational surrogacy dispute can be resolved through the Indian Arbitration Legislation whereas currently India do not follow the transnational surrogacy but the authors of this chapter consider that arbitration can be the best model for resolving the dispute. According to Scott (2020), mediation provides a cooperative setting where both parties can voice their issues and strive for a solution that is agreeable to both. This approach has demonstrated efficacy in resolving conflicts related to custody, financial responsibilities, and postnatal communication between the surrogate and the child in surrogacy disputes. Arbitration, however, entails the involvement of an impartial third party who delivers a final decision that must be followed, after listening to arguments from both parties. Although less adaptable than mediation, this approach offers a conclusive answer, which is vital in situations where the parties are unable to come to a mutual agreement. India now possesses one of the most well-suited arbitration statutes of 1996. The family courts are the first court of instance when it comes to such dispute and in India do not have proper single window mechanism for the resolution. However alternative dispute mechanism is best way to resolve the family disputes (Barbara Mills KC 2024).

## Contextual Background of International Surrogacy

In the year 1944, Professor John Rock Miriam Menkin Lab technician of Harvard University for the first time experimented with fertilizing egg outside human body (Stephen Ruffenach 2009) which was a man-made process of creating a natural offspring same like the process of divine but later this magical process of human made technique turned out as a business all over the globe as many countries it can be witnessed that there are stringent laws for surrogacy and many do not have surrogacy laws yet many countries are still awaiting for their stringent laws. the first child born out of surrogacy is itself is a 47 year old now in 2025 and the concept of Surrogacy was experimented in the year 1944 but with the changing times there are major problems occurring in the process mainly after the time period of mid 80's there were problems relating to the custody of child, legality of child but whatever the timeline it is, there is always legal battle of surrogacy which is mainly between the intended couple, surrogate mothers and child born out of surrogate mothers. On 25th July 1978, Louise Brown (Katharine Dow, 2019) was the first "test-tube baby", was born in Great Britain, United Kingdom the result of the first successful IVF (in vitro fertilization). The concept of surrogacy was experimented scientifically but there is still on-going legal battle for surrogacy tracing back to the historical times of mid 80's in United States where there was legal battle between the surrogate mother and biological mother who refused to hand over the child where the New Jersey court gave the custody to the intended couple.

## An Ancient History of Surrogacy and Niyoga in India

In India the world's second and India's first IVF (in vitro fertilization) baby, Kanupriya alias Durga was born in Kolkata on October 3, 1978. It is also evident in Hindu mythology about Niyoga practices also discussed in Mahabharata (Gail Hinich Sutherland 1990) in which a widow women or wives who do not have children allowed to have children with another man in the family or close relative of the family to continue the family lineage, this was mainly followed in the Brahmanical society for those women who faced challenges with regard to society and financial. In the ancient practices, Niyoga was a practice done to keep the family lineage and the brother or close relative marry the wife of the deceased husband. In the contextual text of the Rig Veda and Yajnavalka, the practice of Niyoga is mentioned. Even in the recent judgment delivered by the Justice Anoop Kumar Dhand in (para 18)[1] the practice of Niyoga Dharma was addressed in the context of surrogacy which was considered as duty (Dharma) regulated by social norms. Henceforth, surrogacy is modern form of Niyog Dharma when a couple can't reproduce due to infertility, they rent a womb of another woman who shall be a close relative according to the new surrogacy regulation legislation of 2021. In Vedic times, surrogacy has a paramount considered to be historically evident that the story of Devki's 7th child Balrama was born through surrogacy from the womb of Rohini. It is evident from Mahabharata that king Pandu and Kunti gave the concept of Niyog in which a woman while facing widowhood or impotency of a couple can appoint someone to bear a child. The modern idea of close relative in the new surrogacy law is not a new concept it is evident from the time of Niyog practice where intending mother gets her biological offspring from brother-in-law to complete the family lineage. Niyoga, when accomplished with mutual agreement, resulted in the birth of strong and legitimate successors. The presence of several examples of surrogacy in these ancient stories indicates a historical embrace of the concept and serves as evidence of the thriving practice of surrogacy in India. In the present era, surrogacy continues to be of great significance for India as it was once acknowledged as the global hub for surrogacy. This is mostly due to legal loopholes and the low expenses in India. Surrogacy has been practiced in India since 1978, and the country is well-known for its high rate of "reproductive tourism" and its growing role as a centre for the fertility industry. Anand, a town in Gujarat renowned for its dairy sector, has also emerged as a prominent hub for the surrogacy industry. (The Indian Express 2014) The surrogacy is not a new practice in India, but it used to be unregulated and lacked oversight due to the absence of regulation. Nevertheless, with the implementation of the surrogacy legislation.

The background history of surrogacy has developed in almost every country which has achieved a significant response starting from each and every country. In the ancient historic times of biblical era the concept was mentioned even in the bible. The popular story of those time a servant who bore a child named Abraham and Sarah named Hagar who is known to be born out of Surrogacy. (Tamar Kamionkowski 2021). In the early twenty century in the year 1930's there was time to trace the Artificial Insemination was incepted then in the year 1950-60 the development of advanced reproductive medicines took place in the market practice for the development of fertility drugs and techniques like artificial insemination set place for the surrogacy to be practiced in the modern era. The time in the year 1970 which achieved the milestone success for the history and development for surrogacy made legal by the attorney named Noel Keane in the United States and the birth of traditional surrogacy took place which is not in practiced with the latest legislation in India and the term traditional surrogacy therefore which means the fathers gametes and surrogate mother was artificial inseminated which made her biological child of the surrogate mother. In the United States of America during the time of 1970's the first time legally recognised agreement related to surrogacy arrangements was done by the Keane (worldwide surrogacy specialist 2021) in which traditional surrogacy was done by the artificial insemination with the intending father's gamete then in the year 1980, Elizabeth Kane in USA, conceived the baby through artificial insemination. The history of gestational surrogacy can be traced back to eighties times especially in the year 1985 where an embryo created through in vitro fertilization was implanted into a surrogate who had no biological link to the child. The surrogate baby who took attention in the eyes of large public was the traditional surrogate mother named Mary Beth Whitehead wanted to keep the child with her but the court held that the intending parents must keep the child in their custody. During the time of 1990s, we can see that there was an improvement of IVF technologies made for the gestational surrogacy which is a welcoming step and more acceptable. In the twenty first century especially in the year 2000's, India became evidently popular for the destination of surrogacy due to best opportunity cost and less stringent legislation leading to blooming industry of surrogacy.

## GLOBAL ANALYSIS OF REPRODUCTIVE CHALLENGES

### The Permissibility of Surrogacy Around the Globe

The global surrogacy is often searched because of the medical reason of infertility, economic affordability and stringent regulations in their own countries. If most of the nation states forbids surrogacy services there would be childless (IP) intending parents in future due to urban lifestyle. There are no global surrogacy laws governing transnational or cross border surrogacy as each state has its own laws and regulations and many of the countries forbids cross border surrogacy. India legalised commercial surrogacy in the year 2002. (Malavika R.) There are several countries where surrogacy is not prohibited but not regulated, countries like Kenya (Fatuma Rashid, 2017) where there is no formal law although commercial surrogacy is allowed and there is legal protection is available. In Malaysia (Nehaluddin Ahmad et., al 2016) where there are no formal law, commercial surrogacy is applicable and legal guidelines are under review in the current status, The Nigerian government (Olanike S Adelakun, 2018) has also not enacted formal law and commercial surrogacy is permissible. The surrogacy contracts are enforceable in Nigerian as there are many countries where surrogacy is strictly prohibited like Cambodia, Denmark, France, Germany, Ireland, Spain, Portugal, Bulgaria and Nepal (Reuters 2023). The best practices and global analysis for commercial surrogacy law which lesser the reproductive challenges for women in the countries are Ukraine and Russia where it is considered as work (Veronika Siegl, 2023) where commercial surrogacy is permitted but after the war many IP's (intending parents) went later to took their biological offspring through surrogacy as Ukraine is considered to be the global surrogacy motherland where surrogacy services are rendered with less stringency only the outbroke of war with Russia made less in demand for the international intending parents (IP) to travel across. Another global fertility destination is Georgia where commercial surrogacy is allowed for heterosexual couples. The Russian government allows surrogacy but religious groups/communities like in India forbids commercial child birth through surrogacy. (Reuters 2023). The European countries like Bulgaria, France, Germany, Italy, Portugal, Taiwan and Spain prohibit all kinds of surrogacy. (India tourism statistics, 2023, Ministry of Tourism, Government of India.) The United States of America also allows commercial surrogacy especially the states like California, Nevada and Illinois, same as Mexico some states like Tabasco, Sinaloa. (Claudia Flores 2023).

*Table 1. Status of Surrogacy around the globe*

| Name of the Country | Legal Status of Commercial Surrogacy | Legal Status of Altruistic Surrogacy |
|---|---|---|
| India | Prohibited from 2021/ Illegal | Legal |
| United States | It varies from State to State | It varies from State to State |
| United Kingdom | Illegal | Legal |
| Canada | Illegal | Legal |
| Russia | Legal | Legal |
| Ukraine | Legal | Legal |
| Georgia | Legal | Legal |
| Greece | Legal | Legal |
| Australia | Legal | Illegal |
| Mexico | Legal | Varies from state to state |

*Note*: Adapted from Reuters (2023).

## Abortion Law

Before the medical and legal specialists, the authors thinks common men should face fewer reproductive challenges as there are few countries which have best practices for abortion laws like Canada (Government of Canada 2024) where abortion is allowed at any stage of pregnancy which is one of the best model framework around the globe whereas in India it allows up to thirty weeks (The Indian Express, Apurva Vishwanath 2024) on the view of two medical practitioners and there many case precedent where even a single woman has to go through reproductive challenges in abortion laws and the best legal framework evident in India for abortion laws is that it allows abortion for those who have foetal abnormality under the Medical Termination of Pregnancy Act 1971. The Netherland government have the same legislation up to twenty-four week of pregnancy and can be terminated in case of abnormalities. The Polish residents have more restrictive beliefs than other Europeans and so as Swedish being supportive and liberal. (Janell Fetterolf et., al). The countries which allow to terminate pregnancies in twelve to fourteen weeks are Germany which also a best model as first step is counselling followed by the waiting period of at least three days also the same model is followed in Spain (Reuters 2024). Therefore, those countries who have adopted mandatory counselling are also one of the best remedial for the reproductive challenges faced by a woman.

## INTERNATIONAL LAW FRAMEWORK ON REPRODUCTIVE CHALLENGES

### International Conference on Population and Development

The international framework (ICPD-Cairo,1994) International Conference on Population and Development deals with the reproductive health, family planning which deals with an overall physical, mental and social well-being. The sexual and reproductive health rights are given under the Beijing declaration and platform for action in the year 1995 which deals with family planning, safe motherhood, STD'S/ HIV, infections in the reproductive tract.

### UDHR (Universal Declaration of Human Rights)

One of the most important international documents which talks about the right to found a family and right to marry under article 16 and right to health under article 25 of the UDHR (Universal declaration of Human Rights.)

### CEDAW-Convention on the Elimination of All Forms of Discrimination Against Women

The United Nation has many international policies, framework and initiatives done for the reproductive challenges for the women. *CEDAW* 1979 is one of the conventions on the elimination of all forms of discrimination against women which is interlinked with article 12 of the convention which directly talks about rights of women which relates to health care services, family planning, maternal health, pre- and post-natal care services during pregnancy and the birth of the child.

## Sustainable Development Goal

The pointer number three of Sustainable Development Goal which deals with reproductive challenges are given under the Goal 3 which ensure healthy lives and make sure that there should be access to sexual and reproductive health care services. The goal five deals with gender equality and empowering the rights of women and girls in which they should get the access to sexual and reproductive health care services.

## UNFPA, United Nations Population Fund

The strategic plan for UNFPA, United Nations Population Fund also promotes the rights of reproductive health, lower the maternal mortality, eliminating the gender-based violence. The right to sexual and reproductive health is also discussed under the human rights council resolutions.

## Subsidiary Organ of United Nations (World Health Organization)

The world health organization which is popularly known as WHO which is targeted from 2016 to 2030 (Global Strategy for women's, children and adolescent's health) ensure that the right to physical, mental health can be realised for women, children and adolescent by ensuring the gender inequality and there should be better quality of sexual and reproductive health services. The International Framework are once made but there is no generic awareness on comprehensive sexual education, reproductive health and rights. The Legal framework and policies in the countries must protect the reproductive rights and discriminate violence against women and there should be proper monitoring, reviewing and analysing the data which address the reproductive health services.

## The Hague Conference and ICMR Guidelines

The guidelines were made for ART (Assisted Reproductive Technology) by ICMR (The Indian Council for Medical Research) which were not enforceable but later after ten years, a conference was organised known as the Hague Conference on Private International Law incepted by the working group of international surrogacies. In 2015, India didn't legislate the laws related to surrogacy but there were constant bills in making for banning the commercial surrogacy and finally in 2016 there was an introduction to the surrogacy regulation bill of 2016 which aims to regulate the surrogacy practices by banning commercial surrogacy and allowing for altruistic surrogacy for the Indian heterosexual couples. Therefore, there were many

Indian scholars who fought for banning the commercial surrogacy in fact the there is a huge research gap in between that the researcher in this thesis have evaluated by interrogating the doctors especially who are dealing with invitro fertilization they demanded that there shouldn't be blanket ban on the surrogacy law whether altruistic or commercial in fact they must be well regulated. The researcher also believes that the Surrogacy (Regulation) Act of 2021 could have been a well-regulated law by allowing all forms of surrogacy especially commercial, altruistic and gestational where the main problem of Indian intended parents could be solved as the researcher argues by quoting the landmark statement of the jurist Jeremy Bentham "greatest happiness to the greatest number" in which a law should be passed only if it is satisfying the wants by minimising the pain. This legislation has no scope for the intending parents, future IVF aspirants to experiment and learn the medical technological advancement and there will no scope of future research on this.

The legalisation of surrogacy in India occurred in 2002. Consequently, commercial surrogacy was permitted in India, however, there was a lack of a comprehensive legal structure to regulate it. This created a new revenue stream for numerous economically disadvantaged women, with the town of Anand serving as a notable illustration of this phenomenon. As a result of the commercialisation of surrogacy, numerous commercial firms and clinics emerged, with some even boasting specialised knowledge in the sector and providing assistance to foreigners. During this course, India assumed the role of the surrogate capital of the world. Poverty was the main contributing factor to the success of surrogacy in India. In 2005, the Indian Council of Medical Research released guidelines on surrogacy, which permitted the determination of monetary compensation by the parties involved. These guidelines prohibit the surrogate from donating her egg and mandate her to surrender all parental rights.

Simultaneously, the Assisted Reproductive Technology (Regulation) Bill, 2008 was being developed. Although not formally introduced to Parliament, the Law Commission undertook a study on surrogacy, resulting in the publication of its 228th Report in August 2009, which recommended the implementation of new legislation to regulate surrogacy.

The 2014 version of the Assisted Reproductive Technology (Regulation) Bill was drafted in response to the Law Commission's suggestion. Regrettably, similar to its antecedent in 2008, this legislation failed to be enacted. In 2015, Jayshree Wad, an activist and lawyer, brought forth a case to the Supreme Court of India, (Hindustan Times 2016) emphasising the dangers associated with the commercial surrogacy sector. Concurrently, the Surrogacy (Regulation) Bill, 2016 was created. In contrast to the 2014 edition, the Lok Sabha approved it in December 2018, but encountered delays in the Rajya Sabha. The 2016 bill was reintroduced as the Surrogacy (Regulation) Bill, 2019 and was passed on August 5th, 2019. The expansion of the surrogacy industry has led to the emergence of negative consequences associated with its commercialisation, which has raised significant concerns among campaigners.

## AN ANALYSIS OF THE BABY MANJI CASE FROM JAPAN TO INDIA.

The case of baby Manji is known as first international dispute arising in India in the year 2008 started from Japan to India which was a benchmark dispute which shook the entire commercial surrogacy industry in India and many people started forbidding this as the factual submission of this case is that a couple from Japan named Dr. Yamada and wife contracted with an Indian surrogate mother from Anand, Gujarat (commonly known as Surrogate Capital of India). The child named baby Manji born at the surrogacy capital, Gujarat in the month of July, meanwhile during the pregnancy the intending parents went through legal separation and the wife of Dr. Yamada refused to take the baby but the intending father wanted the child but the regulations during that time forbid to take the baby as laws related to surrogacy were unclear and not regulated by any legislation until 2021 in India. The legal status of child was questioned under the law known as Indian Guardian and Wards Act, 1890 and the nationality of the child as the intending parents were Japanese and child born in India through a commercial surrogate mother. There were Non-Government Organisation (NGO) who actively took suo moto part in this case challenging the legal and ethical grounds and claimed that the baby was immorally trafficked and the Indian court of Rajasthan gave a temporary restriction for carrying the baby to Japan due to single parents and nationality concerns. However, the apex court of India allowed to carry the child and also stated that commercial surrogacy is permissible and dismissed the claims of the NGO about the trafficking of the child and granted the travel document to the child. Henceforth, this case is a landmark case of International Surrogacy in India but unfortunately the current legal system in India do not permit International commercial surrogacy and only allows altruistic to the Indian heterosexual couples and proper law is formulated in the year known as the Surrogacy Regulation Act of 2021.

### National Legislative Framework on Reproductive Legislations in India

As correctly stated by the Jurist – Jeremy Bentham *"The greatest happiness to the greatest number"* which means that those legislation where maximum people should get the pursuit of pleasure by avoidance of pain as he gave the doctrine of pain and pleasure where the authors connected by interpreting the reproductive statutes in India. The National Legislative framework and policies on reproductive challenges in India are the few beneficial piece of legislation which is a solution to the reproductive problems are Medical Termination of Pregnancy (MTP) Act, 1971, The Maternity Benefit Act, 1961, The Pre-Conception and Pre-Natal Diagnostic Techniques (PCPNDT) Act, 1994, The Surrogacy (Regulation) Act, 2021, The Assisted Reproductive Technology Act 2021. As the author also believes in the importance of Historical School of Jurisprudence where the jurist of this school emphasis in the codification of the legislation and these reproductive laws are well codified in India but not benefiting the requisite parties to the act who seek reproductive legislation as a solution to it. Therefore, the main objectives of these Act are:

## The Medical Termination of Pregnancy (MTP) Act, 1971

It provides safe legal and properly regulated abortion for the married women as marriages are socially accepted in India. The current problem of this Act that it covers the term "pregnant woman" and does not cover the autonomy and reproductive rights of the single, divorced, widowed, women staying in Live-in-relationship where it is very common in urban cities and these woman if they get pregnant have to face social stigma with such stringent legislation where the opening statement and the objectives of the Act states that the termination of pregnancy with the help of RMP (Registered Medical Practitioner) where it is challenging journey for a woman to reach out to a registered medical practitioner not only economically but also due to legal and social battle.

## The Current Scenario of Abortion Cases.

As there are many recent case precedents in India where it is challenging for a woman to reach the doors of the court in these scenarios which is also dealt in a recent case where a civil appeal was filed against the Principal Secretary, Health and Family Welfare Department, Govt. of NCT of Delhi & Anr. in the year 2022 where a single Manipuri girl age of 25 years based in New Delhi India hailing from the background of farmer who can't economically afford to keep the pregnancy and maintain the child without marriage and her male partner refused to marry her and there after knowing the pregnancy in the 22 weeks she sought for abortion which is a reproductive challenge for a woman where the author suggests that the medical professionals should be allowed to abort the pregnancy of a woman in all the circumstances with a written consent form which should be registered by taking an undertaking or an legal affidavit from the woman and her male partner to abort the pregnancy at any stage. These are the basic reproductive rights of a woman but the best practice of the Act is that it covers the age of the pregnant woman who shall be major and the pregnancies to abort in certain challenging situation like rape, sexual assault, any kind of disability and abnormality and the medical board will allow to terminate the pregnancy. Therefore, to remove such discrepancies in the Act and in upcoming cases it is necessary to make a common window solution for all the reproductive legislation dealing with all the issues in these cases of abortion where single, divorce/separated, widowed, live in relationship shouldn't face reproductive challenges to abort her pregnancy as there should be once bodily autonomy right to decide to keep the pregnancy or not as it is a matter of three peoples life despite of social and legal stigma and the pregnant woman definition should be clarified in the legislation.

## The Maternity Benefit Act, 1961

It is a legislation passed by Indian Government which is for the benefit of the pregnant female employee availed before and after child birth. The reproductive challenges in this Act are the definition of *commissioning mother* which only includes natural biological mother whose gametes are used or implanted in another woman. The women availing pregnancy through surrogacy should also be covered in this definition or a separate reproductive legislation where she should avail the maternity benefit and this also infringes the right to equality.

## The Journey of Maternity & Paternity Benefit around the Globe

There are best practices of paternity leave policy like in India only Central Government *married* male can avail the paternity leave for fifteen days, Sweden three months of paid leave for the father, one year in Japan and Germany and India is still fighting for the age-old maternity leave which is only for a natural mother. The latest amendment of 2017 under the Maternity Benefit Act, it is given twenty-six weeks and better facilities for working women like work from home, creche facilities etc. India is growing and shifting towards privatisation leaving behind the government monopolistic employment where the new reproductive challenges for a urban woman is when she is having a government job she get the maternity benefit right after joining the organization but in most case of private entity they allow to give maternity at least after three years of working in the organization which is pragmatically challenging for a woman.

## The Indian Case of Maternity Leave of Urban Employee Through Surrogacy was Declined

Recently in 2024, a female finance officer Supriya Jena in Odhisa, a State in India filed a petition in the High court seeking to avail the benefit of this Maternity Benefit Act of 1961 in pregnancy through surrogacy and the law enacted for surrogacy in 2021. This case is a set precedent where the authors urges for the rights of surrogate for the maternity benefit as she also argued that when an adoptive mother can avail why not a surrogate mother. However, Justice Panigrah of Odhisa High Court interpreted various National and International laws related to it. In India, there are no standard leave policy for the pregnant female working employees and the constant cases, rulings there are battle for the maternity benefit through surrogacy which is also held in the leading case of Chanda Keswani in the year 2020 against the State of Rajasthan (Principal Secretary, Higher Education Government of Rajasthan) as she too sought for the same relief and her petition was rejected on the basis that there is as such no laws and rules made under the same and the term Maternity Benefit definition was widely interpreted by the Judicial system in India. Henceforth, these are reproductive challenges of an urban working women despite of various legislations.

## The Pre-Conception and Pre-Natal Diagnostic Techniques (PCPNDT) Act, 1994

This act the author does not find any grey areas in this legislation as India is one of the countries which is still having patriarchal beliefs of having a male child for succession, inheritance of the property, performing last rituals of life in the graveyard is also done by a male child (son) and there are many cases of female foeticide. Therefore, this Act is well executed legislation aiming to fulfil the objectives of the Act where the intending parents can't determine the sex of the child in any case of natural pregnancy, assisted reproductive technology or even through surrogacy.

## The Surrogacy (Regulation) Act 2021

It is beneficial piece of legislation for the solution to the problem facing reproductive challenges who cannot have their own biological offspring and through the process of surrogacy one can have their biological child. The Surrogacy law prohibits the sale, prostitution and any other exploitation. Under Section 6 of the surrogacy laws, the mother shall give the consent in writing to become a surrogate in whatever the language she understands by telling her all the pros and cons of surrogacy procedure and also, she can withdraw from the procedure before the embryo implantation. The clinics must be registered and the clinics shall not indulge in the with the intermediaries and brokers who deal with surrogate mothers and take a lot of money from the intending parents as well as the clinics. The Act also defines the appropriate authorities and penalties.

### The Assisted Reproductive Technology Act 2021

*The (ART) Act 2021* is the Indian legislation for reproductive technology which monitors the system of ART assisted reproductive technology which oversees the regulation of ART Clinics, Assisted Reproductive Technology (ART) banks for freezing gametes, embryos legalization of surrogacy and banning of commercial surrogacy, counselling and consent for the individuals, donor's rights and recipients, ethical guidelines, challenges and criticism. The best practice of this act is that it has ART clinics banks, it has National and State board for ART and Surrogacy under section 3 & section 6 of this Assisted Reproductive Technology (ART) Act 2021.

## THE INDIAN CONSTITUTIONAL REPRODUCTIVE RIGHTS FOR WOMEN

The Indian Constitution is the supreme law of the land & its objectives are laid down in the Indian Preamble as its *key feature as it gives women equal rights as men.* The Fundamental Rights which are also known as basic rights *under article 14 embodies the general principles of equality before law and equal protection of laws.".* In the Case of Suchitra Shrivastava v Chandigarh Administration AIR 2009 which held right to reproductive choice flows from article 21 which gives the right to life and personal liberty. The (DPSP)'s Directive Principles of State Policies direct the states for securing justice and humane conditions of work and for maternity relief enlisted under article 42 of the Indian Constitution of 1950 which is also a promise towards women in fighting for the reproductive challenges.

The reproductive rights of a women or a reproductive choice of women like surrogacy, abortion, family planning must be protected under the fundamental rights of a women in today's century. The women of today have reached to a certain height in all the sectors for earning their livelihoods and sustainability in their family and society but many women have to still struggle for their reproductive rights even after marriage as there are many social reasons like female foeticide, family pressure for the birth of a child particularly "a boy child" just after the marriage. Even though the educated women can't fight for their reproductive rights from their own in laws and husband in today's time as there is always a pressure from their own family for getting marry at a certain point of time because of their biological age as law and biology are contradictory with each other as we can change laws for the society but we can't change the science which is also rapidly growing with the help of IVF specialist doctors all over the world. The commercial surrogacy is to purchase a womb which was legal in India till 2002. India was one of the surrogacy hub and people from different countries used to hire surrogate women for the purpose of becoming surrogate mother for the commissioning couple. In India, due to poverty, lack of education, unemployment and much other social discrimination, the system of surrogacy was popular in India. The practice of surrogacy was a like a business making process for the brokers who used to supply surrogate mothers to the intended couples and to the surrogacy clinics. This is how the commercialisation was done and the middlemen came into the picture due to commercialisation.

## The Analysis of Government Policies in India

The Indian government adopted certain policies ensuring towards reproductive rights and health services, promoting equality of gender. The policies which related with reproductive health care services, contraception and child care is introduced in the year 2000 as National Population Policy (NPP) and National Family Planning Program (NFPP) which aims to lower the mortality rate of the infants, fertility replacement which is one of the key steps towards the battle of reproductive challenges. The National Rural and Urban Health Mission (NRHM & NUHM) aspires to render the quality healthcare services to rural and urban women which should also cover the surrogates. On the other hand, there is a policy which deals with lowering the neonatal mortality and renders economic assistance to the mothers for the delivery which is also silent in terms for the surrogate mothers and other fertility treatments who aspire to have their own offspring as you may say these reproductive challenges can be fought only by those intending parents who are fortunate and privilege to afford the treatments. In India, there are also policy program for the adolescents reproductive and sexual health which is relevant for not covering the surrogate mothers due to the age criteria. Therefore, it shall be revised from time to time.

## Jurisprudential Interpretation of Reproductive Rights

The authors will focus on reproductive challenges faced by the urban intended married couples, transgender couples, single men and women etc. The reproductive challenges are not only related to abortion laws but also there are many other reproductive laws like Surrogacy (Regulation) Act, 2021. ART Act 2021, Assisted Reproductive Technology 2021. Earlier when there was no laws and regulation for surrogacy it was not universally defined in any of the Act. There are few scholars gave their interpretation to the term Surrogacy. Therefore, now the Surrogacy is defined under section 2(zd) of the Surrogacy Regulation Act 2021. Even after removing the term commercial surrogacy from the Act by prohibiting the means of commercial rented womb, there will always be a life-threatening risk of death for both mother and child whether it is commercial surrogacy or altruistic surrogacy (ethical compensated).

## An Interconnection of Natural Justice and Reproductive Laws from the eyes of Jeremy Bentham and John Austin.

The authors are true believer of Natural School of Jurisprudence where the thought process laid down as law of morals, universal law, law of God but with the changing needs of the time the role of Analytical School also plays it importance especially with the thought process of Jeremy Bentham where he stated "*greatest happiness to the greatest number*" which means that there should be maximum happiness and minimum pain where the large number of society should get benefit from a particular law but in connection with the Surrogacy Regulation Act of 2021 does the intending parents getting out of the pain or the pain got increased. Does the piece of legislation is a beneficial piece of legislation? The authors find out in today's modern world do we get anything free of cost starting from education where there was a time of Gurukul (old school education) and now everything got commercialised, then how the legislators and society expect the children born out of surrogacy should not be compensated (altruistic form) and for the nine months a mother should do natural justice to an intending parent by choosing law of morals.

## An Empirical Study of Indian Urban Residents for Resolving Dispute Through ADR

Hypothesis
The surrogacy dispute in India is settled through alternative dispute settlement mechanism
H0- The surrogacy dispute in India can't be settled through alternative dispute settlement mechanism.
H1- The surrogacy dispute in India can't be settled through alternative dispute settlement mechanism
Research Methodology

The authors have done a significant empirical study involving all the urban stakeholders like medical professionals, Indian Advocates, Law researchers and students about the resolving the reproductive challenges through an alternative dispute settlement mechanism. (ADR).

## Research Findings

The authors suggested well-regulated commercial surrogacy and properly regulated abortion laws as a Reproductive-challenges shall be settled through a dispute settlement mechanism especially through Arbitration or Mediation method of resolving. To successfully embrace surrogate mothers in India, it is essential to adopt a comprehensive strategy that combines forward-thinking legal structures with cultural awareness and public education. India has the potential to establish a more inclusive and supportive framework for surrogate mothers. Ukraine's legal structure, characterised by explicit restrictions, effectively protects the rights of surrogate mothers, intended parents, and the resulting child. This framework could potentially serve as a blueprint for India. India can promote the recognition and appreciation of surrogate mothers by implementing comparable legislative measures, thereby diminishing the social stigma surrounding surrogacy. Furthermore, it is essential to promote a cultural transformation by conducting public awareness campaigns and providing education to alter society perspectives. Highlighting the selfless and empathetic qualities of surrogacy can contribute to altering the prevailing story, fostering tolerance and understanding towards women who serve as surrogate mothers. India may cultivate a conducive atmosphere for the acceptance and appreciation of surrogate mothers by implementing legal reforms and promoting societal knowledge. This would facilitate a more progressive approach to reproductive rights and the formation of families. The increasing acceptability of the practice indicates a rising willingness to embrace it, despite the limitations imposed by the existing legal system. India's conflict settlement systems, including as arbitration, mediation, and the legal system, are well-prepared to address surrogacy disputes. The Surrogacy (Regulation) Act, 2021, and the Assisted Reproductive Technology (Regulation) Act, 2021, establish a comprehensive legal framework that outlines precise standards for resolving disputes that may arise from surrogacy arrangements. These mechanisms guarantee the protection of the rights of all parties involved and facilitate the resolution of problems in a systematic and legally valid manner, which can be achieved through the use of alternative dispute resolution methods outside of the court. India's approach to surrogacy demonstrates a harmonious blend of ethical considerations and the rights of individuals aspiring to become parents. While commercial surrogacy is limited, the legal and social landscape is changing, as more people recognise surrogacy as a valid method of forming a family. Hence, the existence of strong dispute resolution processes guarantees the efficient resolution of issues relating to surrogacy in India. The authors found in their empirical research where they investigated various stakeholders including advocates, researchers, common people, medical professionals' responses were out of 207 responses, 58 percentage of the stakeholders believes that ADR (Alternative Dispute Resolution) can be better solution rather than surrogacy and ART boards constituted in India which is not in execution actively and few common people know about such authorities. Therefore, ADR could be the best proposed mechanism to resolve the disputes.

*Figure 1. Do you think surrogacy disputes can be settled through Alternative Dispute Settlement Mechanism rather than Board?*

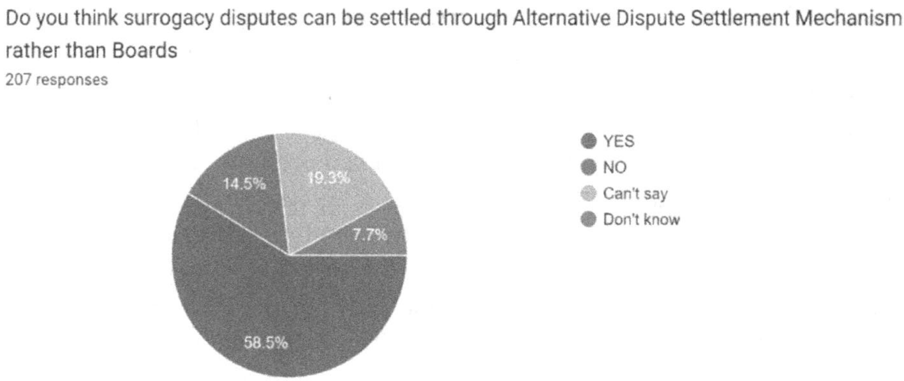


*Note: Authors own empirical research*

## THE VARIEGATED ASPECTS OF REPRODUCTIVE CHALLENGES

### An Ethical Dilemma of RMP's (Registered Medical Practitioners)

As earlier before the surrogacy regulation there were no RMP's and underground commercialization of surrogate industry were carried out with the help of middlemen which is now contemporarily forbidden but the current ethical concerns are the growing IVF/fertility clinics making large sum of money from the IP's (intending parents) who promises the birth of biological children. These IVF treatments are not cost-friendly and many clinics are unethically making monetary benefits.

## An Unethical Behavioral Aspect of the Surrogate Mothers

The authors are not biased about the rights of surrogate mothers as they render a neutral opinion towards the rights of the parties. However, the author witnessed many International and national movies and stories of surrogate women who emotionally involves with intending father and the child where the rights of intending mother get infringed and no single country legally address such rights and penalties.

## The Moral and Legal aspects of IP's (Intending Parents)

The child born through surrogacy is often abandoned in the case of disability. As there are many cases where children having various disability are abandoned and expected to be kept with the surrogate mother or given for adoption.

## The Social Acceptance of those facing Reproductive Challenges

An unmarried single woman who goes through abortion, surrogacy, adoption, live-in marriages are not socially acceptable. The acceptance of surrogate mothers, infertile intending parents, the social status of surrogate children in India are never acceptable. However, there are certain religions in India forbids abortion, surrogacy, adoption and considered as a sin. The Surrogacy is considered as noble profession and work in countries like Ukraine and Russia. (Veronika Siegl 2023). The author is referring another side of coin from a speech delivered by Olivia Maurel at Czech Republic Parliament who was born through surrogacy and she has to fight for the offspring of today's generation born through surrogacy. The mental trauma that Olivia faced for her whole life that she felt abandoned and depressed like an adopted child as she was born through traditional surrogacy where India is having a good practice of 2021 regulated Law for allowing gestational surrogacy.

## An Emotional Aspect and the Rising Death of Surrogate Mother and Child

As India forbids commercial surrogacy and the question here is whether death of a surrogate woman and child isn't possible in altruistic surrogacy as the new law talks about near relative so who are the parties where the insurance coverage of the death or damage could be claimed for child and surrogate mother as death is something which is uncertain during natural birth or any forms of surrogate birth. The onus of pre-natal and post-natal care is also a need of an hour which is now a days covered through Insurance companies.

## A Case Study

A forty-two-year-old woman who delivered twins and later she died due to chronic health issues, a doctor of AIIMS Delhi (Denton S.) highlighted that there is lack of governing laws in India which is still silent in new surrogacy regulation act of 2021.The Another case of USA, where a surrogate mother died (Friends of Lazarus Association) named Michelle in California (CBC-Network 2020) a wife and mother of a child already who died after baby's delivery but India having same practice in the new law of 2021 that surrogate mother should at least have one biological child and medically second time pregnancy can give more complications which should be removed when the term commercialisation of surrogacy already got prohibited.

## Future Consideration and Access to effective remedial Laws: Need of an Hour

The reproductive challenges for women are mainly due to lack of medical, legal, ethical, economic facilities and social acceptance. The urban working woman who economically affords to freeze their eggs (her gametes) can easily find a family at later stages which is growing very popular in urban cities but there are less social and family acceptability. The Surrogacy especially commercial surrogacy and well-regulated abortion laws can be a solution for certain reproductive health challenges for the urban woman despite of her marriage as child is a creature which is not only an essential for a couple but also for a single parent particularly for individuals and couples who are unable to conceive or carry a pregnancy to due to many factors like infertility which is a major cause in today's time also reported by the world health organisation, multiple IVF (in-vitro-fertilization) failures and surrogacy is the best option for those couples but in India challenge to find a near relative as a surrogate mother and same as an orphan child to find a surrogate, genetic disorders, challenges for the LGBTQ individuals, those women who are endangered to carry the pregnancy they also can opt for surrogacy if they can afford the treatment which is also not a cost effective and pre-determined for the procedure as it also depends from the case to case basis.

## CONCLUSION AND WAYS FORWARD

On a concluding note, the authors have analysed various legislation in India as to conclude that the more law the less justice and India having the supreme law of land as an Indian Constitution of 1950 and various other reproductive legislation which is also yet challenging in the Indian courts as there are no single dispute mechanism and the authors suggesting alternative dispute settlement mechanism shall be the best way to resolve the dispute as empirically tested by the authors and doctrinal analysis of today's contemporary times of infertility among the couples or a woman who is unable to reproduce. The Surrogacy and Abortion are codified legislation in India which is key highlight of Historical School of Jurisprudence (Savigny and Bentham). The authors also believe that the rising cases in India and USA, United States of America for the surrogate mother's death and also if a child is not born alive who shall bear the consequences of such circumstances. Here, the author suggests that during the agreement done with the surrogate mother, intended parents and insurance company, registered clinics and others parties related to it. There shall be an *Alternative Dispute Settlement for the reproductive challenges for surrogacy, abortion, IVF procedures etc* where the dispute shall be resolved either through Arbitration, Mediation and Conciliation methods where India having a legislation for this is known as The Arbitration and Conciliation Act 1996 where the Arbitrator shall be appointed by the parties to the dispute to resolve the case within a stipulated time given under the aforesaid Act. The reproductive challenges shall be taught to the students which would enable youngsters to comprehend the concept and help lessen the societal stigma around it. It is imperative for medical providers to prioritise the holistic well-being of surrogate mothers, encompassing both their physical and emotional needs, in order to provide them with optimal care during the surrogacy process and also to provide legal assistance and financial assistance to surrogate mothers to prevent their exploitation and ensure they have access to essential resources. The government and policymakers are responsible for formulating policies that aim to enhance the well-being of surrogate mothers. It is crucial to prioritise tackling the socioeconomic issues faced by these individuals and to ensure that they are not subjected to marginalisation or discrimination. The use of arbitration and mediation to address surrogacy disputes highlights the potential of these procedures to offer efficient, adaptable, and less confrontational outcomes in comparison to conventional litigation. Mediation is highly regarded for its capacity to maintain relationships and promote collaboration, while arbitration provides a conclusive answer when required. Nevertheless, it is crucial to effectively address issues such as unequal distribution of power, the possibility of manipulation, and ethical considerations regarding the protection of private information in order to guarantee equitable and impartial results. As surrogacy progresses as a reproductive choice, it is crucial to conduct additional study and develop alternative dispute resolution (ADR) methods to effectively handle the distinct and intricate challenges that arise in this context.

## REFERENCES

Arbitration and Conciliation Act. 1996., Act, No. 26, Acts of Parliament, 2021 (India).

Bachman, S. (2023). Lessons from Ukraine: Shifting international surrogacy policy to protect women and children. Journal of Public and International Affairs. https://jpia.princeton.edu/news/lessons-ukraine-shifting-international-surrogacy-policy-protect-women-and-children

Baillie, A. (2018). The effectiveness of arbitration in resolving surrogacy disputes: A comparative analysis. *International Journal of Law and the Family*, 32(4), 300–316.

Brodsky, A. (2019). Alternative dispute resolution in family law: Navigating the complexities of surrogacy agreements. *Family Law Quarterly*, 53(2), 147–170.

Brown, L. Louise Brown on 40 years of IVF: 'I was the world's first IVF baby; this is my story'. The Independent [Internet]. 2018 Jul 25 [cited 2024 Jul 17]. Available from: https://www.independent.co.uk/life-style/health-and-families/ivf-baby-louise-brown-story-test-tube-world-first-40th-anniversary-a8455956.html

Center for Reproductive Rights. (n.d.). The world's abortion laws. Available from https://reproductiverights.org/maps/worlds-abortion-laws/

Crosbie, T., & Kirkman, S. (2023). From war to law? The role of the rule of law in international peacebuilding. *International Peacekeeping*, 28(4), 515–537.

Altruistic Surrogacy and Dispute Resolution:Dyer, J. (2020). The role of arbitration in resolving disputes in altruistic surrogacy agreements. *Journal of Family Law*, 58(2), 145–162.

Gilmore, S., & Herring, J. (2017). Mediation in surrogacy: Legal and ethical considerations. *Child and Family Law Quarterly*, 29(1), 25–43.

Johnson v. Calvert, 5 Cal. 4th 84, 19 Cal. Rptr. 2d 494, 851 P.2d 776 (1993).

Khurtsidze, I. (2016). *Legal regulation of surrogacy in Georgia* (Special Edition). European Scientific Journal.

Krawiec, K., & Rampell, A. (2020). Power dynamics in surrogacy arbitration: Legal representation and fairness. *Harvard Journal of Law & Gender*, 43(2), 95–118.

Marinelli, S., Del Rio, A., Straccamore, M., Negro, F., & Basile, G. (2022). The armed conflict in Ukraine and the risks of inter-country surrogacy: The unsolved dilemma. European Review for Medical and Pharmacological Sciences, 26(5646 Malavika R. A Critical Analysis of the Surrogacy Regulation Bill 2016 [Internet]. Feminism in India. 2016 Aug 31 [cited 2024 Jul 17]. Available from: https://feminisminindia.com/2016/08/31/critical-analysis-surrogacy-regulation-bill-2016/

Mason, C. (2016). Challenges in arbitration of surrogacy agreements: Addressing power imbalances and fairness. *International Journal of Law, Policy and the Family*, 30(4), 369–387.

Millbank, J. (2018). Transparency and accountability in ADR processes for surrogacy disputes. *Journal of Legal Ethics*, 41(3), 271–288.

Neel, M. M. (2019). Carrying capacity: Should Georgia enact surrogacy regulation? *Georgia Law Review (Athens, Ga.)*, 54(1), 333–360.

Patton, M. (2021). Hybrid approaches to resolving surrogacy disputes: Combining mediation and arbitration with litigation safeguards. *Journal of Dispute Resolution*, 2021(2), 200–215.

Perdue, M., & Jenkinson, L. (2018). Surrogacy and mediation: A study of outcomes and satisfaction among parties involved in surrogacy disputes. *Journal of Mediation & Arbitration*, 10(1), 55–74.

Reuters. (2023, April 5). Which countries allow commercial surrogacy? https://www.reuters.com/world/which-countries-allow-commercial-surrogacy-2023-04-05/

Arbitration in Family Law:Rivas, C. (2021). Arbitration in family law: An emerging tool for resolving disputes in surrogacy agreements. *Family Law Review*, 12(1), 88–103.

Scott, E. (2020). Mediation in surrogacy disputes: Balancing the interests of the surrogate and intended parents. *Journal of Family Law*, 45(3), 321–345.

Smith, R., & Robertson, J. (2019). ADR versus litigation in surrogacy disputes: A comparative analysis. *Family Court Review*, 57(4), 587–605.

Thompson, S. (2017). Ethical implications of mediation in surrogacy disputes: Ensuring fairness and avoiding coercion. *Bioethics*, 31(6), 420–429.

What are the international surrogacy laws by country? Surrogate.com. Available from: https://surrogate.com/intended-parents/surrogacy-laws-and-legal-information/what-are-the-international-surrogacy-laws-by-country/

Zois, A. (n.d.). In Ukraine and Russia, surrogacy is seen as work. Available: https://www.zois-berlin.de/en/publications/meet-the-author/in-ukraine-and-russia-surrogacy-is-seen-as-work

## KEY TERMS AND DEFINITION

**ADR:** Alternative Dispute Resolution by a way of Arbitration, Mediation and Conciliation.

**ART:** Assisted Reproductive Technology.

**Altruistic Surrogacy:** The surrogacy in which no charges, expenses, fees, remuneration or monetary incentive except the medical expenses incurred on surrogate mother and the insurance coverage for the surrogate mother are given to the surrogate mother or her dependents or her representative.

**Commercial Surrogacy:** - It is also known as Compensated surrogacy which means commercialization of surrogacy services or procedures or its component services including selling or buying of human embryo or trading in the sale or purchase of human embryo or gametes or selling or buying or trading the services of surrogate motherhood by way of giving payment/ Rented womb.

**Gestational Surrogacy:** It is also known as gestational carrier takes place when an embryo created by in vitro fertilization (IVF) technology is implanted in a surrogate.

**IP:** Intending parents

**IVF:** In vitro fertilization

**NFPP-National Family Planning Program:**

**NPP:** National Population Policy

**NRHM & NUHM:** The National Rural and Urban Health Mission

**RMP:** Registered Medical Practitioners

**Traditional Surrogacy:** The surrogate mother eggs are used, making her the biological mother of the child she carries

## ENDNOTE

1 Chanda Keswani vs. State of Rajasthan AIR 2020.

# Chapter 10
# Navigating Human Rights and Ethical Challenges in Compensation Models of Commercial Surrogacy: Comparative Analysis

**V. Chaitra**
https://orcid.org/0000-0002-5983-6123
*Christ University, India*

**K. Hema**
https://orcid.org/0000-0002-3189-0996
*Christ University, India*

## ABSTRACT

*The critics argue that commercial surrogacy would result in commodification of pregnancy, exploitation of economically vulnerable women in the lower social strata and ultimately leads to depersonalised reproduction process. However, the advocates of commercial surrogacy contend that commercial surrogacy provides financial stability to the surrogate mother and is a boon for those infertile parents who want to safeguard their privacy and are reluctant to involve their family members or relatives as surrogate mothers. This research study aims to explore and analyse compensation models in commercial surrogacy arrangements across different jurisdictions in the context of ensuring equitable treatment and protection of human rights of surrogate mothers. In meticulous detail, this study examines the ethical, legal, cultural and economic dimensions, particularly regarding the compensation offered to surrogate mothers for their labour.*

DOI: 10.4018/979-8-3693-7837-3.ch010

## 1. INTRODUCTION

Surrogacy, predominantly a solution for fertility issues, parenthood and recurrent miscarriages is not a recent phenomenon, rather has become a new normal over the past few decades. It has historical roots as different forms of surrogacy have been cited in the biblical reference, *Book of Genesis* as well as in the pages of Indian mythology (Jargilo, 2016). Surrogacy, in the present day, is medically assisted and relatively safer. In the chronological context, the biological father of the child impregnated the surrogate mother, but in 1884, surrogacy was carried on through artificial insemination using eggs of the surrogate mother, thus establishing the genetic link with the child (South California Reproductive Centre, 2016). It was only in the 1980s the IVF embryo transfer was successful (Cohen, 2005), which is also known as gestational surrogacy. In this form of surrogacy, the intended mother is not genetically related to the child as the embryo is created using the egg of the intended mother and sperm of the intended father. The embryo is transferred to the surrogate's uterus who carries and gives birth to the child (Ramalingam et al., 2016). Over the years, altruistic surrogacy (no payment to the surrogate beyond medical expenses) and commercial surrogacy (financial compensation beyond medical expenses) have gained prominence in the field of gestational surrogacy. In the beginning, altruistic surrogacy was permitted in many countries across the globe and commercial surrogacy was widely prohibited. However, with the changing times, commercial surrogacy has been legalised in a few countries and is gradually witnessing increased global acceptance.

There are three common responses to surrogacy adopted by countries globally. While surrogacy is absolutely prohibited in countries like Germany, France and China, both altruistic and commercial surrogacies are permitted in countries like Israel, Russia, Ukraine and a few US states (Yuri Hibina, 2023). However, in the UK, India, Australia, Canada, Hong Kong, South Africa, Greece, and Iceland, only altruistic surrogacy is permitted, while commercial surrogacy is prohibited (Yuri Hibina, 2023). It is comprehensible by these approaches that the legal framework which regulates surrogacy varies widely between countries. Though there are various international conventions to protect child and women rights, there is currently no international instrument that specifically focuses on surrogacy and rights of the stakeholders involved in the process. In the absence of model guidelines that can be relied upon by the countries and each country having a distinct regulatory approach to surrogacy, challenges like establishing parentage, citizenship, inadequate compensation, custody, childrens' rights in transnational surrogacy are inevitable. However, the scope of this paper is restricted to compensation models within the context of commercial surrogacy as this topic has received limited research attention. For the purpose of this research, the term compensation models refers to the compensation structure and multiple components of compensation provided to the surrogate such as medical expenses, health insurance, remuneration for gestation carrier services and other related expenses. This study aims to explore and analyse compensation models in commercial surrogacy arrangements across different jurisdictions by relying upon the relevant statutes and secondary data sources (case-studies, interviews, govt. survey reports, NGO etc) to gain valuable insights and propose policy reforms. The criteria for selecting countries for the study include those where commercial surrogacy is legalised *(Israel, Russia, Ukraine and certain states in the USA).* In meticulous detail, the study also examines the ethical, legal, human rights and economic dimensions, particularly regarding the financial compensation offered to surrogate mothers for their labour.

The paper is structured as follows-

*Section I* provides an introduction to the concept of surrogacy, development of altruistic and commercial surrogacy, critically examines the divisive discourse that inevitably arises due their contrasting approaches. *Section II* critically presents, in particular, human rights and ethical implications of financial compensation in the enforcement of commercial surrogacy contracts. It presents a comprehensive review in the light of international standards and feminist and economics principles. *Section III* explores and discusses compensation models with respect to gestational services across various jurisdictions to compare and contrast the financial compensation under diverse legal systems to understand and analyse their adherence to human rights and ethical principles like autonomy, exploitation, adequate compensation and fairness. *Section IV* provides a conclusion summarising the findings and suggestions for further reforms to guarantee fair treatment and protection of the rights of the surrogate mothers.

## 1.1 Development of Altruistic and Commercial Surrogacy

Gestational surrogacy as we know it today can be traced back to the 19th century, but traditional surrogacy has been mentioned in the biblical pages, Hindu mythologies, and legal codes of various civilizations. The Old Testament at around 2000 BC remarks that Ishmael, son of Abraham and Sarah was born to Hegar, a handmaid of Sarah through traditional surrogacy (Meinke, Sue A, 1988) Hindu mythology boasts of traditional surrogacy where the embryo of Vasudev and Devaki was transferred to Rohini's womb to save the baby from being killed by Kamsa (Niyogi, 1988). In the Mesopotamian civilization, the Hammurabi Code mentions that if the wife gives her husband a maid-servant in cases where she is unable to conceive and the maid bears a child with him, he shall not sell her for money (Paramjit S. Jaswal & Jasdeep Kaur, 2021). Society has always witnessed surrogacy in different forms.

Reproductive services have also been provided for a sum of money from the middle age to modern times (Patel NH et al, 2018).

The first case of artificial insemination was reported in the 1700s when Dr. John Hunter successfully helped an infertile husband in becoming a father by inseminating his wife using a sperm injection, moving away from traditional surrogacy and paving the way for gestational surrogacy. In 1978, a traditional surrogacy agreement was first drafted by a US-based lawyer Keane, but the agreement lacked any clause for monetary compensation to the surrogate (Campbell, Jhonell, 2021). In 1978, gestational surrogacy saw a breakthrough when Louise Brown was born of in vitro fertilisation where the genetic material of the intending parents was transferred to the womb of the surrogate mother (Jessica M. Caamano, 2016). This marked a salient scientific milestone where the surrogate mother delivered a baby with whom she had no biological or genetic link. Two years later, the US witnessed the first commercial surrogacy contract where $11,500 was paid for surrogacy services to Elizabeth Kane (Kane, 1989).

Gestational surrogacy is often considered better than traditional surrogacy on various fronts. In genetic surrogacy or traditional surrogacy, the sperm of the donor or the intended father fertilises the egg of the surrogate mother (Mondal, Verma et al, 2012). Consequently, the baby carries with it the genetic material of the surrogate mother. In contrast, gestational surrogacy involves the artificial fertilisation of the egg and the sperm of the intending parents, and the embryo is placed in the host or surrogate mother's womb. The point of difference between genetic surrogacy and gestational surrogacy is the genetic connection of the baby with the mother or the lack of it (Patel NH et al, 2018). In traditional surrogacy, the surrogate mother is also the biological mother and this arrangement is prone to certain inevitable emotional complexities and legal challenges. The intending parents have no claim whatsoever on the child as she is the biological mother unless she consents otherwise, thus, leaving the room for potential disturbances. However, in gestational surrogacy, the child is born without any genetic link with the surrogate mother, and the parental rights are more definitive and legally certain.

The Baby M (Melissa Stern) case *(109 N.J. 396 (1988)* is the most controversial development in the field of traditional surrogacy and law. Mary Beth Whitehead agreed to be a surrogate mother for the intended parents, Mr. & Mrs. Stern for a consideration of $10,000. Through artificial insemination Mr. Stern's sperms, Beth Whitehead was impregnated, contributed to the genetic material of the child born, establishing her biological connection with the child. The surrogate mother denied handing over the child to the intended parents and litigated for the custody of the child. The New Jersey Supreme Court had ruled that the surrogacy contract was illegal and custody was granted to Mr. Stern with visitation rights to the surrogate mother while registering her name in the birth certificate as legal mother. In the light of these unavoidable issues, many jurisdictions have recognised and legalised gestational surrogacy which is also known as 'IVF surrogacy' as a solution to the infertility problem.

The next significant transition in gestational surrogacy and its legal aspects was when the surrogate mother refused to relinquish her right over the child, though she had no biological or genetic link with the child. In, Johnson v. Calvert *(No. S023721. May 20, 1993)*, the California Supreme Court ruled that when a baby is delivered by a surrogate who has no genetic connection with the baby, the legal parents of the child would be the commissioning couple and not the surrogate mother. Consequently, California became the first state to recognise and validate gestational surrogacy contracts. The early innovations and legal issues in the USA paved the way for reforms in reproductive technology, significantly influencing fertility treatments and surrogacy practices across the globe (*History of IVF: Origin and Developments of the 20th Century | PFCLA*, 2022).

## 1.2 Examining Standpoints: Altruistic v. Commercial Surrogacy

Investigating perspectives on altruistic v. commercial surrogacy is crucial for deconstructing the financial compensation aspects of the latter. In altruistic surrogacy, the surrogate mother is paid for the medical expenses only to the extent of the pregnancy and until the delivery of the child whereas in commercial surrogacy, the surrogate mother is paid a fee over and above the pregnancy and delivery expenses (Blazier J, Janssens R., 2020). Commercial surrogacy is alleged by some to be inherently exploitative of women. However, whether it is exploitative or not is highly debatable. To consider commercial surrogacy exploitative, it's necessary to show that her welfare deteriorates more than what justice allows (Machinton, 1987). If the surrogate's welfare is disproportionately affected by commercial surrogacy, then the same holds for altruistic surrogacy. The payment of money will not neutralise the harm, in case suffered, by the surrogate mother, be it in altruistic surrogacy or commercial surrogacy. The next ethical debate that appears is the underpayment to the surrogate mother. It is argued that the commissioning parents possibly underpay the surrogate mother and exploit her for the services provided (Cara Luckey, 2011). However, the underpayment to the surrogate mothers can be redressed by law. A minimum amount can be prescribed by the law and thus, underpayment in the cases of commercial surrogacy stands resolved (Wilkinson, 2015). Another connected ethical issue would be that poor women are more likely to be exploited than rich women (Meinke, 1988). With informed consent of the health and emotional consequences, if a woman from an economically disadvantaged position chooses to be a surrogate to alleviate her family from poverty, the law should respect her financial decision and autonomy, rather than stand against her and prohibit commercial surrogacy.

The follow-up ethical consideration is the commodification of reproductive services. It is argued that commercial surrogacy commodifies reproductive labour, women and children (Arneson, 1992). Society has normalised the commodification of various types of labour but not reproductive labour because the bond between the mother and the child is considered sacred and emotional. The social conventions, traditions and culture impose the sanctity of women's reproductive labour, but it need not be necessarily a fact (Baumhofer, 2012). Assuming that reproductive labour is somehow special, there is no reason to believe that commodification will devalue its special nature (McLachlan & Swales, 2009). Nevertheless, it is argued in the Kantian philosophy that humans are to be treated as an end in themselves and not as a means. Commercial surrogacy is being criticised for commodifying the human body in the framework of Kantian philosophy, which holds that humans should be viewed as ends in themselves rather than as means to an end. (Kant, 1998). Commercial surrogacy risks undermining the surrogate's intrinsic dignity by treating her body as a means to achieve the intended parents' goal of having a child, reducing her to a vessel for another's benefit, which contradicts the Kantian principle of respecting each individual's autonomy and inherent worth. In the context of commercial surrogacy, persons who consider the surrogate mother solely as a tool to fulfil their desire for a child, regardless of the outcome, are morally responsible for limiting her autonomy and dignity to a transactional service. Even if the outcome—bringing a child into the world—is viewed positively, the ethical implications remain, as Kantian ethics requires that all humans be considered as ends in themselves, with full humanity, rather than being used as instruments to achieve the goals of others. Under Kantian ethics, commercial surrogacy is morally unacceptable because it does not completely respect the surrogate's fundamental dignity and liberty as a human. Kant, additionally states that he who has it in mind to make a false promise to others realizes right away that he intends to utilize another human being only as a means, without the other containing in himself the end (Kant, 1998). Applying this philosophy to commercial surrogacy would imply that in the case of commercial surrogacy, if the intended parents or intermediaries enter into the agreement with promises that do not completely respect the surrogate's rights or autonomy, using her body as merely a means to an objective, they risk violating Kant's moral principle. Similar to making a false promise, they may use the surrogate for their own interests without assuring that her well-being, dignity, and autonomy are equally respected in the arrangement. If people treat others as a means to their ends, irrespective of the favourable result, they must be accountable to the moral arguments (Mark, 2021). Naturally, commodification occurs when there is manipulation of the surrogate to the extent that it deprives her of her dignity, autonomy and liberty as a human and makes her vulnerable before society. Commercial surrogates are dehumanised by the middlemen, agencies and brokers and not by the process itself. If there is a law in force to counter the degrading treatment of surrogate mothers, reproductive services would not be commodified.

Another aspect of the contention is the role of informed consent in commercial surrogacy. Along with the consent being free, it is required that the consent shall be informed consent in cases of surrogacy contracts (Shepherd, 2022). Informed consent dictates that the surrogate mother is aware of all the potential consequences of the surrogacy procedure. However, seeking informed consent from the surrogate mother that she would relinquish her baby upon the delivery is not entirely possible as it is difficult to ascertain the emotional and psychological relationship between mother and child even before the pregnancy (Tanderup M, Reddy S et al, 2015). The doctrine of informed consent presumes that people are capable of predicting whether the medical procedure will be beneficial to them. As long as the surrogate mother is capable of making a rational and informed decision based on the information available to her, her consent must be duly acknowledged (Brandao & Garrido, 2022). Informed consent plays a vital role in both altruistic and commercial surrogacy. If informed consent is sufficient and good enough for altruistic surrogacy, it has to be the case also for commercial surrogacy. Money compensation received in commercial surrogacy does not per se have the potential to vitiate the validity of a surrogacy contract.

Along with informed consent, the critics argue that the surrogate mother's autonomy in commercial surrogacy is weakened. Reproductive autonomy is related to the informed choices made by the woman concerning her deliberate decision to conceive, abort, selectively reduce or use birth control methods (Sifris R, 2016). When a State denies her the right to be a surrogate mother, it imposes restrictions on her reproductive autonomy, considering her incapable of making informed decisions about her reproductive health. Autonomy in the case of surrogacy would include firstly the choice of being a surrogate mother, followed by the decisions during pregnancy, selective reduction, nutrition and diets etc till the delivery of the baby (Munjal & Shankar, 2015). Where surrogate agreements are entered voluntarily, there can be no exploitation and discrimination faced neither by the surrogate mother nor the child (Wertheimer, 1997). Money compensation received by the surrogate mother in cases of commercial surrogacy will not negate her reproductive autonomy and rights. The State by permitting altruistic surrogacy and prohibiting commercial surrogacy is in fact imposing restrictions on her reproductive autonomy, financial independence and other allied rights. A woman's reproductive autonomy and rights have to be protected by the State. However, the State by prohibiting commercial surrogacy is devaluing the reproductive labour of the money like the domestic labour of a woman (Cheney, 2018). The State's inability to allow the surrogate mother to be properly compensated for her reproductive services would amount to not recognising her reproductive autonomy (Menon, 2009).

In examining the diverse standpoints surrounding altruistic v. commercial surrogacy, the authors propose that surrogacy should either be prohibited or permitted without discriminating between altruistic and commercial surrogacy as the former is inherently fair practice than the other as both these arrangements can result in emotional challenges and exploitation of the surrogate unless properly regulated.

## 2. HUMAN RIGHTS AND ETHICAL CONSIDERATIONS OF FINANCIAL COMPENSATION WITHIN THE CONTEXT OF COMMERCIAL SURROGACY CONTRACTS

The global statistics relating to commercial surrogacy has been rising with $14 billion in 2022 and is expected to grow by $129 billion in 2032 (Han, 2023). As few countries have legalised commercial surrogacy, intercountry gestational surrogacy has emerged as a form of medical tourism. The commissioning parents from developed countries like Australia, Canada, and France enter into international surrogacy agreements with the surrogates of developing countries like India, Nepal and Thailand (A/HRC/37/60, 2018). The divergent approaches taken by the countries in regulating commercial surrogacy have resulted in the sale of children, gross violation of human rights, exploitation of developing countries by the developed countries etc. In the absence of international model law, it seems difficult to mitigate human rights violations that transpire out of surrogacy, more so in cases of commercial surrogacy (Engel, 2017). There is clearly a divided opinion on reproductive freedom of women in the context of commercial surrogacy and it requires a multifaceted analysis of human rights, ethical and economic considerations. The inevitable question that arises is whether compensation should be provided to surrogate mothers for their reproductive services which is often met with social disapproval and contested as leading to commodification of human reproduction. In order to effectively regulate commercial surrogacy, it is important to find a right balance between ethical and legal consideration surrounding surrogacy, women's reproductive autonomy and freedom to contract. The courts in certain countries have criticised commercial surrogacy arrangements and compared it to a situation where the surrogate child is equivalent to an ordered and delivered product (Suzanne Griffiths & Logan Martin,, 2006). On the other hand, there are contrasting opinions that the "surrogacy contracts are not for resale, they are for a one-of-a-kind creation (Epstein, 1995). In the context of these conflicting viewpoints, *Section II* of this paper critically presents, in particular, human rights and ethical implications of financial compensation in the enforcement of commercial surrogacy contracts. It presents a comprehensive review in the light of international standards and feminist and economics principles.

## 2.1 Human Rights and Ethical Concerns Related to Financial Payments in Commercial Surrogacy Arrangements

The financial compensation aspect of commercial surrogacy raises critical questions about the commodification of human reproduction, exploitation and coercion, health risks etc. In 1988, the Supreme Court of New Jersey, in a notable decision though invalidated commercial surrogacy, while addressing the moral implications surrounding a surrogacy contract between the biological father and the surrogate mother, however remarked "*that without monetary compensation, surrogacy probably would not survive* (Luckey, 2011) In this judgement the court pointed out various critical concerns such as potential health risks, economic exploitation of women in the lower strata and in closing, the suitability of parents, stressing upon the fact that in adoption, an agency is able to place the child with most suitable parents unlike the commercial surrogacy where the child is often given to the parents who offer to pay the most money to the surrogate (re Baby M, 537 A.2d 1227, 1250 (N.J. 1988)).

A key problem, documented in few studies, is that a surrogate mother is not able to safeguard her own interest because the large sums of money involved in surrogacy can entice a woman without realising the full extent of the physical and psychological effect on her as a surrogate carrier which may result in human rights abuses (Rimm, 2009) There have been instances where surrogate mothers have agreed to unreasonable terms and conditions influenced by their social and educational status. In order to protect the surrogates interests, it is necessary to ensure that they fully understand the implications of their decision. One potential reform highlighted in certain studies, is to restrict surrogacy only to those women who have experienced pregnancy and are fully aware of its health and emotional consequences, thus leading to more informed decision-making, See 750 ILL. COMP. STAT. 47/20 (2005). Illinois has chosen to require that the surrogate mother have at least one child of her own before a surrogacy contract will be valid; (Shanley, 1993) Bromham provides an interesting critical perspective to the issue of exploitation in commercial surrogacy, "*To induce anyone to undertake similar employment without reasonable payment would certainly, in other fields, be regarded as exploitative. With surrogates, the reverse seems true and the payment of a fee to a surrogate seems to be the major factor linking surrogacy with accusations of female exploitation*" (Bromham DR, 1995)

In the context of commercial surrogacy there are two aspects of financial compensation. *Firstly,* in a few jurisdictions, any payment in excess of the medical and health insurances to a surrogate mother under surrogacy contract is not permitted. In these situations, the proponents of this type of commercial surrogacy assert that the intended parents compensate the surrogate mother in terms of medical expenses for gestational services, including the mother's prenatal health responsibilities and such arrangements cannot be considered as economic exploitation and commodification of human reproduction as it simply makes a gift of gestational services and lacks any payment or compensation beyond medical expenses (Tuininga, 2008). *Secondly,* there are few countries which allow compensation beyond medical and insurance expenses, which are often criticised as commodification of human reproduction and economic exploitation of socially and economically weaker sections of women by the rich intending parents to bear their children. A compelling line of argument outlined in an article, cited in this study, is that there are situations where payment from the intended parents to the surrogate is unconnected to the actual child i.e although the intending parents in surrogacy agreements postpone the payment until birth, the legal framework might obligate to make prorated payment to the surrogate mother according to the term of the contract regardless of child's health at birth (Tuininga, 2008). This approach highlights that financial payments are made for the gestational role of the surrogate and not for the sale of a child, thus ruling out the argument of commodification of human reproduction. Further validation can be found in the theory of Macpherson which indicates that in surrogacy matters, women are entitled to be paid for the work of gestation (her capacity to labour) and not for the pregnancy itself (personhood of the woman) (Macpherson & Crawford Brough, 1962).

## 2.2 Commercial Surrogacy and the Jurisprudence of International Conventions

Despite the rise in numbers of commercial surrogacy across the globe, in particular intercountry gestational surrogacy as a form of medical tourism, presently there are no international conventions which directly address the critical concerns surrounding these arrangements. It lacks clear provisions to regulate the financial compensation aspects in surrogacy, leading to a scattered approach across the globe. The International Covenant on Civil and Political Rights 1966 holds that every individual has the "right of self-determination", which enables everyone to "freely determine their political status and pursue their economic, social, and cultural development (Art. 1, ICCPR 1966). In the context of surrogacy, this extends to the bodily autonomy of the surrogate mothers in making informed decisions about their involvement in commercial surrogacy, including the terms and conditions of the contract, financial compensation and their well being etc. The Convention on the Elimination of all Forms of Discrimination Against Women 1979 (CEDAW) requires that the state parties do not discriminate against women in their laws and policies, which can restrict the participation of women, on equal terms with men, in the political, social, economic and cultural life (Art. 13, CEDAW, 1979). State Parties are obligated to grant women, in civil matters, a legal capacity identical to that of men and the same opportunities to exercise that capacity. In particular, they shall give women equal rights to conclude contracts and to administer property and shall treat them equally in all stages of procedure in courts and tribunals (Art. 14 CEDAW, 1979).

The reading of the aforementioned provisions in conjunction indicates that women possess the right to make decisions regarding their reproductive choices and to exercise their contractual rights and freedom. CEDAW also obligates the states to eliminate the prejudices and customary practices that promote gender superiority or inferiority, stereotypical gender roles and to take effective steps to guarantee full and equal enjoyment of social, political, and economic rights for women (Art. 5 CEDAW, 1979).

In addition, the International Covenant on Economic, Social, and Cultural Rights 1966 (ICESCR) also holds that all individuals have the fundamental "right of self-determination" (Art. 1 ICESCR, 1966). ICESCR also mandates the state parties to take steps to recognize the right of everyone to the enjoyment of the highest attainable standard of physical and mental health (Art. 12 ICESCR, 1966). On the basis of the reading of the aforementioned implicit provisions, a woman by virtue of the right to self-determination, economic rights and freedom to conclude contracts can enter into surrogacy agreements and exercise their reproductive choice with access to efficient medical service and medical attention. The European Convention on Human Rights (1954) prohibits slavery and forced labour (Art.4, ECHR 1954). However, commercial surrogacy arrangements do not constitute slavery or forced labour when it is entered into by the parties with mutual consent and benefits. These provisions establish minimum standards for the protection of women who make an informed decision for pursuing their economic and social development and in surrogacy, a complete prohibition of commercial surrogacy would lead to the infringement of a woman's autonomy and self-determination.

## 2.3 Feminist and Economic Analysis of Commercial Surrogacy, Freedom to Contract and Reproductive Rights

For this study, the feminist perspective on commercial surrogacy is very significant to understand the exploitation concerns, reproductive autonomy and the rights of surrogate women. As in-vitro fertilisation has paved the way for more reproductive methods, women are faced with new reproductive choices and challenges. There are differing perspectives on the morality of surrogacy among feminists regarding commercial surrogacy. According to some feminists, it violates human dignity, bodily autonomy, exposes women to potential health risks and, being akin to of slavery or prostitution, consider it to be highly exploitative of women (Ramskold LAH, Posner MP, 2013) (Lieber, 1992). There are also concerns about the likely threat to women's autonomy by the application of new reproductive technologies, by enabling the exploitation of their reproductive capacities to advance the interest of the patriarchal dominated social order (Norma J. Wilder, 1986) . However, liberal feminists who support commercial surrogacy claim that every woman has the right to personal autonomy and reproductive freedom, including the choice to enter into commercial surrogacy agreement as long as it is an informed decision of a competent surrogate mother regarding the potential physical, psychological, social, legal and financial risks (Kerian,, 1997). Ramsey defines exploitation in the context of surrogacy as follows and recognizes that not all surrogacy arrangements are exploitative which can be beneficial to all the parties- "*A person is exploited if they are harmed or treated unfairly by another party and if their choice is compromised. The commissioning couple will receive a much-desired child and the surrogate mother... will have the knowledge that she helped them in a way no other could. She may also receive financial compensation for her role* (Ramsey J., 2006). According to Freeman, women in the past have endured health risks during pregnancy, at a time when obstetric care was less advanced (Freeman M, 1999). This leads to an inevitable question, "Do we comment on the risks to bring a child into the world only now financial gain is mentioned?" (Ramskold LAH, Posner MP., 2013).

Judge Dedov, dissenting in the European Court of Human Rights, criticised that "it is extremely hypocritical to prohibit surrogacy in one's own country in order to protect local women, but simultaneously to permit the use of surrogacy abroad" (Paradiso and Campanelli v. Italy (European Court of Human Rights, Grand Chamber, Application No 25358/12, 24 January 2017). In his application of law and economics theory to the validity of enforceability of commercial surrogacy contract, Judge Richard A. Posner assumes that people are "rational maximizers" of their self interest seeking to maximise their personal benefit and will not enter into surrogacy contracts unless they believe that surrogacy will offer mutual benefits (Richard A. Posner, 1989). Under the lenses of economics and law, a contract should be enforced when it makes two people better off (Kaplow & Shavell, 2002). The parties are the best judges of their own welfare and their desire to enter a surrogacy contract should only be interfered by paternalistic intervention in exceptional circumstances (Hatzis, 2009). When the state forbids payment for contract pregnancy it treats reproductive activity as it has traditionally treated women's domestic labour-as unpaid, noneconomic acts of love and nurturing, rather than as work and real economic contributions to family life (Shanley, 1993).

The multifaceted analysis of commercial surrogacy from ethical, human rights, feminist and economics perspective surrogacy do not entirely rule out the freedom of choice and the freedom to contract of women in surrogacy arrangements. Just as the right to choose surrogacy to become a mother is recognised for the intending parents, the choice to become a surrogate mother as a matter of reproductive choice should be taken into account. However, such contracts can only be detrimental to the interests of women, if they are compelled to enter against their free will without obtaining informed consent. In these circumstances, it is the duty of the state to adopt appropriate measures to ensure surrogacy contracts are fair and voluntary.

## 3. REGULATORY APPROACHES TO COMPENSATION PRACTICES IN COMMERCIAL SURROGACY

Several countries have barred compensated surrogacy within their domestic system in the interest of their female population, however authorise their citizens to obtain surrogacy services from other jurisdictions where commercial surrogacy is legally permitted. This is significant and a global concern as economic imbalance between the countries may result in the exploitation of surrogate mothers in the low income countries. Therefore, it is the need of the hour to regulate commercial surrogacy at the global level rather than prohibiting it in the light of rising numbers of commercial surrogacy as a form of medical tourism. This section of the chapter focuses upon countries which practises commercial surrogacy, to explore and analyse their compensatory practices and determine whether it equitably balances between protecting surrogate mothers' rights, preventing exploitation, fair financial compensation and fostering ethical practices in surrogacy. In this research, the authors have also examined the experiences of surrogate mothers and intending parents in commercial surrogacy permissible countries by relying upon the secondary data sources (case-studies, interviews, govt. survey reports, NGO etc) to gain valuable insights and propose policy reforms. The criteria for selection of the countries for the study-*Compensation practices and guidelines in countries with permissive commercial surrogacy laws (e.g. Israel, Russia, Ukraine and certain states in the USA)*. Little research has been done about the compensation models in the permissive commercial surrogacy legal environments across the globe.

### 3.1 Regulatory Framework

***Israel*** has legalised commercial surrogacy in 1996, only to the residents of Israel under the Embryo Carrying Agreements (Agreement Approval and Status of the Newborn) Law 5756-1996 where in all surrogacy agreements should be approved by the approval committee appointed by the Ministry of Health, which is a seven member committee comprising of three doctors with expert degrees in neonatology, gynaecology and internal medicine, a clinical psychologist, social worker, lawyer, and clergyman (Ministry of Health, Israel). The experts in the panel carefully screen and determine the suitability of the surrogate mother including psychological evaluation, surrogate mothers must be unmarried unless the intending parents are unable to secure a surrogate after all reasonable efforts, in which case married women may be permitted. Surrogates must have prior pregnancy experience and be between the ages of 22 and 39 (Ministry of Health, Israel). The other screening requirements include having not more than four children, not being overweight or a smoker, no Caesarean surgery in the past (Teman, 2019).

The legal environment for commercial surrogacy in ***Russia*** has been very liberal with fewer limitations due to their low birth rate and high infertility rates until recently, in 2022 when it was prohibited for foreign nationals (Svitnev, 2007). The law on commercial surrogacy in Russia is scattered across various federal regulations and the orders issued by the Ministry of Health, i.e Federal Law *On the Fundamentals of Public Health Protection in the Russian Federation" of 21.11.2011 N 323-FZ,* Order of the Ministry of Health of the Russian Federation of August 30, 2012 N 107n *On the order of use of assisted reproductive technologies, contraindications and restrictions on their use* and Order of the Ministry of Health of the Russian Federation of October 30, 2012 N 556n *On approval of the standard of medical aid in infertility with the use of assisted reproductive technologies.* To be a surrogate mother, the woman must be aged 20-35 years old, have at least one biological healthy child of her own, have a satisfactory medical report, informed and voluntary consent to surrogacy related medical procedures, written consent of the husband if married and cannot be an egg donor (Para 3, Article 55, Federal Law On the Fundamentals of Public Health Protection in the Russian Federation). In addition, an individual whether married or unmarried can avail the assisted reproductive technologies(Para 3, Article 55, Federal Law On the Fundamentals of Public Health Protection in the Russian Federation). It also mandates that the embryo used in the surrogacy must not contain any genetic material from the surrogate mother, thus distinguishing it from traditional surrogacies where the surrogate's egg is either inseminated or she acts as an egg donor, are equated with sale of child/commodification and are therefore prohibited under Russian Federation laws (Dushina et al, 2017). The licensed surrogacy clinics in Russia provide the parties not only with commercial surrogacy services but also with representatives of legal organisations and screen every applicant in accordance with the laws of the Russian Federation. These clinics assess the potential parents and surrogate mother to identify their medical conditions, mandatory requirement to undergo psychological evaluation, drug testing, and an interview with specialists and in the event a patient fails an screening, the clinic will refuse surrogacy services(Para 3, Article 55, Federal Law On the Fundamentals of Public Health Protection in the Russian Federation). The state registration process of the birth of a child born to a surrogate mother is a standard procedure recognising the right of the mother to approve the registration of the genetic parents as the child's parents(Article 51, Para 4, Family Code of the Russian Federation) nevertheless this provision allows the surrogate mother to bring claims against the intending parents after the child is born(Snitnev, 2007).

Following the ban on commercial surrogacy and prohibition of surrogacy for foreign nationals in India, Thailand, and Nepal due to abuse of human rights of surrogate mother and the child, ***Ukraine*** became a favourable destination for international commercial surrogacy until Russia's invasion in 2022. It is not that there were no concerns in Ukraine until 2022, as the unethical practices like exploitation, criminal activity of the surrogacy agencies had been highlighted by the various stakeholders and requested the Government to act on those issues (Bobyn, Christopher., 2018). The surrogacy practise is similar to that of Russia, but the distinguishing feature is that the Family Code of Ukraine clearly establishes the maternal and paternal affiliation in cases of surrogacies. It inherently recognizes the commissioning/ intending parents in the surrogacy arrangements as the legal parents of the child (Article 123, Family Code of Ukraine).

In the ***USA*** there is no federal law governing surrogacy and its regulation is left to each state. Among the US States, this study focuses on four specific states, California, Illinois, New York and Washington. In California, the intended parents are recognised as legal parents through pre-birth order obtained by the court or after the birth of the child (California Family Code Section 7960-7962). The legal definition of intended parents /commissioning parents extends to an individual, married or unmarried and same-sex parents (Vaughn, 2012). In Illinois, the Gestational Surrogacy Act lays down the guidelines and procedures to safeguard the interest of surrogate, intended parents and children involved in a gestational surrogacy contract. It recognizes the intended parents as the parents of the surrogate child (Section 15(3), Gestational Surrogacy Act, Illinois, USA). To act as a gestational mother, a woman must be 21 years or more, having at least one biological child, undergone the physical health and mental health assessment, legal consultation and owning a health insurance policy covering medical treatment and hospitalisation expenses, which may be secured by the intended parents on behalf of the surrogate mother (Section 20(6), Gestational Surrogacy Act Illinois, USA). The Child-Parent Security Act (CPSA) validated gestational surrogacy in New York which came into force in the year 2021. This law is significant because it provides the unrestricted right to surrogates to make their own health and welfare decisions, including choosing a healthcare professional, whether to terminate or continue a pregnancy, to have access to comprehensive health insurance and independent legal counsel, wherein all these expenses are to be borne by the intended parents (Department of Health, New York). Revised Code of Washington 26.26A.710 sets out the rights and obligation of the surrogate parties. The eligibility criteria for the surrogate mother is the same as that of New York.

## 3.2 Compensatory Models

Under ***Israeli*** law, a commercial surrogacy arrangement mandates a preconception agreement between the intending parents and surrogate mother which must be approved by the approval committee. The committee may include conditions regarding monthly payments to the surrogate mother to cover expenses involved in the execution of the agreement, legal costs and expenses and insurance premiums and compensation for loss of time, suffering, income, temporary loss of earning capacity, or any other reasonable compensation (Section 6, Embryo Carrying Agreements Law 5756-1996). The provision also specifies that neither party to the surrogacy agreement will receive or offer compensation beyond the payments sanctioned by the approval committee (Section 6, Embryo Carrying Agreements Law 5756-1996). While the artificial insemination for the surrogate mother is publicly funded, like other IVF treatments, the gestational surrogate's fee, amounting to 140,000–150,000 NIS ($39,000–42,000) and other related expenses will be borne by the intended parents (Teman E, 2016)

In ***Russia,*** the surrogate mother can be compensated for actual expenses for medical examinations, travel, absence from work, possible injuries and remuneration for her 'service' (Mouliarova, 2019). Remuneration generally ranges between US$ 15,000 to US$ 30,000, with the upper limit being US$ 100,000 (Svitnev K., 2010).In practice, surrogate contracts in Russia also include certain conditions to limit the surrogate mother's rights to physical integrity/autonomy in the interest of the surrogate child and intending parents, such as prohibitions on pregnancy termination without medical reasons, restrictions on her sexual activity, and the use of alcohol and if a surrogate voluntarily agrees to these restrictions, she is entitled to compensation accordingly, which can be specified in the contract and in a case, the Moscow City Court confirmed that if a surrogate mother breaches these contractually agreed-upon restrictions, the contract may stipulate reduced compensation (Viktoriya Omelchenko, 2011).

The average compensation for the surrogates in ***Ukraine*** ranges between 35,000 to 58,000 USD paid in portions at different stages of pregnancy and after childbirth and the total program cost is determined by the surrogate mother's compensation for the services along with associated expenses, including medical examinations, IVF procedures, pregnancy management, childbirth, medications, and legal support (*Surrogacy in Ukraine:IVMED*) (Dolzhenko,, n.d.). However, the surrogates have reported that companies involved in surrogacy paid them as little as $350 USD (Kitson, 2018) indicating that the compensation paid by the intending parents do not reach the surrogates thus exploiting the surrogate labour only to maximise the companies own interests.

The ***U.S***. News and World Report records that the standard expenses of a gestational surrogacy ranges from $100,000 to $150,000 (Snider, 2020) with California exceeding this limit (Field, 2014). The costs and expenses include various components such as fees paid to the agencies, the surrogate services fee (often $30,000 to $50,000), healthcare costs, insurance costs, legal fees, and other incidental expenses. In addition, the agencies involved in gestational surrogacy can charge high fees. For instance, in California the agencies earn as much as the surrogate mother for their services provided in matching the surrogate with the intended parents with the fees escalating with every IVF attempt (Morrissey, 2015). In Illinois, in addition to reasonable compensation paid for the surrogate, the intended parents must also reimburse for the reasonable expenses including, without limitation, medical, legal, or other professional expenses (Section 25, Gestational Surrogacy Act Illinois, USA). Gestational surrogacy costs can be expensive in New York ranging between between $60,000 and $150,000 which include legal fees, medical expenses, surrogacy agency fees, surrogate's compensation (payments to a person acting as surrogate are limited to the duration of the pregnancy and up to eight weeks postpartum) and other miscellaneous expenses (Department of Health, New York, 2021).

## 3.3 Socio-Legal Implication: Impact on the Surrogate Mothers and Intending Parents

Although there are laws and procedural safeguards in place in countries which practise commercial surrogacy, the experiences of surrogates and intending parents often tell a different story. The authors explored and examined the experiences of surrogate mothers in countries where commercial surrogacy is permitted by analysing secondary data sources such as case studies, interviews, government survey reports, and NGO publications. The findings indicate that commercial surrogacy poses significant socio-legal implication, in particular brought to attention, by experiences where surrogate mothers face long term medical complications and insufficient compensation. For instance, in Illinois a surrogate suffered permanent medical complications, received poor compensation and did not have effective legal representation, thus making the experience of surrogacy either empowering or exploitative dependent on various factors (Berk HL., 2020). According to the American College of Obstetricians and Gynecologists women who undergo multiple gestations are more likely to suffer from adverse health conditions like preeclampsia, gestational diabetes, preterm birth, Caesarean birth, as well as postpartum depression (The American College of Obstetricians and Gynecologists, 2019). Other studies also establish that severe risks include gestational hypertension, anaemia, miscarriage, and postpartum haemorrhage (Stanford's Children Health, n.d.). Throughout this research study, in the examination of the regulatory approaches of selected jurisdictions, the authors did not find any provisions which provided compensation to the surrogates for long-term health consequences following surrogacy. Though the statutes mandate the intended parents to pay for the health insurance of the surrogate, it is obvious that the latter will pay it only for the duration of the pregnancy. In Ukraine, surrogates report forced termination of pregnancies by the intended parents, inadequate compensation, unsafe and unhygienic living conditions provided by surrogacy agencies, poor prenatal and postnatal health care, thus leading to long term chronic health issues (Roache & Everingham, 2018). These instances only indicate that the rights and autonomy of the surrogate is compromised, often leading to economic exploitation due to underpayment. There are also reports of surrogate children with disabilities being abandoned by the intended parents putting the children at risk and leaving them stateless (Horn, 2019). The overall well being of the child born through surrogacy arrangements is undermined in cases of abandonment/neglect by the intended parents consequently leading to lack of legal recognition thus restricting the surrogate child's access to fundamental rights and legal protection in any country. According to the interviewees, on the assertion that children are sold in commercial surrogacy and should be banned, argue that the surrogate mother is not carrying her own child but rather the child of the parents who have contracted to use the company's services, view it as boon for infertile couples (Dushina et al, 2016).

The findings from the analysis indicate that regulations governing compensation in commercial surrogacy are heterogeneous and this will lead to financial exploitation of surrogates, particularly in jurisdictions with a lenient regulatory framework. The jurisdictions analysed in the study do not address the situation where the child is not wanted/abandoned by the intended parents involving disabled children born through surrogacy or in the event of the death or separation of intended parents. These unfortunate circumstances have resulted in surrogate children becoming stateless. In the era of globalisation, it is the need of the hour to protect the rights of the surrogate mother and surrogate children through global cooperation to establish uniform surrogacy standards to mitigate the conflicts that arise due to the different laws in the surrogate and intended parents countries. The Hague Conference Experts' Group on the Parentage/Surrogacy Project is a ray of hope in this regard.

## 4. FUTURE RESEARCH DIRECTIONS

Commercial surrogacy can be further explored to identify the psychological and emotional challenges faced by the surrogate mother in the due course of pregnancy and the delivery of the baby. Selective reduction and abortion poses a challenge in commercial surrogacy in the countries where abortions are banned like in the US, which requires further research. With the differences in the culture, religion, traditions among the States, research has to be conducted to understand the standpoint of each State on commercial surrogacy in the light of the differences. An empirical research can be undertaken to understand the real-life experiences of a surrogate mother in commercial surrogacy to understand the implications of money compensation in the surrogate contracts.

## 5. CONCLUSION

The analysis of the findings of this research stresses the requirement for global standard practices rather than absolute prohibition. Banning commercial surrogacy at the outset might seem like an effective means of addressing legal and ethical questions like underpaying surrogate mothers and exploitation of women, but it consequently lead to illicit practise of commercial surrogacy carried out on the black market which would only increase exploitation and increase allied crimes. Furthermore, resolving human rights abuses linked to commercial surrogacy—like discrimination, exploitation, and child trafficking—needs cross-border cooperation on an international scale. A comprehensive approach to this global issue can be accomplished by having regulation in place covering citizenship and nationality, informed consent standards, clearly laid down the rights and obligations of the parties to surrogacy and standard compensatory practices. By putting these rules into place, we could establish an environment in which commercial surrogacy is carried out morally and lawfully, safeguarding the interests of all parties concerned.

Given the differences in how commercial surrogacy is treated legally around the world—some nations forbid it, while others allow it—there are many obstacles and potential for abuse. Due to this inconsistent approach, the regulatory framework becomes fragmented, increasing the danger of abuse and weakening safeguards for surrogate mothers and their children. The intended couples residing in counties with stringent regulation/ where commercial surrogacy is prohibited may simply avail the reproductive labour from countries with less regulation giving rise to cross border surrogacy disputes in case they abandon the child leaving it stateless.

On the basis of the combined reading of the international conventions such as ICCPR, ICESCR, CEDAW, a woman by virtue of the right to self-determination, economic rights and freedom to conclude contracts guaranteed under these conventions can enter into surrogacy agreements and exercise her reproductive choice with access to efficient medical service and medical attention. These provisions establish minimum standards for the protection of women who make an informed decision for pursuing their economic and social development and in surrogacy, a complete prohibition of commercial surrogacy would lead to the infringement of a woman's autonomy and self-determination. The multifaceted analysis of commercial surrogacy from ethical, human rights, feminist and economics perspective surrogacy do not entirely rule out the freedom of choice and the freedom to contract of women in surrogacy arrangements. However, such contracts can only be detrimental to the interests of women, if they are compelled to enter against their free will without obtaining informed consent. In these circumstances, it is the duty of the state to adopt appropriate measures to ensure surrogacy contracts are fair and voluntary.

The findings of the comparative analysis point out that countries with permissive commercial surrogacy arrangements conduct physical health and psychological evaluation to determine the suitability of the surrogate and also mandate that the compensation to the surrogate from the intended couple cover the entire costs and expenses of surrogacy including various components such as fees paid to the agencies, the surrogate services fee, healthcare costs during pregnancy and few months after child birth, insurance costs, legal fees, and other incidental expenses. However the experiences of the surrogates indicate that they face long term medical complications and insufficient compensation at the hands of intended couples/ surrogacy agencies. To resolve this issue, it is important to have standardised surrogacy contracts indicating compensation rates, medical coverage/insurance for long term health consequences, grounds for reduced compensation to the surrogate etc. In addition, clear guidelines for the operation of surrogacy agencies and independent bodies to monitor their compliance should mitigate the difficulties associated with the compensatory practices across different jurisdictions. The Hague Conference Experts' Group on the Parentage/Surrogacy Project is a crucial development in the light of rise of commercial surrogacy cases as a form of medical tourism and is a ray of hope to address the surrogacy related issues globally and a directive to drafting of domestic legislations.

## REFERENCES


Berk, H. L. (2020). Savvy Surrogates and Rock Star Parents: Compensation Provisions, Contracting Practices, and the Value of Womb Work. *Law & Social Inquiry*, 45(2), 398–431. DOI: 10.1017/lsi.2019.57

Blazier, J., & Janssens, R. (2020). Regulating the international surrogacy market:the ethics of commercial surrogacy in the Netherlands and India. *Medicine, Health Care, and Philosophy*, 23(4), 621–630. DOI: 10.1007/s11019-020-09976-x PMID: 32929622

Bobyn, C. (2018, December 14). *Inside Ukraine's surrogacy industry where Australians are travelling to have a family*. ABC. Retrieved September 8, 2024, from https://www.abc.net.au/news/2018-12-15/inside-ukraines-surrogacy-industry/10614172

Bromham, D. R. (1995). Surrogacy: Ethical, legal, and social aspects. *Journal of Assisted Reproduction and Genetics*, 12(8), 509–516. DOI: 10.1007/BF02212913 PMID: 8589569

Caamano, J. M. (2016). International, commercial, gestational surrogacy through the eyes of children born to surrogates in Thailand: A cry for legal attention. *BUL Rev.*, 96, 571.

Campbell, J. (2021). Gestational Surrogacy Contract Terms Under the 2017 Uniform Parentage Act. *Barry L. Child & Fam. LJ*, 9, 1.

Cohen, J., Trounson, A., Dawson, K., Jones, H., Hazekamp, J., Nygren, K.-G., & Hamberger, L. (2005). The early days of IVF outside the UK. *Human Reproduction Update*, 11(5), 439–460. DOI: 10.1093/humupd/dmi016 PMID: 15923202

Contributor, S. C. R. C. (2016, November 29). https://blog.scrcivf.com/ivf-the-history-and-evolution-of-fertility-treatments

Department of Health. New York. (2021, February 15). *The Child-Parent Security Act: Gestational Surrogacy Agreements, Acknowledgment of Parentage and Orders of Parentage*. New York State Department of Health. Retrieved September 8, 2024, from https://www.health.ny.gov/vital_records/child_parent_security_act/

Department of Health. New York. (n.d.). https://www.health.ny.gov/vital_records/child_parent_security_act/#:~:text=The%20Child%2DParent%20Security%20Act%20(CPSA)%20is%20a%20law,(ART)%20to%20have%20children

Dolzhenko, (n.d.). *Surrogacy Laws In Ukraine*. https://nccconline.org/blog/article/14#:~:text=In%20 addition%20to%20clear%20and,created%20and%20 frozen%20 FET%20 embryos (19/03/2024

Dushina, . (2016). he Legitimation of Commercial Surrogacy in Russia. *Russian Education & Society*, (58), 12.

Dushina, A. D., Kersha, Y. D., Larkina, T. Y., & Provorova, D. D. (2017). The Legitimation of Commercial Surrogacy in Russia. *Russian Education & Society*, 58(12), 789–815. DOI: 10.1080/10609393.2017.1353835

Epstein, R. A. (1995). Surrogacy: The Case for Full Contractual Enforcement,. *Va. L. Rev., 81*.

Field, M. A. (2014). Compensated Surrogacy. *WASH. L. REV., 89*, 1155,1161.

Freeman, M. (1999). Does surrogacy have a future after Brazier? *Medical Law Review*, 7(1), 1–20. DOI: 10.1093/medlaw/7.1.1 PMID: 11658024

Griffiths, S., & Martin, L. (2006). Assisted Reproduction and Colorado Law: Unanswered Questions and Future Challenges. *Colorado Lawyer*, 35(11), 39.

Han, L. K. (2023, March 7). *The commercial surrogacy industry is booming as demand for babies rises*. CNBC. Retrieved September 8, 2024, from https://www.cnbc.com/2023/03/07/womb-for-rent-more-women-are-working-in-commercial-surrogacy-industry.html

Hatzis, A. N. (2009). From soft to hard Paternalism and back: The Regulation of Surrogate Motherhood in Greece [PORT. EcON. J.]. *Portuguese Economic Journal*, 8(3), 8. DOI: 10.1007/s10258-009-0049-5

Hibina, Y. (2023). The advantages and disadvantages of altruistic and commercial surrogacy in India. *Philosophy, Ethics, and Humanities in Medicine; PEHM*, 18(8), 8. DOI: 10.1186/s13010-023-00130-y PMID: 37420245

*History of IVF: Origin and Developments of the 20th Century | PFCLA*. (2022, July 25). Pacific Fertility Center Los Angeles. Retrieved October 19, 2024, from https://www.pfcla.com/blog/history-of-ivf

Horn, A. (2019, August 19). *Damaged babies and broken hearts: Ukraine's commercial surrogacy industry leaves a trail of disasters*. ABC. Retrieved September 8, 2024, from https://www.abc.net.au/news/2019-08-20/ukraines-commercial-surrogacy-industry-leaves-disaster/11417388

Igareda González, N. (2020). I. (2020). Legal and ethical issues in cross-border gestational surrogacy. *Fertility and Sterility*, 113(5), 916–919. DOI: 10.1016/j.fertnstert.2020.03.003 PMID: 32327242

Jargilo, I. (2016). Regulating the Trade of Commercial Surrogacy in India. *Journal of International Business and Law*, 15(2), 12.

Jaswal, P. S., & Kaur, J. (2021). SURROGATE MOTHERHOOD IN INDIA: An Analysis of Surrogacy (Regulation) Act, 2021. *Shimla Law Review*, IV, 257.

Kerian, C. L. (1997). Surrogacy: A Last Resort Alternative for Infertile Women or a Commodification of Women's Bodies and Children. *WIS. WOMEN's L.J., 12*.

Kitson, M. (2018, October 1). *Surrogacy in Spain: The dark side of Ukraine's surrogacy boom | Spain*. EL PAÍS English. Retrieved September 8, 2024, from https://elpais.com/elpais/2018/09/27/inenglish/1538051520_476218.html

Lieber, K. B. (1992). Selling the Womb: Can the Feminist Critique of Surrogacy Be Answered?,. *68 IND. L.J.*, 205.

Luckey, C. (2011). Commercial Surrogacy: Is Regulation Necessary to Manage the Industry. *Wisconsin Journal of Law. Gender & Society*, •••, 26.

Luckey, C. (2011). Commercial Surrogacy: Is Regulation necessary to manage Industry. *Commercial Surrogacy: Is Regulation necWISCONSIN JOURNAL OF LAW. Gender & Society*, 26(2).

Machinton,, N. (1987). urrogate Motherhood: Boon or Baby-Selling - The Unresolved Questions,. *71 Marq. L. Rev., 115*.

Macpherson, C. B. (1962). *The political theory of possessive individualism: Hobbes to Locke*. Clarendon Press.

Meinke, S. A. (1990). Surrogate motherhood: ethical and legal issues.

Ministry of Health. (n.d.). *Surrogacy in Israel*.

Mondal, V.. (2012). Genetic and Gestational Surrogacy: An Overview. *Walailak Journal of Science and Technology*, 9(3), 189–193.

Morrissey, J. F. (2015). Surrogacy: The Process, the Law, and the Contracts,. *WILLAMETTE L. REV., 51*.

Mouliarova, E. (2019). The Legal Regulation of Surrogacy in Russia. *11 ITALIAN J. PUB. L.*

Patel, N. H., Jadeja, Y. D., Bhadarka, H. K., Patel, M. N., Patel, N. H., & Sodagar, N. R. (2018). Insight into Different Aspects of Surrogacy Practices. *Journal of Human Reproductive Sciences*, 11(3), 212–218. DOI: 10.4103/jhrs.JHRS_138_17 PMID: 30568349

Ramalingam, M., Durgadevi, P., Durgadevi, P., & Mahmood, T. (2016). In vitro fertilization. *Obstetrics, Gynaecology & Reproductive Medicine, 26*(7), 200-209. //.DOI: 10.1016/j.ogrm.2016.05.006

Ramsey, J. (2006). Paying for reproduction—The case against paid surrogacy. *The Juridical Review*, 4, 325–349.

Ramskold, L. A. H., & Posner, M. P. (2013). Commercial surrogacy: How provisions of monetary remuneration and powers of international law can prevent exploitation of gestational surrogates. *Journal of Medical Ethics*, 39(6), 397–402. DOI: 10.1136/medethics-2012-100527 PMID: 23443211

Richard A. Posner,. (1989). The Ethics and Economics of Enforcing Contracts of Surrogate Motherhood,. *H.LTH L. & POL'Y.*

Rimm, J. (2009). Booming Baby Business: Regulating Commercial Surrogacy in India, *U. PA.J. INT'L L*, 30, 1443–1444.

Roache, M., & Everingham, S. (2018, September 13). *Ukraine's 'baby factories': The human cost of surrogacy | Women's Rights.* Al Jazeera. Retrieved September 8, 2024, from https://www.aljazeera.com/indepth/features/ukraine-baby-factories-human-cost-surrogacy-180912201251153.html

Shanley, M. L. "Surrogate Mothering" and Women's Freedom: A Critique of Contracts for Human Reproduction. *Signs (Chicago, Ill.)*, 18(3), 618–639. DOI: 10.1086/494822 PMID: 11659996

Sifris, R. (2016). Commercial surrogacy and the human right to autonomy. *Journal of Law and Medicine*, 23(2). PMID: 26939504

South California Reproductive Centre. (2016, November 29). *The Evolution of Fertility Treatments and Development of IVF.* Blog. Retrieved October 18, 2024, from https://blog.scrcivf.com/ivf-the-history-and-evolution-of-fertility-treatments

Stanford's Children Health. (n.d.). *Complications of Multiple Pregnancy.* Stanford Medicine Children's Health. Retrieved September 8, 2024, from https://www.stanfordchildrens.org/en/topic/default?id=complications-of-multiple-pregnancy-85-P08021&sid=

*Surrogacy in Ukraine: Cost.* (n.d.). IVMed. Retrieved September 8, 2024, from https://ivmed.agency/surrogacy-in-ukraine

Svitnev, K. (2010). Legal regulation of assisted reproduction treatment in Russia. *Reproductive Biomedicine Online*, 20(7), 892–894. DOI: 10.1016/j.rbmo.2010.03.023 PMID: 20435519

Tanderup, M., Reddy, S., Patel, T., & Nielsen, B. B. (2015). Informed consent in medical decision-making in commercial gestational surrogacy: A mixed methods study in New Delhi, India. *Acta Obstetricia et Gynecologica Scandinavica*, 94(5), 465–472. DOI: 10.1111/aogs.12576 PMID: 25581093

Teman, E. (2016). *Surrogacy in Israel: state-controlled surrogacy as a mechanism of symbolic control.* Cambridge University Press. DOI: 10.1017/CBO9781316282618.023

The American College of Obstetricians and Gynecologists. (2019). *Women's Health Care Physicians. Multiple Pregnancy*https://www.acog.org/Patients/FAQs/Multiple-Pregnancy?IsMobileSet=false#risk

Tuininga, K. (2008). The Ethics of Surrogacy Contracts and Nebraska's Surrogacy Law. *CREIGHTON L. REV.*, 41, 185.

Viktoriya Omelchenko, V. (n.d.). *Assisted reproduction technologies in Russian Federation.* https://medlawlab.web.auth.gr/wp-content/uploads/2022/03/Assisted-reproduction-in-Russian-Federation-by-Viktoria-Omelchenko.pdf

Wilder, N. J. (1986). Society's Response to the New Reproductive Technologies: The Feminist Perspectives, *S.California Law Review*, •••, 59.

Worldwide Surrogacy Specialists. (2021, November 1). *3 Commercial Surrogacy v. Altruistic Surrogacy.* https://www.worldwidesurrogacy.org/blog/commercial-surrogacy-vs-altruistic-surrogacy

# Chapter 11 Men's Role in Reproductive Health and Rights: Understanding the Involvement and Impact of Men in the Reproductive Health Decisions of Women in India

**Ankita Rituraj**
https://orcid.org/0009-0006-5130-5068
*KLE Technological University, India*

**Ayush Jha**
https://orcid.org/0009-0000-8684-7103
*MATS University, India*

## ABSTRACT

*Reproductive health and rights encompass a broad range of issues, including family planning, maternal health, sexual health education, and access to safe and legal abortion. While these areas are often viewed through a lens that primarily considers women's roles and responsibilities, the involvement of men is equally crucial. Lack of male engagement in reproductive health perpetuates gender inequality. By reinforcing the notion that reproductive health is solely a woman's domain, societal norms continue to marginalize women and restrict their autonomy. This not only affects women's health and well-being but also impedes progress towards achieving gender equality and empowering women in India.*

DOI: 10.4018/979-8-3693-7837-3.ch011

# I. INTRODUCTION

*"Promoting sexual and reproductive health and rights requires challenging harmful and unequal gender power relations by working with men alongside women."* - *Dr. Maria Lohan, UNESCO Chair in Masculinities and Gender Equality at Queen's University Belfast.*

Access to reproductive healthcare remains a global health concern. Gender is a fundamental influence along with decision making power, access to education and earning power which impacts access to choices. (Wegner et al., 2022) While women occupy the centre stage in reproductive health debates, their actions and choices alone do not impact reproductive health outcomes.

Men in most societies, occupy preponderant power in nearly every sphere of life ranging from personal decisions regarding the size of families to the policy and programme decisions taken at all levels of government. (United Nations Population Fund, 1994). The role of men within the family, when examined from sociological and anthropological perspectives, reflects a multifaceted and evolving construct shaped by cultural traditions, economic circumstances, and societal expectations (Coltrane, 1996). Traditionally, men were often viewed as the main providers and the dominant authority figures in the household. Throughout various societies and historical epochs, the responsibilities of men in the family have been deeply rooted in prevailing gender norms and economic frameworks. In most societies, men are expected to assert control over family matters and limit women's autonomy (Kandiyoti, 1988). The understanding of men's roles in reproductive health has been shaped by the historical construction of gender roles. In many societies, men have been perceived as detached from reproductive processes, with women's health, fertility, and pregnancy seen as matters exclusively under the domain of women (Dudgeon & Inhorn, 2004). This viewpoint often stems from traditional patriarchal structures, where masculinity is associated with dominance and authority, while reproductive health is framed as a female responsibility (Greene & Biddlecom, 2000). As a result, women have been the key focus of awareness programs and medical interventions pertaining to reproductive health and men have been sidelined from effectively engaging in policy decisions, interventions and responsibilities. Men and women are equal partners and in realisation of better reproductive health and it is crucial to involve men to play an active and responsible role in matters of maternal health and family planning.

This commitment was first highlighted by the International Conference on Population and Development held in Cairo in 1994. It underlined the role of men in sharing equal burden in achieving better reproductive health for their partners. The National Population Policy of India reaffirmed the same by focusing on promoting a "*gender sensitive, multi sectoral agenda..... For population stabilization, basic reproductive and child care needs*" (Government of India, 2000). Sociologists too, argue that involving men in reproductive health interventions, such as sexual health education and maternal care, can lead to more equitable relationships and better health for both partners (Ashford, 2003). Men who are informed and engaged in reproductive health are more likely to support their partners during pregnancy, childbirth, and postpartum care, reducing risks to maternal and infant health (Mullany, 2006). Modern sociological theories emphasise the importance of shared decision-making between men and women, particularly in areas such as family planning, contraceptive use, and antenatal care, which have significant implications for the health and well-being of all family members (Greene & Biddlecom, 2000). When men actively participate in discussions about contraception and fertility, it can lead to more informed choices, better communication between partners, and reduced rates of unintended pregnancies (Ezeh, 1993)

The national and international commitments have contributed to a visible shift in approach in dealing with reproductive health. The government policies in India aim at instilling awareness in adolescents as well as young adults about their sexual and reproductive health and involving men in conversations on family planning and maternal health. However, despite government policies and interventions, the participation of men in key areas remains low (Population Fund of India, n.d.) It is crucial to involve men in these conversations because implementation of better reproductive health requires involvement of both men and women. In particular, men need to overcome cultural and social barriers to become equal partners in planning families, maternal care, adoption of contraceptives and supporting women's contraceptive choices (Population Fund of India, n.d.)

As societal norms around gender continue to shift and evolve, fostering more equitable partnerships, it is crucial to acknowledge the importance of men's involvement in reproductive health (Dudgeon & Inhorn, 2004) Recognising that reproductive health is not solely a woman's concern, but a shared responsibility, is essential to achieving comprehensive and inclusive healthcare outcomes for everyone (Ashford, 2003). Men's active engagement in reproductive health challenges traditional and harmful gender roles, promotes mutual responsibility, and helps dismantle structural inequalities that hinder progress (Greene et al., 2006). By fostering a culture where men are participants in discussions and decisions around family planning, pregnancy, and sexual health, societies can build healthier families, strengthen communities, and move toward greater social justice (Dudgeon & Inhorn, 2004).

The primary objective of this chapter is to contribute to the discourse on the importance of men and the key role they play in shaping the reproductive rights of their female partners. Part II of the Chapter provides a theoretical framework on the concept of reproductive health, its evolution and various perspectives associated with it. Part III specifically focuses on role of men in family planning by analysing trends and patterns based on the data of National Family Health Survey (2019-2021). Part IV looks into the trends and patterns on use of contraception by men. Parts V and VI identifies the socio cultural barriers in India which limit men from sharing equal responsibility in achieving better reproductive health and rights for women and stories of successful intervention and changes respectively. The chapter ends with a conclusion and recommendations for policy makers for ensuring effective intervention in raising awareness and inclusion of men as equal stakeholders.

## Aims and Objectives

There are four fold objectives of this chapter -

1. To provide a comprehensive overview of the current state of men's involvement in reproductive health and rights.
2. To analyze the impact of male participation on reproductive health outcomes vis a vis their role in family planning and maternal health
3. To identify the barriers to men's active engagement in reproductive health.
4. To make recommendations for enhancing male involvement in reproductive health decisions.

## Methodology

In writing this chapter, the author has relied upon the data collected from The National Family and Health Survey 5, 2022 (NFHS). The NFHS is a detailed and comprehensive survey undertaken by the Government of India which provides rich source of information on key indicators pertaining to family and health across various regions and demographics in India. For this study, the author has analysed relevant data with a particular focus on examining men's attitudes and perceptions toward family planning and use of contraception contraception. This approach allowed for a deeper understanding of the factors that influence male involvement in reproductive health choices.

## Scope

Reproductive Health is a vast concept. It includes various components such as sexual health, family planning, maternal health, health of adolescents, screening and treatment of Sexually Transmitted Diseases (STIs) etc. It is not possible to cover all the parameters sufficiently and lucidly in a chapter, for each of these parameters can warrant an individual chapter of their own. The author, therefore, for the purpose of this chapter, will be analysing the role of men and elaborating upon the trends in male participation in family planning across two broad parameters of family planning and maternal health.

## II. THEORETICAL FRAMEWORK / REVIEW OF LITERATURE

### Understanding Reproductive Health: Conceptual Framework

*"Our current understanding of empowerment has expanded. We believe that power has to be defined not in terms of power over others but in terms of self reliance and inner strength, the ability to determine choices and exercise control over one's own life. This holds true for women as well as men. Just as women need to liberate themselves from patriarchal strongholds, men need to be liberated too, from the patriarchal construct of masculinity." - Social Action for Rural and Tribal Inhabitants of India*

Sexual and Reproductive health is recognised as an indivisible aspect of human rights, with its roots in Right to Health Sexual and Reproductive Health includes the right to life, liberty and security of the person; the right to healthcare and information ; the right of non-discrimination in the allocation of resources to the health services and their availability and accessibility (Shalev, 2000). According to the World Health Organisation, Sexual and Reproductive Health are integral elements of the right of everyone to the enjoyment of the highest attainable standard of physical and mental health (World Health Organization: WHO, 2024). The International Conference on Population and Development (ICPD) in paragraph 7.2 of the Programme of Action, defines reproductive health as a state of "complete physical, social and mental well being…..In all matters related to the reproductive system." (Shalev, 2000). Reproductive health inherently includes the right of men and women to be informed and have access to safe, effective, affordable and acceptable methods of family planning of their choice, as well as other methods of their choice for regulation of fertility which are not against the law (Ki-moon et al., 1994). Reproductive health care is defined as a constellation of methods, techniques and services that contribute to reproductive health and well being by preventing and solving reproductive health problems (Ki-moon et al., 1994). Reproductive health therefore is a part of broader narrative on right to health and human rights. Such rights are already recognised at national and international level.

The United Nations Sustainable Development Goals have explicitly recognised sexual and reproductive health and reproductive rights as essential not only to health, but also gender equality and wider economic and social development (World Health Organization: WHO, 2024). Article 12 of the International Covenant on Economic, Social and Cultural Rights (ICESCR) recognises the right of everyone to the enjoyment of the highest attainable standards of physical and mental health (*International Covenant on Economic, Social and Cultural Rights*, 1966). Convention on Elimination of All forms of Discrimination Against Women (CEDAW), 1978 particularly emphasises on realisation of sexual and reproductive health.

India's legal framework on reproductive health and rights is complex, encompassing various laws, policies, and international commitments. Key legislations include the Medical Termination of Pregnancy (MTP) Act of 1971, which legalises abortion under certain conditions, and the Pre-Conception and Pre-Natal Diagnostic Techniques (PCPNDT) Act of 1994, which prohibits sex-selective abortions and addresses the issue of declining sex ratios (Government of India, 2005). The Indian Constitution, through its fundamental rights and directive principles, also supports the protection of reproductive health and rights. Article 21 of the Constitution of India specifically recognises the fundamental right to life and personal liberty of all individuals. This includes the right to sexual privacy and the ability to make choices for all *(Navtej Singh Johar v. Union of India, 2017)*. Internationally, India is a signatory to several conventions and agreements that recognise and promote reproductive health and rights. These include the International Covenant on Economic, Social and Cultural Rights (ICESCR), the Convention on the Elimination of All Forms of Discrimination Against Women (CEDAW), and the Programme of Action of the International Conference on Population and Development (ICPD). The Constitution of India under Article 51(c) and the judiciary have established that the government has a constitutional obligation to respect international law and treaty obligations (WWW.REPRODUCTIVE RIGHTS.ORG, 2021).

## Evolution of Reproductive Health and Rights in India

In India, reproductive health has traditionally been viewed through the lens of population control rather than individual rights. Post-independence, the government initiated various family planning programs aimed at controlling population growth, often prioritising these over the reproductive rights and health of individuals. In fact, India was among the first countries of the world to develop a legal and policy framework on reproductive rights and health guaranteeing access to abortion, family planning and access to contraception (WWW.REPRODUCTIVE RIGHTS.ORG, 2021). The concept of reproductive health has its roots in the broader framework of maternal and child health (MCH), which was a focus of early public health initiatives post-independence (*Promoting Men's Involvement in Maternal and Child Health*, 2016). The MCH programs primarily targeted women, aiming to reduce maternal and infant mortality through better healthcare services. These programs, however, largely ignored the role of men in reproductive health, treating reproduction as a woman's domain. The introduction of family planning programs in the 1950s marked the beginning of state intervention in reproductive health. India's family planning program, the first of its kind in the world, was initially focused on population control rather than reproductive rights. The infamous forced sterilization campaign during the Emergency (1975-1977) further entrenched the idea of reproductive health as a matter of controlling female fertility. Men were largely excluded from these initiatives, with vasectomies being promoted only sporadically and often coercively.

In 1971, the Parliament of India enacted a Medical Termination of Pregnancy Act, 1971, *MTP Act, hereinafter*- a first of its kind law in the country granting women the right to terminate their pregnancies under certain circumstances. Though with its own limitations, this law marked a departure from the prevalent community based approach to the rights based approach. The MTP Act was further amended in 2021 to make it more comprehensive and responsive to the needs of the women. In 2009, the Supreme Court of India expressly recognised that " a woman's right to make reproductive choices is a dimension of her personal liberty as understood under Article 21 of the Indian Constitution" (*Suchita Srivastava v. Chandigarh Administration, 2009;*Pillai, 2024).

The laws and the judicial decisions in India recognise the reproductive rights of women and attribute supremacy and autonomy to women in making those choices. Despite the progression of law, enjoyment of reproductive rights and access to reproductive health choices remain difficult for women. The sexual and reproductive health outcomes are shaped by "social determinants" that refer to social norms and structures that stigmatise, oppress or marginalised persons on account of their sex, sexual orientation or gender identity, marital status, age, ability or caste, ethnicity or minority status (SAMA Resource Group for Women and Health & Partners for Law in Development, 2018) Historically, there has been little to no focus on involving men as competent stakeholders in this process and the policymakers largely remained indifferent to the role of men and the influence they have over the reproductive decisions of women. In fact, men controlling the reproduction and sexual choices of women were and still remain a well accepted norm in India. The prevailing socio - cultural structure and lack of awareness has thus led to inaccessibility of these rights for women as well erosion of their reproductive health and well being. A highest possible attainment of reproductive health and solid rights based framework can emerge only with inclusion and involvement of men in these matters. The role of men from being controllers and drivers of choices for women must transform into equal partners empowering women to make their own choices.

## Gender Roles and Reproductive Health: Understanding the Dynamics

Gender roles, deeply embedded in cultural, social, and economic systems, have a profound impact on various aspects of life, including reproductive health. There is widespread recognition of the importance of gender norms and their application to the field of sexual and reproductive health as rigid and traditional gender roles often dictate the terms in which intimate sexual activity and reproduction takes place (*Gender Norms and Sexual and Reproductive Health*, n.d.). In India, where traditional gender norms are pervasive, these roles significantly shape the reproductive health experiences of individuals, particularly women. Religion often plays an important role in creating and upholding these structures. Though India has one of the most dynamic and liberal constitutions of the world, its liberal values do not inherently translate into the working of the social structures and impact gender based power dynamics. The social structure including the power dynamics of the genders is deeply pervaded by the religious and cultural beliefs.

## Masculinity and Reproductive Health: Cultural and Psychological Perspectives

Masculinity, a complex and multifaceted concept, has profound implications for reproductive health. In many societies, including India, traditional notions of masculinity play a significant role in shaping men's attitudes towards sexuality, contraception, family planning, and healthcare. Masculinity is described as a socio-culturally constructed concept that is in many cultures characterised by physical strength, self sufficiency, emotional toughness, risk taking and dominance; men earn their status on an ongoing basis through competition and demonstration of these qualities (Agochukwu & Wittmann, 2019). Men are also attributed with certain types of psychological dispositions, with gender specific kinds of behaviour, simply on the basis of their sex (Johnson, 2012). Studies point to the ascribed character of a culture of masculinity that valorises and rewards physically aggressive, competitive, achievement oriented attitudes and behaviour in men (Johnson, 2012). Hegemonic Masculinity is defined as 'configuration of gender practice which embodies the currently accepted answer to the problem of legitimacy of patriarchy which guarantees (or taken to guarantee), the dominant position of men and subordination of women (Lorimer et al., n.d.). Hegemonic masculinity also requires men to avoid engaging in thoughts, behaviours or emotions that are socially construed as feminine (McDermott et al., 2019) Part of the reason for difficulties in access to reproductive health and realisation of rights arise due to significant variation in cultural understanding of these experiences - in how different groups of men and women encounter, define, understand and experience reproduction and reproductive health challenges (Dudgeon & Inhorn, 2004). Masculinity and the traits associated with it can therefore lead men to engage in behaviours that put their health, as well as the health of their partners, at risk. For example, the stigma associated with condom use, particularly in casual or extramarital relationships, can result in unprotected sex, increasing the risk of STIs and unintended pregnancies (Verma et al., 2001). It can also make men susceptible to controlling the size of their families, forcing women to carry unwanted pregnancies etc. As stated previously, masculinity is socio- culturally constructed and is not equivalent to male biological sex. From a psychological standpoint, masculinity is not hard -wired due to genes and hormones, and it is not inescapable (Levant, 2020). Men can retain their gender identities without confirming their thoughts, behaviours and actions to unhealthy masculine forms (Levant, 2020). Sociologists and psychologists have emphasized on the fact that masculinity reflects societal standpoint on men rather than an individual man's perception of himself. However masculinity becomes an inherent part of one's personality due to cultural perpetuation to the extent that it often comes across as purely biological and therefore feels inescapable.

The influence of masculinity on reproductive decision-making can have significant implications for reproductive health outcomes. For instance, men who adhere to traditional masculine norms may prioritise their desire for large families over their partners' health and well-being (Jejeebhoy & Sathar, 2001). This often results in coercion and pressure on women to have more children and a complete neglect for the risks associated with child births and frequent and multiple pregnancies, especially in India where the state aided health infrastructure is inadequate and private healthcare too expensive to be afforded by a vast majority of population. Moreover, the lack of male involvement in reproductive health discussions can lead to a disconnect between partners, where men are unaware of or indifferent to their partners' reproductive health needs (Jejeebhoy & Sathar, 2001).

## The Concept of Shared Responsibility in Reproductive Health: A Feminist Approach on Reproduction and Family

In developing new frameworks for a new reproductive health paradigm, attention has been drawn to the absence of men from previous reproductive health initiatives and the need to incorporate men into new reproductive health frameworks (Dudgeon & Inhorn, 2004). Men's role in affecting women's reproductive health is multifaceted and often lacks the sharing of equal responsibility. Shared responsibility in reproductive health refers to the idea that both men and women should equally participate in decisions and actions related to reproduction. This concept challenges the traditional notion that reproductive health is solely a woman's domain and instead advocates for a collaborative approach where both partners share the responsibilities of contraception, pregnancy, childbirth, and parenting.

Historically, family was considered to be the part of the private sphere which was free from state intrusion. Feminists have long resisted the division of public from private where men were essentially treated as 'public' and women 'private'. Feminists share the view that contemporary families are not only realms of choice but also realms of constraints (Satz, 2013). They also agree that gender hierarchy in our society is unjust, although they differ on what they take its sources to be (Satz, 2013). Family structures, according to certain sections of feminists, are the linchpin of gender injustice. Despite the strides made by feminists over the years, the family structures across the globe are based on unequal division of labor and resources. Globally women are still disproportionately engaged in taking up the responsibility of child care and parenting. The World Health Organisation estimates that women perform three quarters (76.2%) of unpaid care work, dedicating an average of 4 hours and 25 minutes per day as compared to 1 hour and 23 minutes put in by men (*The Missing Piece: Valuing Women's Unrecognised Contribution to the Economy*, n.d.). The Time Use Survey, released by the National Statistical Office in 2020, estimates that 81.2% of women in India aged between 15-59 are engaged in unpaid care work, compared with 26.1% of men, higher than the global average (Bharathram, 2023). Feminists opine that since women spend disproportionately higher time in unpaid care work, they are less likely to take up economic opportunities outside home and depend on their male counterparts for financial support. Women's financial independence, thus allows them to be subjected to physical, sexual, reproductive and psychological control by their husbands/ male partners (Satz, 2013). The existing structure also conditions young children to ape the same in future generations. American sociologist, *Nancy Chodorow,* has stated that girls identify better with their same sex nurturing parent and boys identify with the parent who is 'absent' and feel more individualised from a young age (Chodorow, 1978). Mothering is therefore reproduced across generations through an unconscious mechanism, which leads to generations sharing unequal reproductive and family responsibilities (Chodorow, 1978). The patriarchal structure of power, leading to the gender division of labor, thus, leads to distinct expectations and behaviours from both men and women and creates barriers in realisation of shared reproductive responsibility, which is primarily viewed as a woman's domain.

## III. MEN'S ROLE IN FAMILY PLANNING

Family planning is the process by which individuals and couples predict and achieve the number, spacing and timing of the children they desire (Abebe et al., 2023). Family planning encompasses the services, policies, information, attitudes, practices and commodities, including contraceptives, that give women, men, couples and adolescents the ability to avoid unintended pregnancies and choose whether and/or/when to have a child (Starbird et al., 2016). India was the first country in the world to have launched a National Programme for Family Planning in 1952 (*Family Planning*, n.d.) and ever since it has been a key component of the reproductive health policies. Positive involvement of men is crucial for such programmes to succeed and meet their targeted impact since it also enables women to make choices beneficial to them and to the family. Involvement of men is also important not only to enhance the effectiveness of contraceptives but also promote shared responsibility and gender equality.

Despite the emphasis on family planning in India's public health agenda, the involvement of men has historically been limited. This has led to a disproportionate burden on women to manage contraception and reproductive health, which is further compounded by cultural, social, and economic factors.

### Early Family Planning Initiatives in India

According to T.J Samuel, The development of present policy of family planning and population control by the Indian Government falls into four distinguishable categories - (i) The period of indifference (before 1945) (ii) The period of neutrality (1947 - 1952) (iii) The period of experimentation (1952 - 1961) (iv) The beginning of the policy of population control (1961 - 1962) (Samuel, 1966)

The history of family planning in India dates back to pre-independence times. The British Government remained largely indifferent to the population explosion in India. However, Indian social reformists and educators played an important role in advocating for the cause of family planning and population control in India. Pyare Kishen Wattal was one of the first advocates of family planning in 1916 (Cassen, 1978). The formal history of family planning began in India with the work and initiatives of Ragunath Dhondo Karve in 1925. Karve was in favour of sexual liberation of men and women from the shackles of morality, customs and law (Lele, 2023). He was also opposed to the then existing social structures where women's bodies were treated as the property of their husbands and they had no control over their choices, including the choice of reproduction and family planning. Karve was also in favour of selling contraceptives as a measure of birth control (Lele, 2023). His ideology stemmed from his viewpoint on women as individuals capable of making choices about their body and sexuality. He opened a family planning clinic in Bombay in 1926 (Shah et al., n.d.). His views cost him his position as a Professor at a reputed university.

On Governmental level, Mysore Government opened a birth control clinic in 1930 and two years later i.e. in 1932, the Government of Madras opened a family planning clinic in the presidency (Shah et al., n.d.). The All India Women's Conference established a Family Planning Centre in 1937, which is now known as the family planning association of India (*AIWC : All India Women's Conference*, n.d.). The Indian National Congress and stalwarts like Gandhi and Jawaharlal Nehru supported it. Gandhi advocated for birth control through abstinence and self control. The views of others in the Indian National Congress were more pragmatic. The views of Samuel, as stated earlier, may therefore not be entirely correct since the indifference to population growth was by the British who saw India's population explosion as a symbol of prosperity. India did have a policy on family planning before independence, although its expanse may have been limited.

The general population of India largely remained unacquainted with the idea of family planning, even after independence. The onus completely fell upon the newly formed government of independent India to limit the growing population. The first chapter of India's family planning began in the year 1951 - 56 with the adoption of First Five Year Plans. The focus was to promote planned parenthood models as practiced in the West and establish family planning clinics (Maharatna, 2002). Dr. S. Radhakrishnan, in his inaugural address at the Third Conference on Planned Parenthood in Bombay in 1952 stated that - *"if you subject women to frequent childbirths you will be guilty of cruelty to human beings, you will be making difficult marriages which otherwise might have been successful. If, therefore, your attention is to safeguard the health and happiness of family life you must determine the time of child birth, space the arrival of the children. I take it, to determine this, is to plan a family."* The Second Five Year Plans (1956- 1961), too emphasized on reduction of population as an important consideration for elevated standard of living. The Third Five Year Plans (1961-66) too focused on population stabilization. The focus shifted on creating awareness in which health workers were to visit women of child bearing ages to motivate them to limit the size of their families (Maharatna, 2002). In 1952, the Indian Government initiated what would become in the 1960s, the largest government sponsored family planning programme in the world (Ledbetter, 1984). The government stressed upon the importance of family planning for 25 years, and splurged large sums of money on it but soon realized that merely spending large sums had not been effective to meet the targeted goal (Ledbetter, 1984). During the period of emergency in India, the Indira Gandhi Government extensively promoted the use of IUD (intrauterine device), which was promoted as being a safe and reversible method. IUD was accepted by over 800,000 Indian women in 1965-66 and another 900,000 in 1966 - 67 (Gwatkin, 1979). However, the move backfired and a large number of women suffered adverse health consequences as a result of IUD use, which was hastily put into use by the then government. Due to the then existing socio-political circumstances and in a bid to retain power, forced sterilisation were performed. Forced sterilisations had become so rampant that some of its targets remember the emergency as '*nasbandi ka waqt*' (the era of sterilization) (Williams, 2014).

At the cusp of the 21st century, India adopted the National Population Policy of 2000. Its objectives were to address the unmet need for contraception, bring down the total fertility rate to replacement rates and to stabilise the population by 2045 (Chiinhauching et al., 2022). The Population Regulation Bill, 2019 was introduced in the Parliament of India, to penalise couples who had more than two children. This bill was however withdrawn in 2022. Various provincial governments too have introduced multiple laws aiming at family planning. However, the available data on fertility rates suggest that the brunt of these reformatory estimates will be borne by the oppressed and the burden for sterilization will be loaded especially on women (Chiinhauching et al., 2022). It is important to understand that family planning initiatives in India were never driven by the rights based approach. Rather, family planning was often looked upon as a poverty alleviation measure.

## Trends in Male Participation on Family Planning

### Defining Family Planning

The approach of the government has undergone a change. Especially after Cairo, the policies of the government focus on ensuring reproductive health of women and engaging men in ensuring better reproductive outcomes for all. Family planning is a vast concept. For the purpose of this chapter, the author will be elaborating upon the trends in male participation in family planning across three parameters -

i) Men's knowledge about methods of contraception
ii) Men's share in modern methods of contraception
iii) Perceptions of Men on Family Planning

**Men's Knowledge About Methods of Contraception.** One of the significant steps in realisation of better reproductive health is timely access to information. According to the data released by National Family and Health Survey - V (NFHS) in 2022, about 78% of men between the age of 15-49 were exposed to family planning measures/ messages. There is universal knowledge about at least one method of contraception across all men, whether married or unmarried, between the age of 15-49 years (Government of India, 2022). Amongst the modern methods of contraception, condom remains the most popular method with 96.2 percent of men reporting to know about it. NFHS V data also suggests that 91.8 percent of all men within the age group of 15-49 know about female sterilization, however the knowledge among men about male sterilization is relatively less at 84.3 percent.

*Figure 1. Depicts knowledge of contraception in men and women in India (2019-2022)*

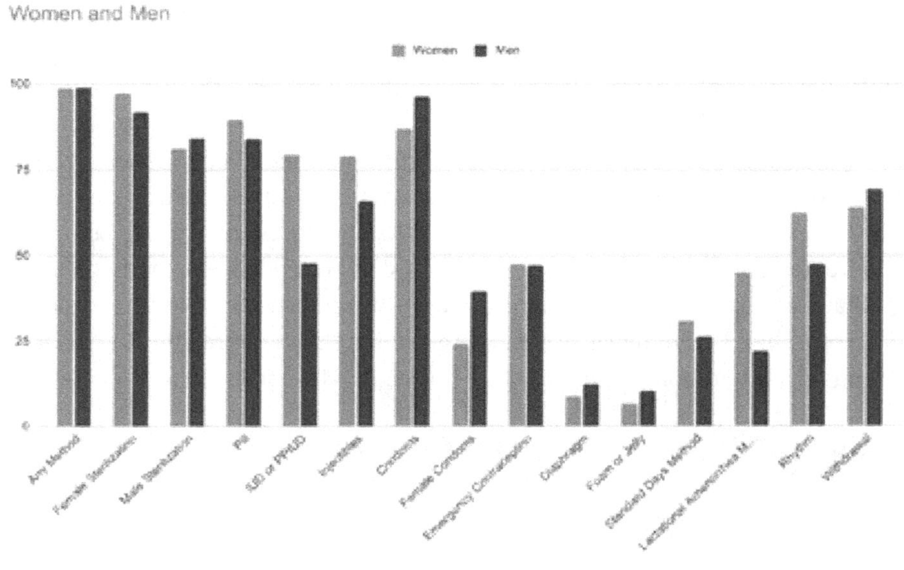


*Source - Based on the report of NFHS V, Government of India (2019-2022)*

Including all traditional and modern methods of contraception, the mean number of methods known by women is 8.1 and the mean number of methods known to men is 7.5.

Women, though slightly, have a better exposure to methods of contraception than men. The fact that women know more methods than men might reflect the traditional focus on women in family planning programs. Women are often the primary targets of these programs, leading to higher levels of awareness and knowledge about different contraceptive options. Men's slightly lower awareness may indicate a need for increased efforts to educate men about contraception, particularly about methods that are less well-known or those that men might not traditionally consider.

**Men's Share in Modern Methods of Contraception.** Modern Contraceptive Prevalence Rate is measured by the percentage of women who report using a modern method (themselves or their partner) to delay or avoid pregnancy (NFHS-5, 2021).

The data by NFHS V also reveals that women have a higher share in use of modern methods of contraception. Female sterilization alone comes up to 37.9 percent of all contraceptives used. Male sterilization, although it's safer and easier, remains at 0.3 percent (Pandey, 2022).

*Figure 2. Share in use of contraception by men and women*

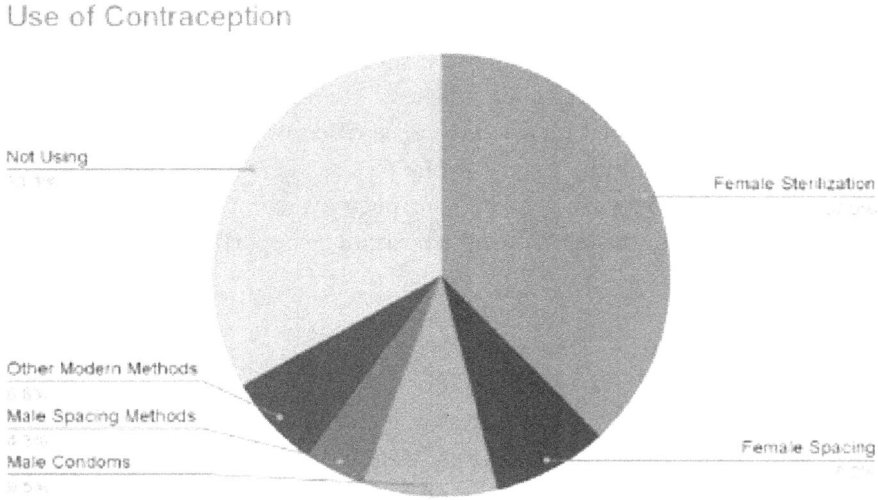


*Source - Based on the data of NFHS V, Government of India (2019-2022)*

The data by NFHS V points out that men in India have high knowledge about different methods of contraception. This however, does not translate to a higher use of contraception among men and the burden falls largely on women. A study conducted by Abhinav Pandey from 2017-19 across various Indian states shows that about 50 percent of men consider contraception to be a woman's business and that a man need not worry about it (Pandey, 2022). Though there is an overall increase in the use of contraception amongst Indians, the sharing of burden between men and women largely remains unequal.

**Perceptions of Men on Family Planning and Use of Contraception by Women**. Since men are dominant decision makers in India, it is prudent to discover knowledge, perception and attitudes of men (Balaiah et al., 1999) on family planning and use of contraception. According to the data by NFHS V, 75 percent women and 78 percent of men had exposure to various messages on family planning in the last few months (The People's Archive of Rural India, n.d.). The survey reports that if men aged between 15-49 years were given a chance to choose their family size, they would want to have an average of 2.1 children, similar to the response of the women in that age group (NFHS-5, 2021b). Among currently married men with three or more children (with at least one son), 83 percent of them do not want any more children.

The same survey also reports that 35.3 percent of surveyed men aged between 15-49 years feel that use of contraception is women's business and men have nothing to do with it. The same survey also reports that 19.7 percent of surveyed men aged between 15-49 also believe that women who use contraception may become promiscuous.

This represents a dichotomous situation, where men on one hand, are positive on limiting the size of their family and have sufficient knowledge about contraceptives but on the other hand their share on use of contraceptives is not only low, but also coupled with a negative viewpoint on use of contraception by women. This attitudinal problem, stemming from various factors such as socio-cultural conditioning, lack of education and a gendered perspective on reproduction and sexuality hinders meaningful engagement of men in becoming supporting and equal partners in family planning.

## IV. MEN AND MATERNAL HEALTH

The World Health Organisation defines Maternal Health as the health of women during pregnancy, childbirth and postnatal period (World Health Organization: WHO, 2019). A series of important events and changes, physical, emotional and social, occur before, during and well after the forty weeks of gestation and the first year of childbirth (Noursi et al., 2021). These changes, although natural, can be stressful, and they have health consequences, across a woman's life course. (Noursi et al., 2021)

Maternal Health has been a key focus of the public health initiatives in India for a long time. The responsibility for maternal health has largely fallen on women, but there is an increasing awareness of the important role that men can play in this area. As partners, fathers, and community members, men have the potential to make a meaningful impact on maternal health. Their active involvement can lead to better health outcomes for both mothers and their children.

### Policy Initiatives on Safeguarding Maternal Health in India

The Government of India adopted the Reproductive, Maternal, Newborn, Child and Adolescent Health (RMNCH) framework in 2013, it essentially aims to address the major causes of mortality and morbidity, among women and children (Government of India, n.d.). The Ministry of Health and Family Welfare launched the *Pradhan Mantri Surakshit Matritva Abhiyan* which provides for a fixed day for assured, comprehensive and quality antenatal care free of cost to pregnant women on every 9th day of every month (*Maternal Health*, n.d.). *The Janani Shishu Suraksha Karyakram* entitles every pregnant woman to free delivery, including for cesarean section, in public health institutions along with provision of free transport, diagnostics, medicine, other consumables, diet and food (*Initiatives for Pregnant Women*, n.d.) The Government of India has also set up more than twenty five thousand deliveries across the country and has established Maternal and Child Health Wings (MCH) for care of both the mother and the child. Birth Delivery Rooms have been established in remote and tribal areas to facilitate institutionalised deliveries and access to better healthcare facilities.

Apart from running various schemes and policy initiatives to ensure better maternal health, the Government of India back in 1971 had enacted the Medical Termination of Pregnancy Act. The objective was to provide for termination of certain pregnancies by registered medical practitioners (Parliament, 1971). The suggestion for such a legislation was given by the Shantilal Shah Committee which submitted its report in the year 1966 stating that high mortality rates among women were a strong plea for an abortion law (Shantilal Shah Committee, 1966). The argument stems from the fact that due to restrictive abortion laws, women who do not want the pregnancy to continue will resort to means which are gravely damaging to their health and their life (Jha et al., 2023).

Even though focus on maternal health has been a key component of the larger public health initiatives in India, involvement of men in these initiatives has remained limited. A comprehensive maternal health requires participation of both men and women.

## Trends in Male Participation in Involvement in Maternal Health Before, During, and After Pregnancy

Healthcare services during pregnancy and childbirth and after delivery are important for the survival and well being of both the mother and the infant (*National Family and Health Survey*, 2021). The National Family and Health Survey points out various parameters for evaluating maternal health care in India.

**Male Involvement in Antenatal Care**. Antenatal care is essential for maternal health, offering a critical opportunity to monitor the well-being of both the mother and the developing foetus while also identifying and addressing potential complications. When men actively participate in antenatal care, their involvement can significantly improve the health outcomes for both mothers and their babies.

As per the data by the NFHS V, on an average about 78.2 percent of men aged between 15- 49 years were present for any kind of antenatal services. Antenatal care under the NFHS Survey included services such as measuring weight, blood pressure, taking samples of urine and blood, examination of abdomen related issues, vaginal bleeding and convulsions. The data also suggests that the fathers involvement in antenatal care drops as more children are born. The involvement of fathers stands at 81 per cent at the time of antenatal care for their first born. The number drops to 77.7 percent at the time of birth of 2nd and 3rd child and drops significantly at 62.1 at the time of birth of the 4th child and more. NFHS also shows that education has a significant impact on male involvement in ensuring maternal health. On an average 84.9 percent of fathers with more than twelve years of schooling showed involvement in antenatal care as compared to 60.6 percent of fathers who had no schooling.

About 15.3 percent of women surveyed stated that they did not receive any form of antenatal care either because the man did not think that it was necessary or did not allow it.

*Figure 3. Involvement of fathers in antenatal care*

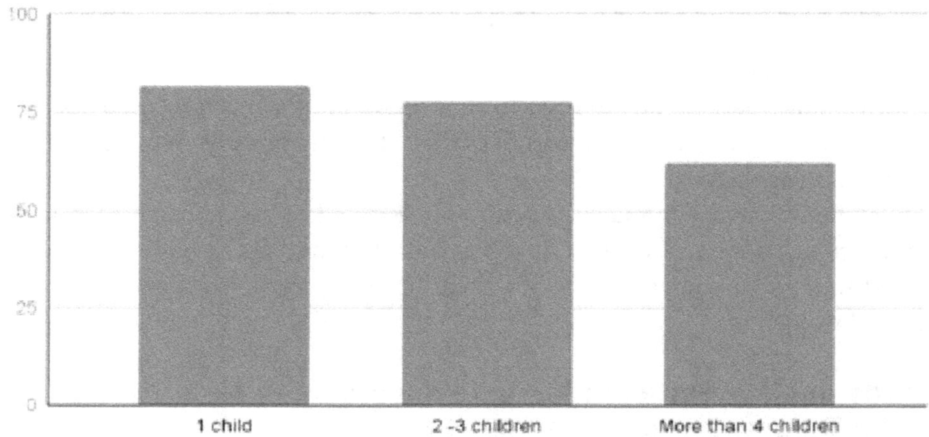


*Source - Based on the data of NFHS V, Government of India (2019-2022)*

*Figure 4 . Involvement of fathers in antenatal care*

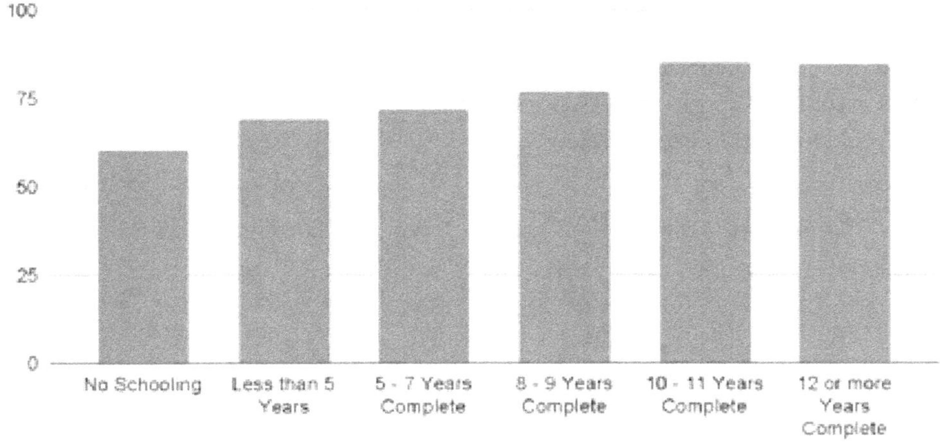


*Source - Based on the data of NFHS V, Government of India (2019-2022)*

**Male Involvement during childbirth and postnatal care.** Following childbirth, women require ongoing care to fully recover and to tend to their newborns. Assistance with household tasks, offering emotional support, and postnatal check-ups are crucial. These aspects are vital for tracking the mother's recovery, identifying any postpartum issues, and ensuring the baby's healthy development (World Health Organisation, 2015). Most maternal and infant deaths take place in the first month of birth due to lack of care after childbirth. Men can play a crucial role in this period. Many studies have revealed the merits of male partner involvement in maternal health; relief of stress, pain and anxiety during delivery; increased access to antenatal and postnatal services; improved maternal mental health and increased contraceptive usage (Aliesio L et al., 2009). The available evidence indicated that approximately two hundred ten million women became pregnant each year with thirty million (15 percent) developing life threatening complications resulting in death, of which the majority of maternal deaths, are attributed to low male involvement (Abie et al., 2023).

As per the NFHS V data, about 72.2 percent of the fathers between the age of 15-49 years stated that a healthcare provider or a worker spoke to them about the importance of delivery at a healthcare centre. 79.1 percent of men stated that a healthcare worker or a service provider spoke to them about the importance of nutrition of the mother during pregnancy and 61.1 percent of men reported that they were advised for family planning or delaying the next child.

61.3 percent of fathers between the age group of 20-49 years reported that someone explained to them the importance of breastfeeding the child immediately after birth. 60.25 percent of men in the same age group reported about being explained the importance of keeping the child warm immediately after birth. On an average, 64.5 percent of fathers in India reported about receiving some kind of information about childbirth and postnatal care.

*Figure 5. Information on child delivery and postnatal care given to men*

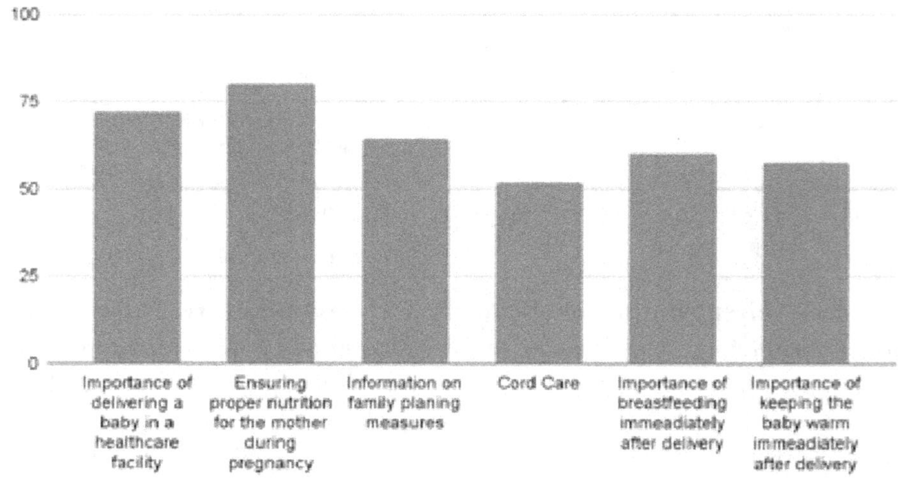


*Source - Based on the data of NFHS V, Government of India (2019-2022)*

Statistics show that men in India are being made aware of the importance of care before, during and after childbirth. More than fifty percent of all men surveyed were given some kind of information about child birth and importance of postnatal care. However, awareness alone does not transform into involvement. While Indian men are generally aware of the importance of antenatal and neonatal care, their involvement still remains low owing to socio-cultural barriers.

## Case Studies of Successful Male Engagement in Family Planning Programs

In India, family planning has long been seen primarily as a woman's responsibility. However, several innovative programs have begun to challenge this perspective by actively involving men in the decision-making process. These efforts have shown that when men are informed and engaged in family planning, the positive impacts reach far beyond just the couples themselves, benefiting entire communities. By looking at successful examples from Maharashtra, Bihar, and Uttar Pradesh, one can see how these programs have resulted in shared responsibility in family planning decisions. *Promoting Change in Reproductive Behaviour of Adolescents (PRACHAR) Project by PathFinder International is one such project.* PRACHAR project (meaning 'promote' in Hindi) between 2001 to 2013, in Bihar, the third most populous state in India with the objective to build local capacity to deliver comprehensive behaviour change programming to delay the age of marriage and promote the healthy timing and spacing of pregnancies among adolescents and young couples (Pathfinder International, n.d.). The project was implemented in three stages in more than 1000 villages. PRACHAR identified the traditional gender norms and values inculcated in the youth. The purpose was to implement gender transformative activities and initiate reflection and dialogues on issues such as gender equitable norms within marriage, empowering girls to delay age of marriage and reproductive health responsibilities for both men and women (Pathfinder International, n.d.). The activities were administered in a gender synchronised form, where both men and women were engaged together to build mutual trust and confidence. The combined results pointed to a shift in change in attitude, especially pertaining to higher use of contraception and delay in the age of marriage, when both men and women are engaged in such conversations (Pathfinder International, n.d.).

*Men Matter: Engaging Men in Reproductive Health Goals (2016),* is an initiative by the Family Planning Division of Ministry of Health and Family Welfare, Government of India which recognises reproduction as a dual commitment and not solely a woman's responsibility (Rishi et al., 2016). Through this initiative, the Government of India, recognises that gender inequality and gender related barriers as key determinants of reproductive health, and therefore promotes gender equality in all areas of programming (Rishi et al., 2016). Men Matter initiative has involved men as allies, initiators and torch bearers of upliftment. Its implementation across various Indian states has resulted in better involvement of men in safeguarding reproductive rights of women, especially regarding maternal health and use of contraception.

The KARMA Project, led by Engender Health, aimed to strengthen institutional capacity for sustainable delivery of quality postpartum and post abortion family planning in two Indian States of Karnataka and Maharashtra (EngenderHealth, n.d.). The KARMA Project was built on the gains achieved through the Men as Partners (MAP) Project (EngenderHealth, n.d.). The goals of the project were to enable men to obtain accurate and relevant information on family planning and maternal care, to enable them to use male contraception or support their partners to use their choice of female contraception. They also aimed at enabling men to extend emotional support to their spouses while using contraception or going through the process of childbirth. The initiative reached more than 2 million men either directly or indirectly, out of which more than seventy percent of them, reported learning new information and ways of involvement in use of contraception and antenatal and postnatal care.

## V. SOCIO-CULTURAL BARRIERS TO MALE INVOLVEMENT

### Traditional Gender Roles and Masculinity

Family Planning is fraught with social and gender norms at various levels which influence the intimate space of the couple as well as impact all other stakeholders of the ecosystem; the most common norms being related to masculinity, marriage and fertility (Seth et al., 2020). The terminology - 'men as partners' has been used explicitly to describe men in a supporting capacity and not as co-equals with women, who are assigned the primary responsibility as autonomous individuals in reproductive decision making (Wentzell & Inhorn, 2014). In India, the notion of men not being co-equals to women is structured in a manner where men occupy the superior status in the social, political and the family hierarchy and often dictate terms to women, including control over their reproductive choices.

Masculinity is a form of gender, variously defined as an identity, a social role, a form of power and is typically, not exclusively associated with men (Mankowski & Smith, 2016). A patriarchal perspective sees men as the centre of rationality and normality (*Masculinities*, 2022). Masculinity lays down a normative context for behaviour of men (Seth et al., 2020). It establishes the ways of behaviour and thinking for men. Men, for example are expected to be the providers to their families and are expected to refrain from display of emotions. Men are also conditioned not to engage in activities considered to be feminine such as cooking, taking care of the children and the household etc. Men are often socialised to believe that reproductive health is a "women's issue" and that their primary role is to provide financially rather than engage in discussions about contraception, family planning, or childbirth. Sex within marriage is also gendered in India. Men occupy a dominant position in their demand for sex and women as subservients are expected to fulfil this demand. The scope for denial of sex is narrow since Indian laws do not penalise marital rape. Men therefore are also conditioned to control the sexuality of women and protect the notion of honour connected to female sexuality. Gender roles therefore accord men a dominant role in all social and familial institutions. Men often evaluate themselves on these specific markers of masculinity and an inability to perform as per these notions becomes a cause of distress for them *(Khan et al., 2008)*.

## Religious Influences on Male Involvement

Religious teachings about gender roles can also influence men's participation in reproductive health. Various religions recognise the superior status and role of men in the family and accord them powers to regulate all matters associated with women and children; including reproductive choices.

Manusmriti, an ancient religious Hindu text, is a code which covers a wide variety of rules and principles on marriage, funeral, adoption, social structure etc. It also contains codes on women and wives, hospitality, pollution and purification, administrative and juridical matters and the text therefore has a high value and belief in the Indian Hindu Community till today (N. M. & Kuruvilla, 2022). Manusmriti contains verses on regulations of reproductive rights of women. It provides that control of sexuality and reproductive rights must vest with men alone and the women have a duty to bear children, more specifically sons. A woman who does not bear children or whose children have died, deserves to be replaced by another wife. Verse 9.81 states that - "*A barren wife may be superseded in the eighth year; one whose children have died, in the tenth; one who bears (only) daughters, in the eleventh; but one who says unpleasant things (may be superseded) immediately*" (www.wisdomlib.org, *2018).*

Manusmriti also rejects abortion and condemns a woman who undergoes abortion. Verse 90:5 states that - *No ritual of libation should be poured for those who are [90:5] nor for women who have joined a heretical sect, or who live on lust, or have abortions, or harm their husbands, or drink liquor"* (N. M. & Kuruvilla, 2022). Manusmriti thus provides for subordination of women by men in all aspects of life, including reproduction, the reminiscent of which still deeply pervade Indian society. Other religions practiced in India like Islam and Christianity, too provide for skewed gender dynamics, largely working in favour of men and robbing women of choices. As a result of this socio- cultural fabric and lack of awareness and sensitisation on gender politics and structures, the reproductive health government programs in India have predominantly focused on female sterilisation as the primary method of contraception, often neglecting male participation. This gendered approach to family planning reflects broader societal norms that view reproduction as a woman's responsibility. Traditional gender roles often lead women to prioritise family needs over their health, impacting maternal health outcomes (Ramanathan, 2002).

## Education Levels and Economic Factors

The Nobel Prize winner Indian Economist, Amartya Sen, states that - " *If we continue to leave vast sections of the people of the world, outside the orbit of education, we make the world not only less just but also also less secure*" (United

Nations, n.d.). Education levels significantly impacts thinking patterns and decision making, including reproductive choices. Economic status may also impact how men view family planning and use of contraception by women. The data by National Health and Family Survey V in India clearly establishes link between higher level of education and better awareness and use of contraception by men. 36.3 percent of men who had more than twelve years of schooling used contraception as compared to 27.6 percent of men with no schooling. Similarly men belonging to the lowest wealth quintile showed less use of contraception as compared to men belonging to middle through highest wealth quintile (NFHS 5, 2022). Educated men also have far better exposure to family planning messages through radio, television and print media as per the NFHS V data. Men belonging to economically well off families also tend to have better perception about contraception and family planning.

Lack of education and economic resources can limit the access to knowledge and information which leads to men holding on to incorrect information and traditional ways, thereby limiting their involvement as partners in reproductive health and family planning.

## VI. CONCLUSION AND POLICY RECOMMENDATIONS

Understanding men's role in reproductive health and rights of women is at the core of furthering gender equity in the 21st century. For decades, reproductive health has been considered a woman centric issue with women as the key beneficiaries and stakeholders in the matter. However, reproductive health outcomes are impacted not only by the actions of women, but also by men. Traditionally, the responsibility of family planning and use of contraception has largely fallen upon women. Men have been sidelined from effectively engaging in policy decisions, interventions and responsibilities. Traditional gender based roles and patriarchal society, coupled with lack of education and awareness have impeded men in being equal partners and realisation of better reproductive health and it is crucial to involve men to play an active and responsible role in matters of maternal health and family planning.

Tackling the socio-cultural barriers that hinder men's involvement in reproductive health requires thoughtful, multi-pronged strategies that resonate with local contexts and respect cultural nuances. After a careful consideration of literature and the prevalent socio-cultural practices in India, **the author makes observations and recommendations to engage men more effectively in reproductive health, ultimately fostering a more inclusive approach to health and well-being -**

- **Effective Sex Education to inculcate value of equality and responsibility**. Schools should have effective sex education and awareness programmes. This helps in inculcating the values of equality and shared responsibility from a young age. Sex

Education, if properly administered can challenge the existing gender norms and can lead to better involvement in family planning and use of contraception from a young age. However, the general perception about imparting sex education is negative. Unfortunately in India, neither government, NGOs or the civil society are broadening their perspectives and believe that exposure to sex education can lead to risk taking behaviour and promiscuity in children *(M. K. Pandey & Rao, 2023)*. There is no government mandated policy for implementation of sex education programmes in India. This needs to change. India needs to come up with a comprehensive sex education programme to create awareness and sensitisation about reproduction and sexuality and the target should not only be adolescent girls but adolescent boys. The Author recommends for a government mandated sex education policy for adolescent boys and girls which should aim at fostering gender equity and dismantling traditional and unscientific notions about reproduction and family planning.

- **Community-based engagement through workshops and seminars.** Workshops and seminar can play a key role in increasing awareness about the importance of male involvement in reproductive health decisions. To be truly effective, these sessions must be culturally sensitive, addressing the specific beliefs and practices within each community that discourage male participation. By engaging with men in their own environments and acknowledging their cultural contexts, these initiatives can foster meaningful change and encourage greater involvement in reproductive health matters. Additionally, for such programmes to succeed, training and sensitisation of volunteers and staff is crucial who are the primary agents in dissemination of information to the target groups.
- **Development of scientific temper.** Scientific temper is key to progress. Education enables development of scientific thinking and access to quality education needs focus. Without education and awareness, both men and women continue to hold on to traditional and patriarchal ideas of reproduction and family planning. Evidence has shown that more years of education has a positive impact on use of contraception and perception of family planning messages of men. (NHFS V, 2022). Programs offering economic support, such as vocational training, job opportunities, and financial literacy education, can help ease the financial pressures that often discourage men from engaging in family planning. When men have a stronger economic foundation coupled with education, they are likely to feel more confident and capable of participating in reproductive health decisions alongside their partners. Education in India is largely privatised and access to good quality education is expensive with majority of Indian population unable to afford it. The government run primary and secondary education system is in rots and needs a massive overhauling, if it were to inspire any changes in the society. The curriculum pitched by the government should mandatorily include modules on critical thinking and gender equality.

- **Altering Couple Dynamics Through Couple Counselling.** Indian society accords power to men and their families in deciding the reproductive choices of women. Women, rather being an active participant and stakeholders are often play the subsidiary role in such dynamics. This inferior positioning becomes even more precarious due to illiteracy and lack of financial opportunities for women. Placing men and women at equal footing requires structural changes in the Indian family system. One way of establishing boundaries and fostering trust is through couples counselling where clear and effective communication can enable men in understanding their role as equal partners in making reproductive choices. Family counselling may also enable other family members to understand and acknowledge their roles in supporting equal choices for women.

## REFERENCES


Abebe, M., Tebeje, T. M., Molla, W., & Melaku, G. (2023). *Male involvement in family planning services*. IntechOpen., DOI: 10.5772/intechopen.111949

Abie, A., Belay, G., Asmare, E., Ayalew, N., Feyisa, W., & Kassie, N. (2023). Male partner involvement in postnatal care service utilization and associated factors: A community-based cross-sectional study in Motta district, Northwest Ethiopia. *PLoS One*, 18(1), e0276477. DOI: 10.1371/journal.pone.0276477

Agochukwu, N. Q., & Wittmann, D. (2019). Stress, depression, mental illness, and men's health. In Elsevier eBooks (pp. 207–221). https://doi.org/DOI: 10.1016/b978-0-12-816665-9.00010-x

AIWC. All India Women's Conference. (n.d.). https://www.aiwc.org.in/achievements.html#:~:text=In%201932%2C%20AIWEFA%20 established%20Lady,Indian%20 Council%20 for%20 Child%20 Welfare.

Aliesio, L. D., E, V., E, A., & R, A. (2009). The Positive Effects of Father's Attendance to Labour and Delivery : A Quasi Experimental Study. International Nursing Perspectives, 9. https://www.researchgate.net/profile/Ercole-Vellone/publication/236679605_The_positive_effects_of_father's_attendance_to_labour_and_delivery_A_quasi_experimental_study/links/00463526ea2d2d7fce000000/The-positive-effects-of-fathers-attendance-to-labour-and-delivery-A-quasi-experimental-study.pdf

Ashford, L. (2003). *The importance of reproductive health to development: Linking fertility, poverty, and population growth*. Population Reference Bureau.

Balaiah, D., Naik, D. D., Parida, R. C., Ghule, M., Hazari, K. T., & Juneja, H. S. (1999). Contraceptive knowledge, attitude and practices of men in rural Maharashtra. *Advances in Contraception*, 15(3), 217–234. DOI: 10.1023/a:1006753617161

Bharathram, S. M. M. (2023, October 19). The measure of the working woman. The Hindu. https://www.thehindu.com/opinion/op-ed/the-measure-of-the-working-woman/article67435724.ece#:~:text=India's%20first%20 national%20Time%20 Use,compared%20with%2026.1%25%20of%20men.

Cassen, R. H. (1978). Health and family planning. In Palgrave Macmillan UK eBooks (pp. 145–209). https://doi.org/DOI: 10.1007/978-1-349-06522-6_3

Chiinhauching, S. Alam, S. N., Bhutia, S. P., Singh, S. P., & PARLIAMENT LIBRARY AND REFERENCE, RESEARCH, DOCUMENTATION AND INFORMATION SERVICE. (2022). Population control in India. In PARLIAMENT LIBRARY AND REFERENCE, RESEARCH, DOCUMENTATION AND INFORMATION SERVICE, PARLIAMENT LIBRARY AND REFERENCE, RESEARCH, DOCUMENTATION AND INFORMATION SERVICE. https://loksabhadocs.nic.in/Refinput/New_Reference_Notes/English/15072022_141200_1021205175.pdf

Chodorow, N. (1978). The reproduction of mothering. In University of California Press eBooks. https://doi.org/DOI: 10.1525/9780520924086

Coltrane, S. (1996). *Family Man: Fatherhood, Housework, and Gender Equity*. Oxford University Press.

Dudgeon, M., & Inhorn, M. (2004). Men's Influence on Women's Reproductive Health : Medical Anthropological Perspectives. Social Science and Medicine. https://marciainhorn.com/wp-content/uploads/docs/inhorn-article-mens-influence-womens-reproductive-health.pdf

EngenderHealth. (n.d.). [Enhancing Male Engagement in Family Planning: Lessons Learned from EngenderHealth's Broadening Accountability of Men Campaign in Karnataka and Maharashtra]. In EngenderHealth (pp. 1–3). https://www.engenderhealth.org/wp-content/uploads/imported-files/Enhancing-Male-Engagement-in-Family-Planning-Lessons-Learned-from-EngenderHealths-Broadening-Accountability-of-Men-Campaign-in-Karnataka-and-Maharashtra.pdf

Family Planning. (n.d.). National Health Mission. https://nhm.gov.in/index1.php?lang=1&level=2&sublinkid=821&lid=222

Gender norms and sexual and reproductive health. (n.d.). Align Platform. https://www.alignplatform.org/gender-norms-and-sexual-and-reproductive-health#:~:text=and%20romantic%20relationships-,Women%20and%20girls%20are%20conditioned%20to%20prioritise%20purity%20and%20modesty,employ%20control%20over%20their%20partners

Government of India. (2005). National Health Mission: Framework for Implementation. https://nhm.gov.in/

Government of India. (2022). National Family and Health Survey V. https://dhsprogram.com/pubs/pdf/FR375/FR375.pdf

Government of India. (n.d.). Collaboration with and Commitments from Industry. https://main.mohfw.gov.in/sites/default/files/26953755641410949469%20%281%29.pdf

Government of India. (n.d.). Maternal Health. National Health Mission. https://nhm.gov.in/index1.php?lang=1&level=2&sublinkid=822&lid=218

Greene, M. E.. (2006). Involving men in reproductive health: Contributions to development. UN Millennium Project. Ezeh, A. C. (1993). The influence of spouses over each other's contraceptive attitudes in Ghana. *Studies in Family Planning*, 24(3), 163–174.

Greene, M. E., & Biddlecom, A. E. (2000). Absent and problematic men: Demographic accounts of male reproductive roles. *Population and Development Review*, 26(1), 81–115.

Gwatkin, D. R. (1979). Political will and family planning: The implications of India's emergency experience. *Population and Development Review*, 5(1), 29. DOI: 10.2307/1972317

Initiatives for pregnant women. (n.d.). https://pib.gov.in/PressReleaseIframePage.aspx?PRID=1843841

IPPF. (2014). Stories of Gender Justice and Sexual and Reproductive Health and Rights. International Planned Parenthood Federation. https://www.ippf.org/sites/default/files/web_ippf_menboyscollection.pdf

Jejeebhoy, S. J., & Sathar, Z. A. (2001). Women's autonomy in India and Pakistan: The influence of religion and region. *Population and Development Review*, 27(4), 687–712. DOI: 10.1111/j.1728-4457.2001.00687.x

Jha, A., & Rituraj, A. Assistant Professor of Law, School of Legal Studies, The Neotia University, West Bengal, & Visiting Faculty, School of Legal Studies, The Neotia University, West Bengal. (2023). X v. Principal Secretary, Health and Family Welfare Dept, Govt. of NCT of Delhi & Anr. In CMR UNIVERSITY JOURNAL FOR CONTEMPORARY LEGAL AFFAIRS (Vol. 5, Issue 1, pp. 315–320).

Johnson, P. (2012). Sexism. In Elsevier eBooks (pp. 84–90). https://doi.org/DOI: 10.1016/b978-0-12-373932-2.00296-9

Kandiyoti, D. (1988). Bargaining with patriarchy. *Gender & Society*, 2(3), 274–290.

Khan, S. I., Hudson-Rodd, N., Saggers, S., Bhuiyan, M. I., Bhuiya, A., Karim, S. A., & Rauyajin, O. (2008). Phallus, performance and power: Crisis of masculinity. *Sexual and Relationship Therapy*, 23(1), 37–49. DOI: 10.1080/14681990701790635

Ki-moon, B., Osotimehin, B., & United Nations. (1994). Programme of action. In International Conference on Population and Development (20th Anniversary Edition). United Nations Population Fund. https://www.unfpa.org/sites/default/files/pub-pdf/programme_of_action_Web%20ENGLISH.pdf

Ledbetter, R. (1984). Thirty years of family planning in India. *Asian Survey*, 24(7), 736–758. DOI: 10.2307/2644186

Lorimer, K., McMillan, L., McDaid, L., Milne, D., Russell, S., & Hunt, K. (n.d.). Exploring masculinities, sexual health and wellbeing across areas of high deprivation in Scotland: The depth of the challenge to improve understandings and practices. *Health & Place*, 50, 27–41. DOI: 10.1016/j.healthplace.2017.12.002

Maharatna, A. (2002). India's Family Planning Programme: An Unpleasant Essay. *Economic and Political Weekly*, 37(10), 971–981. http://www.jstor.org/stable/4411847

Mankowski, E., & Smith, R. (2016). Men's Mental Health and Masculinities. In Elsevier eBooks (pp. 66–74). https://doi.org/DOI: 10.1016/b978-0-12-397045-9.00182-8

Masculinities. (2022, December 2). Gender Matters. https://www.coe.int/en/web/gender-matters/masculinities

Maternal health. (n.d.). UNICEF. https://www.unicef.org/india/what-we-do/maternal-health

McDermott, R. C., Pietrantonio, K. R., Browning, B. R., McKelvey, D. K., Jones, Z. K., Booth, N. R., & Sevig, T. D. (2019b). In search of positive masculine role norms: Testing the positive psychology positive masculinity paradigm. *Psychology of Men & Masculinity*, 20(1), 12–22. DOI: 10.1037/men0000160

Mullany, B. C. (2006). Barriers to and attitudes towards promoting husbands' involvement in maternal health in Katmandu, Nepal. *Social Science & Medicine*, 62(11), 2798–2809.

N. M. N., & Kuruvilla, M. (2022). The Sexual Politics of the Manusmriti: A Critical Analysis with Sexual and Reproductive Health Rights Perspectives. In Journal of International Women's Studies (Vol. 23, Issue 6, pp. 21-). https://vc.bridgew.edu/jiws/vol23/iss6/3

NFHS-5. (2021). Men's participation in family planning & reproductive health in India. https://india.unfpa.org/sites/default/files/pub-pdf/brief3_-_mens_participation_in_fp_and_rh.pdf

Noursi, S., Clayton, J. A., Bianchi, D. W., & Fink, D. (2021). Maternal morbidity and mortality. *Journal of Women's Health*, 30(2), 145–146. DOI: 10.1089/jwh.2020.8851

Office of Population and Reproductive Health. Bureau for Global Health, Sanicki, A., Betron, M., Brown, J., Greene, M., Hardee, K., Kapungu, C., Martinez, L., Shattuck, D., Skinner, J., Underwood, C., & Van Lith, L. (2018). Essential considerations for engaging men and boys for improved family planning outcomes [Report]. https://www.usaid.gov/sites/default/files/2022-05/Engaging-men-boys-family-planning-508.pdf

Pandey, B. G. (2022, June 27). NFHS-5: Why birth control remains a woman's burden in India. https://www.bbc.com/news/world-asia-india-61906015

Pandey, M. K., & Rao, T. S. (2023). Sexuality education in India yet remains a Taboo—An attempt to Dust-Off. *Journal of Psychosexual Health*, 5(1), 11–12. DOI: 10.1177/26318318231155993

Parliament. (1971). THE MEDICAL TERMINATION OF PREGNANCY ACT, 1971 [Legal]. In THE MEDICAL TERMINATION OF PREGNANCY ACT, 1971. https://www.indiacode.nic.in/bitstream/123456789/1593/1/A1971-34.pdf

Pathfinder International. (n.d.). PRACHAR: Advancing young people's sexual and reproductive health and rights in India. In Pathfinder International. https://www.youthpower.org/sites/default/files/YouthPower/files/resources/Prachar%20report.pdf

Pillai, G. (2024). *India's Push-and-Pull on Reproductive Rights*. Verfassungsblog., DOI: 10.59704/41b437064b3e88d3

Population Fund of India. (n.d.). Men's Participation in Family Planning & Reproductive Health Learnings and opportunities for India. https://india.unfpa.org/sites/default/files/pub-pdf/brief3_-_mens_participation_in_fp_and_rh.pdf

Promoting Men's Involvement in Maternal and Child Health. (2016). https://men-care.org

Ramanathan, M. R. (2002). Women's Health and Reproductive Health Services in India: Balancing Rights, Responsibilities, and Needs. *Studies in Family Planning*.

Rishi, G. Government of India, Kashyap, I., National Technical Support Unit - Family Planning (NTSU-FP), & Ministry of Health and Family Welfare (MoHFW). (2016). Men Matter: Engaging men in India's reproductive health goals. https://nhm.gov.in/images/pdf/programmes/family-planing/Campaing/Coffee_Table_Book.pdf

SAMA Resource Group for Women and Health & Partners for Law in Development. (2018). Country assessment undertaken for National Human Rights Commission by: SAMA Resource Group for Women and Health, Partners for Law in Development: Status of human rights in the context of Sexual Health and Reproductive Health Rights in India. https://nhrc.nic.in/sites/default/files/sexual_health_reproductive_health_rights_SAMA_PLD_2018_01012019_1.pdf

Samuel, T. J. (1966). The development of India's policy of population control. *The Milbank Memorial Fund Quarterly*, 44(1), 49. DOI: 10.2307/3349038

Satz, D. (2013). Feminist perspectives on reproduction and the family. Plato Stanford. https://plato.stanford.edu/entries/feminism-family/#3

Seth, K., Nanda, S., Sahay, A., Verma, R., & Achyut, P. (2020). "IT'S ON HIM TOO" PATHWAYS TO ENGAGE MEN IN FAMILY PLANNING. International Centre for Research on Women. https://www.icrw.org/wp-content/uploads/2020/06/Couple-Engage-Evidence-Review.pdf

Sexual & reproductive health. (n.d.). United Nations Population Fund. https://www.unfpa.org/sexual-reproductive-health

Shah, K. T., Bhende, A. A., & Kanitkar, T. Lucknow university, Pillai, A. P., Mahalanobis, P. C., Mukerjee, R., Sapru, P. N., Bhose, S. J., Yeatts, W. M., Datta, R., & Chandrasekhar, S. (n.d.). HISTORY OF FAMILY PLANNING IN INDIA. http://ir.unishivaji.ac.in:8080/jspui/bitstream/123456789/3652/9/09_Chapter%203.pdf

Shalev, C. (2000). Rights to Sexual and Reproductive Health: The ICPD and the Convention on the Elimination of All Forms of Discrimination against Women. *Health and Human Rights*, 4(2), 38. DOI: 10.2307/4065196

Shantilal Shah Committee. (1966). Report of the Committee to study the question of legalisation of abortion. Government of India. https://dn790000.ca.archive.org/0/items/dli.ministry.20283/1266.pdf

Starbird, E., Norton, M., & Marcus, R. (2016). Investing in family planning: Key to achieving the sustainable development goals. *Global Health, Science and Practice*, 4(2), 191–210. DOI: 10.9745/ghsp-d-15-00374

Storming the Citadels of Poverty. Family Planning under the Emergency in India, 1975-1977 on JSTOR. (n.d.). www.jstor.org. https://www.jstor.org/stable/43553297

The Missing Piece. Valuing women's unrecognized contribution to the economy. (n.d.). UNDP. https://www.undp.org/latin-america/blog/missing-piece-valuing-womens-unrecognized-contribution-economy#:~:text=At%20the%20global%20level%2C%20women,1%20house%20and%2023%20 minutes.

The People's Archive of Rural India. (n.d.). National Family Health Survey (NFHS-5), 2019-21: India. People's Archive of Rural India. https://ruralindiaonline.org/en/library/resource/national-family-health-survey-nfhs-5-2019-21-india/

United Nations. (n.d.). Education as the Pathway towards Gender Equality | United Nations. https://www.un.org/en/chronicle/article/education-pathway-towards-gender-equality

United Nations Population Fund. (1994). Programme of action of the International Conference on Population and Development. https://www.unfpa.org/sites/default/files/event-pdf/PoA_en.pdf#

Verma, R. K., Schensul, S. L., & Schensul, J. J. (2001). Risk, perception, and condom use among married men in Mumbai, India. *International Family Planning Perspectives*, 27(3), 138–145.

Wegner, M. N., Landry, E., Wilkinson, D., & Tzanis, J. (2022, August 25). Men as partners in Reproductive Health: From Issues to action. Guttmacher Institute. https://www.guttmacher.org/journals/ipsrh/1998/03/men-partners-reproductive-health-issues-action

Wentzell, E. A., & Inhorn, M. C. (2014). Reconceiving masculinity and 'men as partners' for ICPD Beyond 2014: Insights from a Mexican HPV study. *Global Public Health: An International Journal for Research, Policy and Practice*, 9(6), 691–705. DOI: 10.1080/17441692.2014.917690

World Health Organization. (2015). Postnatal care guidelines. In Postnatal Care for Mothers and Newborns: Vol. April 2015 (p. 2) [Report]. https://www.who.int/docs/default-source/mca-documents/nbh/brief-postnatal-care-for-mothers-and-newborns-highlights-from-the-who-2013-guidelines.pdf

World Health Organization. WHO. (2019, September 23). Maternal health. https://www.who.int/health-topics/maternal-health#tab=tab_1

World Health Organization. WHO. (2024, April 10). Sexual and reproductive health and rights. https://www.who.int/health-topics/sexual-and-reproductive-health-and-rights#tab=tab_2

WWW. REPRODUCTIVE RIGHTS.ORG. (2021). Reproductive rights in India: the current situation. In Reproductive Rights in India: The Current Situation [Report]. https://reproductiverights.org/sites/default/files/documents/Reproductive-Rights-In-Indian-Courts.pdf

www.wisdomlib.org. (2018, February 16). Manusmriti Verse 9.81. https://www.wisdomlib.org/hinduism/book/manusmriti-with-the-commentary-of-medhatithi/d/doc201444.html

Chapter 12

# Complexities of Assisted Reproductive Technology: Exploring Legal Framework, Ethical Debate, and Religious Beliefs

**Upasana Khattri**
*O.P. Jindal Global University, India*

**Rajat Shandilya**
https://orcid.org/0009-0004-6262-8132
*O.P. Jindal Global University, India*

**Sanyukta Saxena**
*O.P. Jindal Global University, India*

## ABSTRACT

*Assistive Reproductive Technologies (ART) has become topic of discussion in the recent times. The introduction of ART in the field of medical science has been subject to controversies. Various laws and guidelines to address the issues related to ART but due to its rapid advancement ART requires re-evaluation. The paper will analyse the existing legal framework, religious beliefs and the ethical issues surrounding the topic of ART. The progressive increment in the use of these techniques ranging from but not limited to vitro fertilisation, genetic editing and surrogacy has brought remarkable change in the field of human reproduction. As it is a common saying the every coin has two sides, same is the case here as on a positive note, this particular*

DOI: 10.4018/979-8-3693-7837-3.ch012

*advancement by the way of ART has given hope to many individual and couples who are aspiring to be parents but are unfortunately suffering from infertility and genetic disorders and on the contrary, this specific advancement can be held to be the reason behind the rise of multiple ethical, legal, and religious concerns and challenges.*

## INTRODUCTION

*And God blessed them, and God said unto them, Be fruitful, and multiply, and replenish the earth and subdue it.*

*—Holy Bible: Genesis 1:28*

The process of reproduction is the fundamental cycle of life. Keeping in mind the principle of letting every human the right to enjoy his life to the highest physically and mentally attainable health standard; infertility stands on the way. Family is considered to be the basic unit of a society. Recognizing family as a social entity acknowledges the fact that they are socially created and defined, and the structure of the family varies across cultures. Every individual and couples has the basic human right to decide and plan about having children. All the major human right instruments have protected right to marry and have family. Universal Declaration of Human Rights (UDHR) 1948 provides that "men and women of full age without any limitation due to race, nationality or religion have the right to marry and found a family". Giving birth to a child is the natural outcome of sexual intercourse between men and women. This arrangement of pregnancy and birth of a child is socially accepted through the institution of marriage. Therefore, the involvement of technology or a third party is not required. However, there are many couples facing difficulty in giving birth to a child through the biological process. This situation is medically termed- infertility. Infertility is a situation in which a couple is unable to conceive naturally even after one year of unprotected sexual intercourse or is unable to carry the pregnancy to a full term (Anwar 2016). Infertility is a global issue with an 8% to 10% rate of effect on the couples worldwide and 3.9-16.8% overall prevalence of primary infertility in India. It has been recognized as a disease by the World Health Organization which needs to be addressed. The issue of infertility mitigates gender inequality. The patriarchal society generally presumes the female to be infertile rather than the male; which negatively impacts the social life of the female leading them down the way of harassment, divorce, violence, low self-esteem, depression and social stigma. These problems need to be addressed and challenges need to be overcome. Although the issue of infertility is a growing concern, the availability, access and quality to intervene infertility is a challenge to most of the countries. The root cause to this lies in the ignorance of policies of countries to address infertility as a disease. In Indian society, the inability to reproduce a child is either a social stigma or a curse from the divine god. The infertile couples look for different opportunities to resolve this reproductive issue. ART has become a ray of hope for infertile couples. Before ART came into the picture, either adoption or remaining childless was the available option. However, with advancements in reproductive technologies, the infertile couple can select from various options available including in-vitro fertilization, and artificial insemination. Moreover, surrogacy is the most popular and widely practiced method (Valentina A, 2019). These methods help in human procreation of without sexual intercourse.

## METHODOLOGY AND RESEARCH QUESTION

The authors have adopted critical, descriptive, comparative and analytical approach to formulate this book chapter. The authors will analyse the problem with the help of periodicals, law books, electronic articles, legal framework, and judicial precedents pertaining to the issue. The authors has selected bibliographic databases to identify secondary sources ranging from text books, bar review, scholarly articles and legal encyclopaedias. The book chapter aims to answer the following research question: What are the legal, ethical and religious challenges of ART. How legal frameworks will address the legal, ethical and religious dilemmas posed by ART.

### Definition: Assistive Reproductive Technologies (ART)

Technologies shapes every aspect of human life. The term ART is general terms which includes those techniques that artificially assist in to conceive when couples and individuals face difficulties with natural conception. ART is the application of laboratory or clinical technology to gametes (human eggs or sperm) and/or embryos for the purposes of reproduction. Any "procedure or method designed to enhance fertility or to compensate for infertility" outside the customary connotation of reproduction can be categorized as ART. (Blank. R, Merrick. J,1995)

ART refers to all medical techniques used to help a woman become pregnant, excluding intercourse. Both of these developments have revolutionized the field of reproductive medicine, bringing hope to millions around the world. And yet, while the term ART is fairly recent, its history and search for solutions to infertility have been going on for millennia. The progression from ancient fertility treatments to the modern day marvels we know has very much mirrored key scientific breakthroughs, technological innovations, as well as societal and ethical discussions. No other scientific field has made such remarkable progress as ART, evolving from prohibition to acceptance, and from research to clinical practice. The swift advancement of ART and related methods is driven by the social and scientific environment that fosters its growth.

## Early Notion of Fertility

The desire to overcome infertility and control reproduction is as old as humanity itself. For much of history, infertility was often misunderstood, and treatments were based on superstition, folklore, and religious practices.

1. **Ancient Civilizations**: The quest to combat infertility and manage reproduction is as old as mankind. Throughout history infertility has been a mystery, with treatments consisting of superstitious or magical beliefs and religious practices. The first written record of treating infertility comes from ancient Egyptian, Greek, and Roman civilizations in which several methods for treating male impotence were described. To the ancient Egyptians, fertility was extremely important and they turned to herbal remedies, esoteric rituals or animal products that were thought to have powers promoting fertilization. Some of the earliest medical theories about infertility came from Greek physicians such as Hippocrates (460-370 BCE), who, however, based their interpretations on very limited knowledge of reproductive anatomy. Aristotle (384-322 BCE) wrote extensively about reproduction, although he incorrectly believed that men contributed the "form" and women the "matter" in procreation. (Hippocrates, 1931)
2. **Religious Interpretations**: In many of the past societies and civilizations, the problem of being infertile was attributed to being punished by Gods or also the 'Test of Faith' Notably, religious texts as the Bible have mention of stories of infertile women like Sarah, Rachel, and Hannah, who suffered from infertility first but their eventual pregnancies were seen as divine blessings by the Almighty. Religious and spiritual rituals were often part of fertility treatment in these early cultures, reflecting the belief that fertility was closely tied to divine intervention.
3. **Medical Theories of the Middle Ages**: During the Middle Ages and the Renaissance periods, the than existing knowledge medical knowledge surrounding human reproduction remained confined and limited. An unfortunate occurrence which was common during the stated period was that that infertility was the female only and it was she was said to be the ultimate reason of not being able to have a child or in other words, childlessness. Treatments during these periods were still primarily herbal or spiritual, with little scientific understanding of the underlying biological processes involved in conception. (Jacquart, & Thomasset, 1988)

## THE EMERGENCE OF SCIENTIFIC DISCOVERIES AND THE FOUNDATIONS OF ART

The basis or foundation for modern day ART was laid by the means of key scientific discoveries globally in the 17th through 19th centuries. These discoveries changed the perception of human reproduction and allied disciplines and carved out a the way for future technological advancements.

1. **Discovery of Sperm Cells**: It was in the year 1677, that Dutch scientist Antonie van Leeuwenhoek made a use of a microscope to observe and study human sperm cells for the very first time. This discovery was a significant milestone in reproductive science, as it uncovered the role of male gametes in the process of human fertilization. Although sperm cells had been identified, it would take more than a century to fully understand their function in human reproduction. (Leeuwenhoek, 1677.)
2. **Discovery of the Egg Cell**: In the year 1827, the German scientist Karl Ernst von Baer is credited for the discovery of the mammalian egg cell (ovum), thereby, completing the scenario of human fertilization. The discovery of both sperm and egg cells established the basis for understanding the process of conception, leading scientists to consider the possibility of intervening in this process through medical techniques. (von Baer, K. E. (1827)
3. **Artificial Insemination**: The 18th century witnessed the first successful experiments in artificial insemination, where sperm was introduced into a woman's reproductive system without any sexual intercourse. It was the year 1790, when a Scottish surgeon John Hunter reportedly performed the first artificial insemination in humans, flagging the inception of a medical approach to identifying and addressing male infertility. By the late 19th century, artificial insemination was becoming more widely practiced, though it remained a controversial procedure. (Hunter, 1786).

### The Birth and Inception of Modern ART

It is a well acknowledged fact that early medical advancements focused on artificial insemination but the 20th century witnessed unprecedented advancements in ART, particularly with the development of In Vitro Fertilization (IVF) and related technologies.

1. **First Animal IVF Experiments**: In 1959, a Chinese-American scientist Min Chueh Chang conducted an experiment and in the same line successfully carried it off by fertilizing rabbit eggs in a pre-adjusted laboratory setting, marking the

conduction of the first successful animal based IVF experiment. This breakthrough demonstrated that it was possible to fertilize eggs outside the body, and it laid the groundwork for future attempts at human IVF. (Chang, 1959)

2. **The First Test-Tube Baby**: The most significant breakthrough in ART occurred in 1978 with the birth of Louise Brown, the world's first "test-tube baby. The birth of Louise was the result of IVF, a procedure that was developed by British scientists Robert Edwards and Patrick Steptoe who was a physiologist, and Steptoe, who was a gynaecologist, worked on IVF for over a decade, despite facing multiple scientific and ethical challenges. Their success marked the beginning of a new era in reproductive medicine and earned Robert Edwards the Nobel Prize in Physiology or Medicine in 2010. (Edwards & Steptoe 1980)
3. **Early IVF Success and Expansion**: After the birth of World's first IVF baby Louise Brown, IVF rapidly saw its expansion in other countries. In 1981, the first IVF baby was born in the United States of America (USA) who was Elizabeth Carr, the baby was born at the Eastern Virginia Medical School, under the care and supervision of Dr. Howard Jones and his team. By the 1990s, IVF clinics had become established in many parts of the world, offering hope to couples struggling with infertility. Advances in laboratory techniques, hormone treatments, and embryo transfer procedures steadily improved IVF success rates. (Jones & Jones 1981).

## Notable Developments in ART Techniques

As the IVF became more widely used, additional ART techniques were brought in place to address specific fertility related challenges. These innovations have widened the possibilities for conception and have made ART accessible to a wider range of patients. The concerned developments are as follows:

1. **Intracytoplasmic Sperm Injection (ICSI)**: During the time of early 1990s, Belgium based researchers Andre Van Steirteghem and Paul Devroey developed the technique of ICSI, a technique where a single sperm is injected directly into an egg to aid fertilization process. The process of ICSI was initially brought in to treat male infertility, specifically in cases where sperm count was low or the sperm quality was poor. Today, ICSI is commonly used alongside IVF to improve fertilization rates, especially for couples experiencing severe male infertility. (Van Steirteghem, 1992).
2. **Egg and Sperm Donation**: Yet another significant development in ART was the use of donor eggs and sperm. While the sperm donation had been an on-going since the early 20th century, the very first successful pregnancy from a donated egg happened to be successfully executed in the year 1984. Donor gametes have

since then, have played an important role in the ART, aiding individuals who are unable to produce viable eggs or sperm to have children. Egg and sperm donation also opened the door for LGBTQ+ individuals and single parents to build families through ART. (Sauer, 2001).

3. **Surrogacy**: Surrogacy is a process which involves a woman executing a pregnancy for a different or couple, and it became a convenient option for ART in the decade of 1980s. Surrogacy can be either the traditional one) or gestational in nature. Gestational surrogacy, made possible by IVF, has allowed couples facing uterine or other fertility challenges to have biological children. (Brinsden, 2003).
4. **Preimplantation Genetic Diagnosis (PGD)**: In the 1990s, scientists developed a process which came to be known as PGD, a technology based procedure which allowed the creation of embryos through IVF to be screened and monitored for genetic disorders before being implanted in uterus of the woman. PGD, as a technique, is used by couples who have a history of genetic diseases to make sure that their child is free of any inherited medical conditions. Although PGD has been a major breakthrough in preventing genetic diseases, it has also raised ethical concerns about the potential for selecting non-medical traits, such as sex or physical characteristics. (Handyside, 1990).

## Reproductive Rights and Issue of Infertility

Every individual is entitled to fundamental right of reproduction without discriminating infertile couples. Now important question that arises is whether right to reproduction includes procreation of child with the help of Assistive Reproductive Technologies (ART) or whether reproductive rights include access to ARTs (Pillai, 2014). The concept of Assistive Reproductive Technologies (ART) has gain lots of attention worldwide. Though, international legal framework has failed to given recognition to right to access to ART but it is inherent part of right to reproduction. This inherent recognition of right to access to ART is necessary for the infertile couple to enjoy right to reproduction. Moreover, the right to access to ART can be considered as a facet of other well established human rights such as right to marriage; right to find a family; right to privacy; right to procreation, right to control the number and spacing of their children and right to enjoy benefits of scientific and technological advancements (Pillai, 2021).

Since 1978, more than 9 million infants have been born worldwide through ART procedure to give joy of parenthood to infertile couple. In 2018 the reproductive market has earned the profit of $12.5 billions and is likely to grow. But there is no uniformity in access to ART treatment. In India infertile couple do not have access to ART treat due to financial constraint.

## Assisted Reproductive Technologies: A Comparative Analysis

Various countries around the world have responded in different ways over the aspect of ART by the means of their legal framework. This segment of the chapter makes an attempt to do a Comparative Analysis. among various countries over the same point. Notably, countries like the United States of America (USA), India, Canada and European Union has brought in place a codified legal framework for the purposes of ART while taking lessons from their respective social and cultural factors present in the society. The various countries of the world have majorly accepted Altruistic Surrogacy. Regarding ART, the International Committee Monitoring Assisted Reproductive Technologies (ICMART) is the organization defining ART worldwide. WHO endorsed the responsibility of preparing a 'Glossary on ART Terminology' for the international meeting on 'medical, ethical and social aspects of assisted reproduction' (Zegers-Hochschild 2006). The analysis of the legal framework among the above listed companies is as follows:

### Canada

ART covers within its ambit, a wide range of medical procedures aimed at helping individuals and couples in achieving pregnancy when unfortunately, natural conception doesn't take place. In Canada, the primary legal framework governing ART is specific and is the Assisted Human Reproduction Act (AHRA) which was passed in the year 2004. The AHRA thereby establishes national standards for ART and highlights the ethical, legal, and social issues related to assisted reproduction. This segment throws light on the main provisions of the Canadian law over the point of ART and is as follows:

### Assisted Human Reproduction Act in Canada (AHRA)

The Assisted Human Reproduction Act was brought in enacted with the purpose of regulating and monitoring ART in Canada, making sure that medical practices in the field are in line with public health and safety standards and also at the same time, addressing ethical concerns. The AHRA specifically lays down and regulatory standards that are aimed at protecting the health and well-being of individuals involved in the process ART.

Main Provisions of the Assisted Human Reproduction Act (AHRA)

1. *Prohibition of Commercial Surrogacy*: Under the ambit of AHRA, one of the main features which even India has now, is that commercial surrogacy is banned. Also, surrogate mothers don't really receive any compensation beyond reasonable costs and expenses that are directly related to pregnancy, such as the medical costs and also legal fees. Surrogacy arrangements must be altruistic, and paying a surrogate for her services constitutes a criminal offense punishable by fines and imprisonment.
2. *Prohibition on the Sale of Gametes and Embryos*: The AHRA bans the commercial sale or purchase of human sperm, eggs, or, for that matter, embryos. Similar to surrogacy, the donation of gametes must be altruistic, and donors may only be compensated for reasonable expenses incurred during the donation process.
3. *Informed Consent*: Another crucial feature of AHRA is that it makes it compulsory that consent should be obtained from all parties which are involved in ART procedures. This means that individuals undergoing treatment, as well as donors and surrogates, must be fully informed about the risks, benefits, and possible outcomes of the procedure before giving their consent.
4. *Prohibition on Certain Genetic and Reproductive Technologies*: Also, The AHRA prohibits specific questionable practices, such as human cloning and germ line genetic alteration. These prohibitions reflect ethical concerns over the manipulation of human life and the potential societal impacts of such technologies.
5. *Regulation of ART Clinics*: The AHRA also makes it mandatory that fertility clinics and professionals should follow strict rules and standard regulations in the management of human gametes and embryos. Clinics must maintain high medical standards, and failure to comply with these regulations can result in penalties, including license revocation and criminal charges.

## The Legal and Ethical Challenges Associated with AHRA

The AHRA was judiciously crafted and implemented to address ethical concerns related to ART, but, notably, it has faced criticism from various groups. One segment of debate involves the ban on commercial surrogacy and gamete sales. Critics of AHRA argue that these restrictions restrict individuals' autonomy, more specifically for those who may not have access to surrogacy or donation without any financial incentives. Proponents of the AHRA counter that commercializing human reproduction risks exploitation, especially of vulnerable women who may be coerced into becoming surrogates or donors for financial gain. (Baylis, 2011) Moreover, the Act driven restrictions on a certain amount of genetic technologies, such as germline modification, have seen controversy. Advances in genetic screening and manipulation could potentially allow for the correction of inherited diseases, raising questions about whether the AHRA's prohibitions should be revisited in light of scientific progress. (Baylis, Françoise, 2019)

## Notable Enforcement and Regulatory Gaps

Even after the AHRA provides for a comprehensive framework, enforcement, still, has been a significant challenge that the country has faced. The AHRA initially established the Assisted Human Reproduction Agency of Canada (AHRAC) to ensure compliance with the Act. However, unfortunately, AHRAC was dissolved in the year 2012, leaving regulatory oversight scattered. Since then, Health Canada has assumed responsibility for enforcing the AHRA, but there have been few prosecutions for violations such as illegal payments to surrogates or the sale of gametes.

The fundamental difficulty in enforcement is because of the nature of ART transactions, which can be really difficult to monitor. For example, informal surrogacy agreements may be entered into without any formal documentation, and some individuals may travel internationally to bypass Canadian laws. This has led to calls for better oversight mechanisms and clearer guidelines for surrogacy and ART clinics. (Van Beers, Britta, 2021)

## United States

The United States of America has one of the most permissive regulatory frameworks for the purposes of ART worldwide, allowing diverse ART practices, including the practice of In Vitro Fertilization (IVF), sperm and egg donation, and also surrogacy. Notably, unlike many countries that have centralized regulations, the legal framework in the U.S. is scattered as the ART is being regulated at both the federal and state levels respectively. This regulatory diversity throws light over the complexity of balancing ethical concerns, individual rights and also, lastly, technological advancements in the field of modern reproductive medicine.

### *Federal Regulations on ART*

The U.S. federal government is not responsible for directly regulating ART with reference to legal restrictions on procedures like surrogacy or IVF. However, certain federal agencies in U.S.A play significant roles in ensuring safety, ethical practices, and consumer protection as well.

1. *Centres for Disease Control and Prevention (CDC) and the Fertility Clinic Success Rate and Certification Act (FCSRCA)*: The CDC plays a crucial role in monitoring specifically, the ART success rates through the *Fertility Clinic*

*Success Rate and Certification Act (FCSRCA) of 1992*, which mandates fertility clinics to report their success rates on annual basis. The CDC also compiles and publishes this data to maintain transparency and help consumers to make informed decisions. However, this act does not regulate clinic practices, focusing instead on transparency for consumers.

2. *Food and Drug Administration (FDA)*: The FDA is responsible for regulating certain aspects of ART, specially related to the screening and handling of human reproductive tissues. The *Human Cells, Tissues, and Cellular and Tissue-Based Products (HCT/P) Regulation* ensure the safety of donated sperm, eggs, and embryos, making sure that they are free from communicable diseases. The FDA also regulates the storage and transportation of reproductive tissues to ensure their viability and safety.
3. *American Society for Reproductive Medicine (ASRM) and the Society for Assisted Reproductive Technology (SART)*: Whereas, the ASRM and SART are not governmental bodies, they do set important ethical and professional standards for ART practices in the U.S.A. ASRM rolls out ethical guidelines for reproductive medicine, addressing issues ranging from compensation for egg donors, ethical concerns related to surrogacy to the management of multiple pregnancies. On the other hand, SART is responsible for working closely with the CDC to provide accreditation for fertility clinics. Though compliance with ASRM and SART guidelines is voluntary, they play a crucial role in self-regulation within the industry.

### *State-Level Regulation of ART*

It is a well acknowledged fact that because of the absence of comprehensive federal legislation regulating ART, state laws, notably, play a significant role in determining the legality of ART procedures.

Surrogacy Laws: It is true that, surrogacy laws in the United States vary widely from state to state. While some states, such as California, are highly permissive and have clear legal frameworks that allow both gestational (where the surrogate carries a genetically unrelated child) and traditional (where the surrogate's egg is used) surrogacy the same is not true with few of the other states. California also recognizes surrogacy contracts and ensures that intended parents have full parental rights from birth, making it a popular destination for surrogacy agreements. (David, 2021)

As mentioned above that there are different laws for different states, states like Michigan bans compensated surrogacy, making it to be criminal act to enter into a paid surrogacy arrangement. Some states have no specific laws governing surrogacy, leading to legal ambiguities and potential disputes over parental rights. For example, New York only legalized compensated gestational surrogacy in 2021 under the Child-Parent Security Act, a significant shift from its previous ban.

## Ethical Concerns and Legal Debates

The lack of a uniform federal law regulating ART in the U.S. has led to ongoing ethical debates about issues such as surrogacy, genetic screening, and the commercialization of reproductive materials.

1. *Commercial Surrogacy and Exploitation Concerns*: One of the primary ethical concerns is the commercialization of surrogacy, particularly in states that allow compensated surrogacy. Critics argue that surrogacy can lead to the exploitation of economically disadvantaged women, who may feel pressured to become surrogates for financial gain. However, proponents of compensated surrogacy contend that it offers a legitimate opportunity for women to help others while being fairly compensated for their time and effort. (Bonnie, 2020)
2. *Egg and Sperm Donation*: The commercialization of egg and sperm donation also raises ethical questions. Although the FDA regulates the safety of donated reproductive materials, there are no laws limiting the compensation that donors can receive. This has led to concerns that high compensation could encourage donors to overlook the medical risks associated with the donation process. Additionally, the anonymity of donors in some cases has sparked debates about the rights of donor-conceived individuals to know their genetic origins. (Ball, 2021)
3. *Preimplantation Genetic Diagnosis (PGD)*: The use of PGD to select embryos free from genetic disorders has led to debates about "designer babies." While PGD is primarily used to prevent serious genetic conditions, its potential use for selecting non-medical traits, such as gender, raises ethical questions about the extent to which reproductive technology should be used to "enhance" future generations. (Spar, 2019)

### India

India, without a doubt has been a prominent pillar in the global Assisted Reproductive Technology (ART) landscape, specifically in the field of surrogacy and (IVF). ART offers hope to couples and individuals experiencing infertility, but it also raises considerable Legal, social and ethical concerns. In response to these concerns, India has formulated a legislation to regulate ART the *Assisted Reproductive Technology (Regulation) Act, 2021* and the Surrogacy (Regulation) Act, 2021. These laws establish the foundation and detailing of for ART practices, address issues of consent, and also safeguard the rights of all the stakeholders.

### *Surrogacy (Regulation) Act, 2021*

The Surrogacy (Regulation) Act, 2021, was enacted along with the ART Act to address the expanding market of commercial surrogacy in India. Before the enactment of this law, India was known to be a global hub for surrogacy due to its cheap costs and the easy availability of surrogates mothers. However, concerns over the exploitation of poor and marginalized women led to the need for stricter regulation.

### *Key Provisions of the Surrogacy Act*

1. *Ban on Commercial Surrogacy*: The Act bans commercial surrogacy, which involves paying a surrogate for carrying a pregnancy. Only altruistic surrogacy, where no monetary compensation is provided apart from medical expenses, is allowed. Violating this provision is punishable by fines and imprisonment.
2. *Eligibility for Surrogacy*: The Act doesn't allow surrogacy to married heterosexual couples who have been married for at least five years and have verified infertility. The couple must also be Indian citizens apart from foreign nationals and non-resident Indians (NRIs) from engaging in the practice of surrogacy setup within India. Like the ART Act, the Surrogacy Act excludes same-sex couples and unmarried partners from accessing surrogacy.
3. *Rights of the Surrogate*: The Act rolls out provision for protection for surrogate mothers, ensuring that they have the right to terminate their pregnancy under certain special conditions. Surrogates are also entitled to medical insurance and reasonable reimbursement for expenses related to the pregnancy.
4. *Legal Parentage*: Potential parents are granted immediate legal parenthood of the child born through surrogacy. This provision simplifies the process of establishing parentage, reducing legal complications that could arise from traditional adoption procedures.

### *Legal Challenges concerning ART in India*

Whenever any law is formed and enacted, the principles, legislative intent, and balance between rights and duties are considered as the fundamental essentials of the same. However, when it comes to surrogacy laws, the ethics, beliefs, and principles, clash with the interests of parties entering into the surrogacy setup thus making it difficult to single handedly frame the laws governing the same. The ART legislations in countries like Latin America and Mexico has recognised infertility as a disease; while in India, the case is different, here, Infertility exists but is not termed as a disease.

*The 228 Law Commission Report on Assisted Reproductive Technologies: The Take of the Law Commission of India*

The 228th report of the Law Commission of India was published in the year 2009, it flags an important milestone in the legal regulation of Assisted Reproductive Technologies (ART) in India. The concerned report by the Law Commission is titled as '*Need for Legislation to Regulate Assisted Reproductive Technologies*' and addresses the need for a she increasing need for a solid codified legal framework to govern ART practices, which had been rapidly increasing in India. The report provides a comprehensive review of ART practices, including in vitro fertilization (IVF), surrogacy, and sperm/egg donation, and proposes a series of legal reforms to ensure ethical and regulated application of these technologies (Law Commission of India, 2009).

ART has radicalized and revolutionized reproductive medicine by opening new avenues for conception and family growth and planning. However, the quick development of these technologies has taken over heavily the existing legal and ethical frameworks, leading to concerns about the protection of the concerned stakeholders The 228th Law Commission Report was commissioned in response to these concerns and aims to address the gaps in regulation by recommending a detailed legal framework for ART practices (Law Commission of India, 2009).

## MAIN RECOMMENDATIONS OF THE REPORT

1. *Regulation of ART Clinics and Banks*: One of the prominent recommendations of the report is regarding the establishment of a regulatory body to monitor ART clinics and sperm/egg banks. The report emphasizes the need for a national registry of ART clinics and banks, which would ensure that these institutions adhere to established standards of practice and ethical guidelines (Law Commission of India, 2009, pp. 20-25).
2. *Consent and Confidentiality*: The report highlights the importance of informed consent in ART procedures. It makes a recommendation that all the concerned stakeholders must provide a formal written consent prior to any ART procedure is carried out. Furthermore, the report stresses the need for strict confidentiality regarding the identity of donors and the details of the ART procedures (Law Commission of India, 2009, pp. 30-35).
3. *Ethical Considerations*: The report highlights certain ethical issues related to ART, such as the status of embryos, the use of (PGD), and commercialization of ART procedures and services. It proposes that ethical guidelines be developed to address these issues and ensure that ART practices are conducted in a manner

that respects human dignity and rights (Law Commission of India, 2009, pp. 40-45).

4. *Surrogacy Regulations*: The report also addresses the legal and ethical consequences of surrogacy, including the need for clear and specific legal agreements between the surrogate mother and the commissioning parents. It recommends that surrogacy arrangements be regulated to prevent exploitation and ensure that the rights of all parties involved are protected (Law Commission of India, 2009, pp. 50-55).
5. *Dispute Resolution*: Over the point of dispute resolution, arising from ART procedures, the report advances the idea of the establishment of a specialized tribunal to handle matters related to ART. This tribunal would provide a mechanism for resolving conflicts in a fair and timely manner (Law Commission of India, 2009, pp. 60-65).

## IMPACT AND IMPLEMENTATION

The 228th Law Commission Report has had a crucial impact on the legal landscape of ART in India. Its recommendations have laid the foundation for subsequent legislation aimed at regulating ART practices in India. For example, the Assisted Reproductive Technologies Act introduced in 2020 is largely based on the recommendations of the recommendations of the 228th Report This Bill seeks to establish a regulatory framework for ART services, including the creation of a National ART and Surrogacy Registry, and the formulation of standards for ART clinics and professionals. (Ministry of Health and Family Welfare, 2020).

### Criticisms and Challenges

It is quite unfortunate that despite being comprehensive in nature its comprehensive nature, the 228th Law Commission Report has faced unwelcoming response and criticism from various segments. Some stakeholders contend that the recommendations may turn out to be overly stringent and could potentially limit access to ART services for individuals and couples who are in need of the same. There are also concerns about the practical implementation of the proposed regulatory framework, given the diverse and complex nature of ART practices (Kumar & Das, 2011).

Moreover, there are demands for more inclusive and comprehensive consultations with concerned stakeholders, including patients, ART practitioners, and legal experts, to ensure that the regulatory mechanism is both effective and equitable. Critics also emphasize the need for continuous review and adaptation of the regulations to keep pace with technological advancements and evolving societal norms. (Sharma, 2013).

The 228th Law Commission Report represents a critical juncture in the regulation of Assisted Reproductive Technologies in India. By addressing key issues related to the ethical, legal, and practical aspects of ART, the report thus provides a valuable base for developing a comprehensive and strong regulatory framework. The report serves as an important reference for policymakers and stakeholders involved in the regulation and governance of ART practices. As India continues to take positive strides in the field of reproductive medicine, the on-going deliberation upon the legal framework will be essential to ensure that ART practices are carried out in an ethical, equitable, and in the best interests of all the stakeholders.

## The Assisted Reproductive Technology (Regulation) Act, 2021

The Assisted Reproductive Technology (Regulation) Act, 2021 (ART Act) is a landmark legislation in India which is aimed at regulating and supervising the field of assisted Reproductive Technologies (ART). It is a well acknowledged fact that the Act came into force on December 18, 2021, and its main objective of the same was to establish a regulatory framework for ART services, ensuring their ethical and regulated use, while safeguarding the rights of patients, donors and also children born through ART, along with surrogate mothers. The Act also addresses several concerns that had seen light in the largely unregulated ART market in India, including surrogacy, sperm/egg donation and IVF.

ARTs has been globally used and in the same line, in India too to help individuals and couples experiencing infertility. However, the rampant commercialization of ART services, along with with the lack of clear legal and ethical framework, raised several issues. These included issues of exploitation and harassment of women (particularly surrogate mothers), unethical practices by clinics, and a lack of safe-guards for the children born through ART. The introduction of the ART Act aimed to provide much-needed regulation to address these concerns and ensure the safe and ethical use of reproductive technologies (Rajya Sabha, 2021).

Before the enactment of the ART Act, the area of ART in India was governed and regulated by a set of guidelines issued by the Indian Council of Medical Research (ICMR) in 2005, which unfortunately lacked binding nature in the eyes of law. The ART Act, therefore, marks the first specific and comprehensive legal framework governing ART in India (ICMR, 2005).

## Key Provisions of the ART Act, 2021

1. *Setting up of Regulatory Authorities*: One of the main feature features of the ART Act is that it calls for the establishment of a regulatory framework to monitor and supervise ART clinics and banks in India The Act mandates the formation

of a National Board, State Boards, and National Registry to regulate ART services (The ART Act, 2021, Sec. 3-6). The National Board will therefore advise the Central Government on policy matters and set minimum basic standards for clinics. The State Boards are tasked with implementing these standards and ensuring compliance, while the National Registry will maintain a central database of ART clinics, banks, and service providers (ART Act, 2021, Sec. 9).

2. *Registration and Regulation of the ART Clinics and Banks*: The ART Act requires all ART clinics and banks to be registered with the National Registry and mandates compliance with the standards set by the National Board (ART Act, 2021, Sec. 14). All clinics must adhere to strict guidelines regarding the collection, handling, and storage of gametes, embryos, and other related biological material. Additionally, the Act stipulates regular inspections of clinics and banks to ensure compliance with prescribed standards (ART Act, 2021, Sec. 15-20).
3. *Informed Consent and Confidentiality*: The ART Act takes due care of the aspect of informed consent and confidentiality. It ensures that individuals undergoing ART procedures are provided with complete and transparent information regarding the entire process. Patients, donors, and surrogate mothers must be informed about the risks, costs, and potential outcomes of the ART procedures before they consent (ART Act, 2021, Sec. 24-25). Furthermore, confidentiality regarding the identities of donors and the details of the ART procedure is strictly protected, and ART clinics are prohibited from disclosing such information without consent (ART Act, 2021, Sec. 26).
4. *Protection of Donors, Patients, and Children Born Through ART*: The Act also aims to safeguard the rights of donors, ART patients, and the children taking birth by the process of ART. It prohibits the sale, purchase, or trade of gametes and embryos, as well as any form of exploitation of donors, especially women (ART Act, 2021, Sec. 29). It also includes provisions to ensure that the child born through ART is legally recognized and has the same rights as a biological child of the commissioning parents (ART Act, 2021, Sec. 31).
5. *Prohibition of Certain Practices*: The Act completely bans several unethical practices, including sex selection, the use of gametes without consent, and the exploitation or harassment of surrogate mothers or donors. It also bans any advertisements related to the sale or purchase of gametes or embryos (ART Act, 2021, Sec. 32-35). Violations of these provisions can result in severe penalties, including imprisonment and fines (ART Act, 2021, Sec. 37-38).
6. *Penalties and Punishments*: The ART Act also specifies strict penalties for individuals and clinics that violate the provisions of the Atc. Unregistered clinics, for example, can be fined or imprisoned for up to ten years, and more severe penalties are imposed for practices like sex selection or gamete trading (ART

Act, 2021, Sec. 37). By setting penalties like these, the Act aims to curb unethical practices and ensure that ART services are made available in a responsible and legal manner.

The ART Act of 2021 is anticipated to bring in significant positive changes in the area of reproductive technologies in India. It lays down a clear legal framework, addressing the rights of all parties involved and ensuring that ART procedures are conducted ethically. By regulating ART clinics and banks, the Act also aims to control unethical practices that were previously widespread due to a lack of monitoring.

Moreover, the Act provides for better protection for women, specifically those who act as donors or surrogate mothers. By banning the commercialization of gametes and embryos and mandating the requirement of the informed consent of all stakeholders, the Act reduces the risk of exploitation. It also ensures that the children born through ART have the same legal rights as biological children, resolving any potential ambiguities regarding parentage. (ART Act, 2021, Sec. 30-31).

The monitoring and regulation of ART services might also be of great help may also help improve the quality of care provided to the concerned patients. By setting basic minimum standards for clinics and mandating regular inspections, the Act ensures that ART procedures are performed.

Despite its strengths, the ART Act has also faced considerable criticism. Some stakeholders believe that the Act's strict provisions might make ART services less accessible, particularly for lower-income individuals and couples. The requirement for registration and adherence to high standards may increase the cost of ART services, potentially placing them out of reach for many people who could benefit from them (Saxena, 2022).

Additionally, some critics have pointed out that the Act does not adequately address the emotional and psychological aspects of ART procedures, particularly in relation to the children born through ART and their parents. (Bhattacharya, 2022). Objections have also been brought up about the Act's provisions concerning surrogacy, which is addressed in the Surrogacy (Regulation) Act, 2021 which was passed in and around the same time. These two acts, although complementary, have caused some confusion in their implementation and interpretation. (Rajya Sabha, 2021).

Conclusively, it is safe to say that The Assisted Reproductive Technology (Regulation) Act, 2021 is a crucial legislation which is aimed at bringing much-needed regulation to the field of reproductive medicine within India. By setting out clear and specific guidelines for ART clinics, donors, patients, and children born through ART, this very Act strives to make sure that ART procedures are conducted in an ethical, safe, and regulated manner. While there are multiple challenges in its implementation, the Act represents a significant step forward in protecting the rights and interests of all stakeholders.

## ETHICAL AND RELIGIOUS CHALLENGES OF ART AMONG DIFFERENT RELIGIONS

ART have duly transformed the landscape of infertility treatment over the years, offering hope to couples and individuals who struggle to conceive naturally. These technologies, which include procedures like In Vitro Fertilization (IVF), Artificial Insemination (AF) and surrogacy, have become widely popular in India. However, the ethical, religious and moral implications of ART are also an inseparable part of the same concept, especially in a country as diverse and multicultural as India. Indian society is deeply influenced by religion, and religious beliefs, in the same line, shape people's attitudes and decisions regarding medical interventions like ART.

Major religions in India, like Hinduism, Islam, Christianity, Sikhism, and Buddhism, offer different viewpoints and narratives on the use of ART. These perspectives often raise ethical challenges. This segment explores the ethical and religious challenges presented by ART in the context of India's religious diversity, focusing specially on how different religions view and respond to the use of reproductive technologies.

### Hinduism and ART: A Complex Relationship

Hinduism is considered to be one of the oldest religions that the world has ever seen and when it comes to its take on ART, Hinduism has a complex relationship with ART. Hindu scriptures, particularly the *Vedas* and the *Dharmashastras*, place a high value on procreation and the continuity of family lineage, which is considered a duty of married couples. (Banerjee, 2015) In Hindu religion, the want to have children is not only a personal aspiration but also a religious obligation upon couples and families for continuing one's lineage. One major issue is the status of the embryo. In Hinduism, life is believed to begin at conception, and the embryo is often considered sacred.(Chaudhary, 2014) This raises concerns fundamentally about the moral permissibility of practices such as selective embryo implantation and the elimination of unused embryos in IVF techniques. Furthermore, Hinduism traditionally values natural procreation within the marital bond, and third-party involvement, such as sperm or egg donation, is seen as problematic, as it may introduce concerns about *gotra* (clan identity) and lineage. (Sanyal, 2013). Also, surrogacy presents ethical dilemmas in Hinduism. While some interpret religious texts to suggest that surrogacy has been made permissible, the counter argument to the same is that it violates the natural sanctity of reproduction. However, the modern commercialization of surrogacy, which often involves financial transactions, is viewed as exploitative and unethical. (Chaturvedi, 2018).

## Islam and ART: Strictures on Third-Party Involvement

In Islam, procreation is also highly valued, and infertility is generally seen as a condition that should be treated, making ART a permissible medical intervention in many cases (Ali & Ahmed, 2016). However, Islamic ethics and value system as learnt from the Quran, *Hadith* (sayings of the Prophet), and the concerned Islamic jurisprudence, specifically impose strict guidelines on ART, particularly regarding third-party involvement. According to most Islamic scholars, ART procedures like IVF are permissible as long as they involve only the husband and wife, without the use of donor gametes. (Rizvi, 2015).

On surrogacy, most Islamic scholars, particularly in Sunni jurisprudence, reject the practice of surrogacy because it involves the introduction of a third party into the marital bond, which is viewed as akin to adultery (*zina*). (Siddiqui, 2017).However, there is a divergence of opinion in some Shia sects, where surrogacy may be considered permissible under strict conditions, provided that the surrogate does not have a genetic link to the child. (Rahman, 2018).

In Islam, The moral and religious integrity of ART practices in Islam, therefore, hinges on maintaining lineage and avoiding third-party involvement. (Ali & Ahmed, 2016).

## Christianity and ART: Moral Constraints Rooted in Doctrinal Teachings

Christianity in India is represented by various sects such as Catholicism, Protestantism, and Orthodox Christianity, sees ART with moral caution. The Catholic Church, in particular, holds firm views against many forms of ART, primarily because they involve the manipulation of human embryos and often lead to the destruction of unused embryos, which is viewed as morally equivalent to abortion (John Paul II, 1987). The Catholic Church teaches that life begins at conception, and thus, any action that results in the destruction of embryos is considered gravely sinful. (Williams, 2019) Also, it is important to mention that Protestant ethical teachings emphasize individual conscience and the interpretation of Biblical teachings on family and procreation. (Thomas, 2015)

Also, within Christianity, surrogacy, especially commercial surrogacy, remains a divisive issue. Many Christian denominations argue that surrogacy commodifies human life and reduces children to products of a contractual agreement, which is contrary to Christian teachings about the dignity of human life and the sanctity of family bonds. (Williams, 2019).

## Judicial Landscape Over the Point of ART

ART, including the In Vitro Fertilization (IVF), surrogacy, and other fertility based treatments, have been significantly transformative for individuals and couples facing infertility. However, on the flip side, it should also be noted that these technologies raise complex legal and ethical issues as well which lead to these type of matters going to court for the purpose of their resolution. In the same line, India along with various other countries globally is not new to the scene over this point. This segment provides an overview of the landmark Indian and international case laws related to ART, emphasizing on the legal challenges surrounding parentage, custody, rights of children born through ART and also the regulation of surrogacy among others

## National Level

India has made unprecedented advancements in the field of medical sciences in the recent past and in the same line, with its advanced medical infrastructure it has become a global centre for ART specially surrogacy. However, the legal framework concerning ART has been dynamic in nature as it has taken an evolving shape with courts playing a key role in addressing and resolving the matters of dispute over the point. Some of the landmark cases are as follows:

### 1. Baby Manji Yamada v. Union of India, (2008) 13 SCC 518

This landmark judgement was delivered by the judiciary when a Japanese couple arranged and commissioned a surrogate mother in India, but the couple got separated before the child's birth. The father asked for custody of the child, but the legal question that came up for consideration became complicated by the absence of the mother. The case went up to the Supreme Court of India which ruled in favour of the father's custody. The judgment also highlighted the lack of a solid regulatory framework for surrogacy in India at that time and emphasized on the need the need for legal clarity regarding ART. The case led to important discussions on surrogacy laws in India and the rights of children born through surrogacy. It also duly highlighted the need for specific comprehensive legislation to regulate surrogacy arrangements, eventually leading to the Surrogacy (Regulation) Act, 2021.

### 2. Jan Balaz v. Union of India (2010) SC Guj 1045

This case was related to a German couple which commissioned surrogacy in India. The surrogate mother gave birth to twins, but, many legal issues arose when the couple intended to take the children back to Germany. Notably, The Gujarat High Court granted Indian citizenship to the twins, relying on the argument that under Indian law, a child who born to a surrogate mother on Indian soil will be Indian citizens. However, Germany did not legally recognize surrogacy, and as a matter of fact, the couple could not take the children to Germany without resolving their legal status. This case was unique in the sense that it highlighted the complexities that arise in cross-border surrogacy setup and the challenges of conflicting legal mechanism over ART.

### 3. ABC v. The State (NCT of Delhi) (2015) 10 SCC 1

Though not directly an ART case, the *ABC* case was significant for ART-related issues concerning the rights of single women. The petitioner was an unwed mother who wanted to register as the sole guardian of her child without disclosing the father's identity. The Supreme Court ruled that the mother had the right to be recognized as the sole guardian of her child without revealing the father's identity. This ruling has implications for ART, as it grants autonomy to single mothers, including those who may use ART methods such as sperm donation to conceive.

## International Level

After discussing the Indian Scenario, it also becomes essential to adequately discuss the international scenario as well. Internationally, the ART has posed considerable legal challenges, particularly concerning parenthood, surrogacy, and the rights and privileges of children born through the assistance of technologies. Over the same point, multiple countries have addressed these issues through judicial precedents, shaping the global legal landscape over the point of ART.

### 1. Johnson v. Calvert, 5 Cal. 4th 84, 851 P.2d 776 (California Supreme Court 1993)

This matter was one of the earliest surrogacy disputes the United States. The aspiring parents, Mark and Crispina Calvert, hired a surrogate who was Anna Johnson, to surrogate their child using the Calverts' egg and sperm. Surprisingly, after the birth, a dispute arose when Johnson claimed parental rights over the new-born child. The California Supreme Court, in this case, ruled in favour of the parents, holding that the genetic relationship between the child and the Calverts was fundamentally responsible for determining parenthood. The court also laid emphasis over the fact that the intent of the concerned parties was also laid down in the surrogacy contract. This case is also responsible for establishing the "intent-based" model of surrogacy in the jurisprudence of the United States of American which is now widely followed in surrogacy arrangements, specifically in cases concerning ART.

## 2. Baby M Case 109 N.J. 396, 537 A. 2d 1227 (New Jersey Supreme Court 1988)

In this case of Baby M, where the concerned surrogate mother, Mary Beth Whitehead, decided to possess the child after birth with her having signed a well formulated surrogacy contract. The aspiring father, William Stern, and his wife thereafter sought custody of the child. The court rejected the validity of the surrogacy contract on the contended grounds that it conflicted with public policy but awarded custody to the Sterns based on concerned child's best interests. However, the court allowed Whitehead the Right to visit. This case adequately highlighted the concerned ethical and legal challenges of surrogacy and stressed upon the difficulties that the courts face in balancing the rights and obligation concerning the aspect of ART.

## 3. Mennesson v. France Application no. 65192/11 (European Court of Human Rights, 2014)

The European Court of Human Rights (ECHR) addressed the issue of surrogacy in the case of *Mennesson v. France*. In this case, a French couple got involved in the process of surrogacy in United States, where it was legal, and the child was born through the process involved in ART. However, as a matter of fact, France did not recognize the process of surrogacy as legal and denied legal recognition of the parent-child relationship, resulting in difficulties in the concerned child's legal status in France. The ECHR held that the French government's denial violated the child's right to respect for private life under the ambit of Article 8 of the European Convention on Human Rights.

## 4. Re G [2006] EWHC 2019 (Fam)

This particular UK case involved an Israel based couple who took assistance of surrogacy setup in California. After the child's birth, the couple moved forward and applied for a custody order in the UK. The UK court had this important question in front of it for consideration which was regarding the couple's domicile and the applicability of UK's surrogacy laws. The court granted the order, recognizing the parents' legal rights to the child.

## CONCLUSION

Change in the lifestyle and increase in the stress level has made pregnancy challenging and complicated. ART has emerged as an effective tool in addressing infertility disorder in men and women. While it has been boon for many couples suffering from infertility but it has raised some legal, ethical and religious debate which society must address. ART is a dynamic field which keeps on changing. The legal framework is not able to keep pace and address all challenges constantly emerging in the field. To effectively address the evolving legal, ethical and religious challenges associated with ART we are required to enhance the existing legal framework. The given suggestion and recommendation aims at providing comprehensive approach in resolving these complexities. There must a uniform law clearly defining status of embryo, rights of parents and role of donors and surrogates. The clarity in legal framework will help in resolving conflicts and protect the rights of the parties. The laws which govern ART practices must enhance transparency and accountability and must ensure that ethical standards are followed. The regular audit of the clinic will ensure in maintaining quality and safety. The clinic must provide the success rate of ART procedures. The government must formulate policies and programme for low income population to increase the accessibility of ART procedure and provide health insurance plan for ART treatment which help in reducing the burden of the family seeking ART assistance for pregnancy. The psychological and emotional support must be given to the patient through counselling services to cope up with challenges arising out of ART. There is a need of organising round table conferences by ethicist, healthcare team, lawyers for discussing legal and ethical challenges arising out of ART.

The ethics committee should be established for reviewing the complex cases of ART and provide guidelines. The workshop on ART should be conducted representing people from different faith sharing their views and focusing on developing mutual understanding and respect. The enforcement of these recommendation and strategies, stakeholders will create more friendly, ethical and respectful environment for patient as well as for their families opting for ART. It is the duty of the physician to monitor the issues related to ART and they must ensure that while delivering the services related to ART social and moral responsibility is not overlooked.

Tough the challenges of ART cannot be underestimated but its rewards is great. The reward is happy family.

## REFERENCES


Ali, S., & Ahmed, Z. (2016). Islamic Perspectives on Assisted Reproductive Technology (ART) and Ethical Challenges. *Journal of Islamic Ethics*, 3(1), 45–60.

Anwar, S., Anwar, A. (2016). Infertility: A Review on Causes, *Treatment and Management. Women's Health & Gynaecology*, no. 2(6), pp. 1–5

Ball, R. (2021). *Egg Donation and the Ethics of Compensation* (Vol. 18). Reproductive Ethics Review.

Banerjee, S. (2015). Hindu Ethics and Assisted Reproductive Technologies: A Study in Reproductive Ethics. *Indian Journal of Ethics in Medicine*, 9(2), 23–34.

Baylis, F. (2011). The Ethics of Commercial Surrogacy, *Journal of Medical Ethics*, vol. 37, Baylis, Françoise, 2019. Human Germline Gene Editing: The Trouble with 'Designer Babies, *Journal of Medical Ethics*, vol. 45, Bhatia, Rekha, 2021. Surrogate Rights and Legal Protection in India, *Journal of Family Law*, vol. 9, no. 3, Chang, M. C. (1959). Fertilization of Rabbit Ova in vitro. *Nature*, 184(4694), 466–467.

Chaturvedi, M. (2018). Surrogacy and Assisted Reproductive Technologies: Ethical Challenges in Hinduism. *The Journal of Hindu Studies*, 12(3), 120–136.

Chaudhary, R. (2014). Ethical Dilemmas in Assisted Reproductive Technology in Hinduism. *Journal of Reproductive and Genetic Ethics*, 10(4), 89–95.

Edwards, R. G., & Steptoe, P. C. (1980). *A Matter of Life: The Story of a Medical Breakthrough.* Hutchinson.

Gupta, Kavita, 2022. *Legal Parentage under Indian Surrogacy Law,* Indian Journal of Legal Studies Handyside, A. H. et al. (1990). Pregnancies from Biopsied Human Preimplantation Embryos Sexed by Y-Specific DNA Amplification. *Nature,* 344(6268), 768-770.

Hippocrates. (1931). *Hippocratic Writings.* (Translated by J. Chadwick and W. N. Mann). Penguin Classics. Originally written in 400 B.C.E.

Hunter, J. (1786). Observations on the Inflammation of the Internal Coats of Veins. *Transactions of a Society for the Improvement of Medical and Chirurgical Knowledge.*

Indian Council of Medical Research. (2005). *National Guidelines for Accreditation, Supervision and Regulation of ART Clinics in India.* Retrieved from https://www.icmr.nic.in

Jacquart, D., & Thomasset, C. (1988). *Sexuality and Medicine in the Middle Ages*. Polity Press.

John Paul, I. I. (1987). *Donum Vitae: Instruction on Respect for Human Life in its Origin and on the Dignity of Procreation*. Congregation for the Doctrine of the Faith.

Johnson, D. (2021). Surrogacy Laws in California: A Model for the Nation, *Journal of Family Law*, vol. *29,* Jones, H. W., & Jones, G. S. (1981). Elizabeth Carr: The First American IVF Baby. *Fertility and Sterility*, 35(1), 1–2.

Kumar, R., & Das, P. (2011). Ethical and legal issues in assisted reproductive technologies. *The Journal of Reproductive Medicine*, 56(2), 79–85. DOI: 10.1037/jrm0001

Law Commission of India. (2009). Need for Legislation to Regulate Assisted Reproductive Technologies *(Report No. 228). Retrieved from*https://lawcommissionofindia.nic.in

Leeuwenhoek, A. (1677). *Observationes D. Anthonii Leeuwenhoek, de Natis e semine genitali Animalculis*. Philosophical Transactions of the Royal Society.

Ministry of Health and Family Welfare. (2020). *Assisted Reproductive Technologies (Regulation) Bill, 2020*. Government of India. Retrieved from http://mohfw.gov.in

Pathak, A. (2021). LGBTQ+ Access to ART: The Indian Legal Context, *Journal of Reproductive Rights*, R.H. Blank & J.C. Merrick, (1995) Human Reproduction Emerging Technolog*ies, CQ Press, Washington, 1995,* Rahman, A. (2018). Islamic Bioethics: The Shia Perspective on Surrogacy and Assisted Reproductive Technologies. *Middle East Journal of Reproductive Ethics*, 15(4), 200–214.

Rizvi, H. (2015). Assisted Reproductive Technologies in Islam: Legal and Ethical Perspectives. *Journal of Islamic Law and Society*, 22(2), 76–92.

Sabha, R. (2021). *Parliamentary Debates on The ART (Regulation) Bill, 2021*. Government of India.

Saha, M. (2022). Social Impacts of ART Regulation in India, *Asian Bioethics Review*, vol. 13, Sanyal, P. (2013). Assisted Reproductive Technologies in the Context of Hindu Family Life and Ethics. *Hindu Ethics Journal*, 5(1), 98–108.

Sauer, M. V. (2001). Reproductive Donation: An Overview of Egg and Sperm Donation and Surrogacy. *Human Reproduction Update*, 7(1), 1–5.

Saxena, P. (2022). Impact of ART Regulation on Accessibility and Affordability in India. *The Journal of Reproductive Medicine*, 25(2), 104–116.

Sharma, D. (2021). Regulating Assisted Reproductive Technology in India: A Critical Overview, *Indian Journal of Medical Ethics*, vol. 7, no. 2, Sharma, S. (2013). Legal and ethical considerations in ART regulation. *Indian Journal of Medical Ethics*, 10(4), 234–238. DOI: 10.20529/IJME.2013.061

Siddiqui, N. (2017). Surrogacy in Islamic Jurisprudence: A Review of Sunni and Shia Perspectives. *Journal of Muslim Family Law*, 29(3), 80–94.

Spar, D. L. (2019). *The Baby Business: How Money, Science, and Politics Drive the Commerce of Conception*. Harvard Business Press.

Srinivas, A. (2021). The Legal and Ethical Complexities of Surrogacy in India, *Indian Law Journal*, Steinbock, Bonnie. 2020. Surrogacy: Exploitation or Empowerment? *Bioethics*, 34, •••.

Surrogacy (Regulation) Act. (2021). Government of India. The Bible (King James Version), Genesis 16:1-2, 21:1-7. *Samuel*, 1, 1–20.

Thomas, A. (2015). Christian Ethics and Modern Medicine: A Protestant Perspective on Assisted Reproductive Technologies. *Theological Studies*, 68(2), 145–161.

Vasilieva, V.A., Stefanyshyn, N.B., Skhab-Buchynska, T.Ya. (2019). Surrogate Motherhood: Analysis of the Basis of the Legislation of Ukraine and Foreign Countries. *Journal of Advanced Research in Law and Economics*, no. 9(6), pp. 2176–2189. DOI: (in English).DOI: 10.14505//jarle.v9.6(36).33

von Baer, K. E. (1827). *De Ovi Mammalium et Hominis Genesi*.

Williams, R. (2019). The Ethical Dimensions of Assisted Reproductive Technology in Christianity. *Christian Bioethics Journal*, 15(3), 125–138.

# Chapter 13
# Human Genome and Embryo Editing:
## Featuring Global Standards for Ethical, Legal, and Social Issues

**Bhupinder Singh**
https://orcid.org/0009-0006-4779-2553
*Sharda University, India*

**Laeeq Razzak Janjua**
https://orcid.org/0000-0002-1948-5859
*WSB University, Poland*

**Hind Hammouch**
https://orcid.org/0000-0002-5897-1649
*University Sidi Mohamed Ben Abdellah, Fez, Morocco*

## ABSTRACT

*Genome and embryo editing technologies are transformative, carries critical implications for the reproductive justice of women. Although these developments offer great promise for health benefits, they raise major ethical, legal and social challenges. The other ethical questions involve the possibility of "designer babies" where genetic traits could be chosen according to societal prejudices, which may serve only to deepen gender inequality. There is a global divide in regulations, with some countries legally allow gene editing under specific guidelines and others the opposite. From a social perspective, the technology can create schisms especially in access to these interventions making marginalized women further behind. It is essential to set worldwide standard that will allow genome and embryo editing only in the interest of reproductive justice, women's rights, rehabilitation community*

DOI: 10.4018/979-8-3693-7837-3.ch013

*equality and due care not to harm this field.*

## 1. INTRODUCTION

Reproductive medicine has undergone a radical transformation because to recent fast advances in genetic science and technology. The intentional modification of genetic material via human genome and embryo editing has enormous promise for curing genetic illnesses, improving human characteristics, and even treating infertility. These revolutionary advancements do, however, have important moral, legal, and societal ramifications that should be thoroughly considered and handled (Alsubai et al., 2023). The lack of a single, worldwide regulatory framework for modifying human genomes and embryos has led to a fragmented environment. various measures have been taken by various nations, ranging from stringent laws to more lax rules. This lack of consistency creates worries about the possibility of abuse and uneven access to these technologies in addition to impeding international cooperation (Chen et al., 2023). For the human genome and embryo editing technologies to be used responsibly and equitably, global governance guidelines must be established. This study examines the complicated world of human genome editing and embryo editing, examining the need for international governance norms and the moral, legal, and societal concerns related to reproductive justice. The development of genetic technology has created new opportunities and brought up difficult issues with relation to the editing of human genomes and the morality of embryonic stem cell research. In addition to emphasizing the need for international norms to guarantee the ethical and responsible use of these technologies, this presentation will provide a thorough analysis of the existing situation, with a special emphasis on the defense of women's rights and the maintenance of reproductive justice (Krishnamoorthy et al., 2023).

A new age in reproductive medicine has emerged with the development of human genome and embryo editing tools, bringing with it both unparalleled potential and moral conundrums. As gene-editing techniques—most especially, CRISPR-Cas9—become more sophisticated, the international community must work quickly to develop comprehensive guidelines governing the moral, legal, and societal implications of these revolutionary technologies. This study explores the complex interactions between the human genome, embryo editing, and the larger context of reproductive justice (Kuranga et al., 2023). The idea of reproductive justice, which includes the freedom to have or not bear children as well as the opportunity to raise children in secure and nurturing homes, offers a prism through which to assess how genome editing may affect various communities (Khan et al., 2023). In light of the international character of scientific research and medical therapies, investigating global standards is essential. This introduction lays the groundwork for a thorough examination by highlighting the need of strong governance to negotiate the tricky waters of genome and embryo editing and make sure that scientific discoveries are consistent with moral standards and preserve social values (Simões-Marques et al., 2023).

The capacity to alter genetic material at the molecular level is at the heart of the human genome and embryo editing concepts, which have significant ramifications for both human existence and medicine in the future (Annoni et al.,2023). With the use of precise modifications to the DNA sequence within the cells, human genome editing makes it possible to improve certain features or fix genetic abnormalities. This capacity also applies to embryos, allowing for interventions during the most formative phases of development (Singh & Kaunert,2024). The groundbreaking gene-editing instrument CRISPR-Cas9 has become a major force in this area. The prospect of curing genetic disorders and developing therapeutic approaches coexists with concerns about unexpected effects and ethical issues surrounding designer babies. While scientists work through the complexities of science, society must negotiate the moral, legal, and social ramifications of using this technology responsibly. The review of the human genome and embryo editing highlights the potential for significant medical advancements but also poses important ethical and social problems about the manipulation of life itself (De Giovanni, 2023).

## 1.1 Objectives of the Chapter

The purpose of this study is to further the scholarly conversation, provide policymakers with information, and direct future genome editing research with an emphasis on moral, legal, and social issues in the framework of reproductive justice (Obiuto et al.,2023).

- **Analyze Existing Technologies:** Give a summary of the human genome and embryo editing techniques that are already in use, with an emphasis on techniques like CRISPR-Cas9 and the implications they have for genetic manipulation.
- **Examine Global Governance Frameworks:** Look at the current national and international legal frameworks that control the altering of the human genome and embryos. Examine these frameworks' advantages and disadvantages in handling moral, legal, and social challenges.
- **Examine the Ethical Implications:** Go over the ethical issues surrounding the altering of the human genome and embryos, such as worries about designer babies, unforeseen outcomes, and possible social effects.
- **Assess Legal state:** Taking into account current court decisions and disputes, assess the legal state of genome and embryo editing in different nations. Talk

about the potential and difficulties of developing unified international legal norms.

- **Examine Social and Cultural Aspects:** Investigate how genome and embryo editing may affect society, with a particular emphasis on problems like inequality, prejudice, and healthcare access. Examine how the public's views, beliefs, and cultural influences have shaped the conversation around these technologies (Singh et al.,2024).
- **Define Reproductive Justice:** Explain what reproductive justice is, including how it relates to the modification of the human genome and embryos. Examine the ways in which genome editing technology might help or hurt reproductive justice.
- **Identify Future Directions and Challenges**: Determine the gaps and difficulties in the existing global governance framework pertaining to genome and embryo editing. Talk about possible areas for development and the need of changing standards.

*Figure 1. Displays the objectives of this chapter*

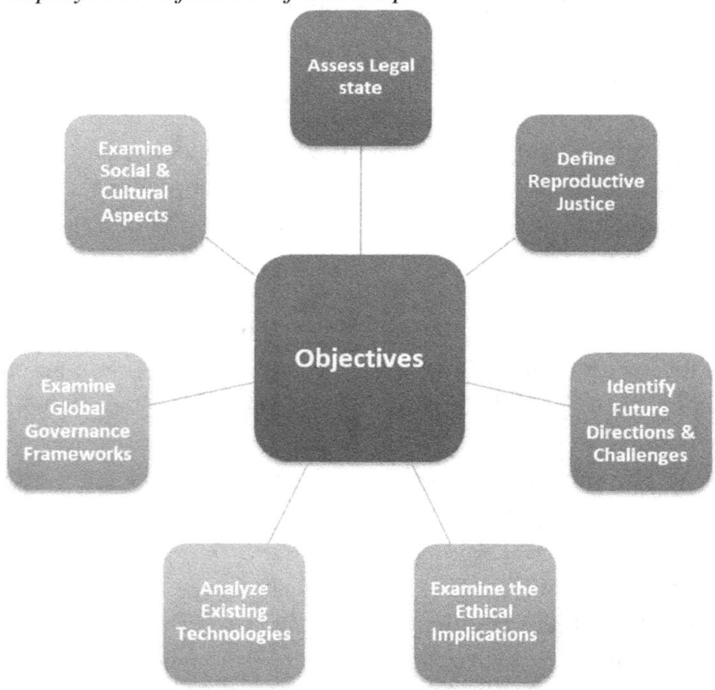


*(Source: Original)*

## 2. TECHNOLOGIES FOR EDITING EMBRYOS AND THE HUMAN GENOME

The field of genetic engineering has made significant strides with the development of the human genome and embryo editing technologies, which have the potential to drastically alter human health and the basic structure of life. Leading the charge in these technologies is the groundbreaking CRISPR-Cas9 system. Bacteria naturally possess a defensive mechanism called CRISPR, which stands for Clustered Regularly Interspaced Short Palindromic Repeats. This technique has been used by scientists to accurately target and edit certain DNA sequences in animals, allowing for the molecular alteration or correction of genes. The required genetic alterations are then either introduced or the current sequence is disrupted by subsequent cellular repair processes (Esposito et al., 2023). With this degree of accuracy, genetic modification might possibly eradicate inherited disorders or improve desirable features in creatures, among other far-reaching effects. These technologies may be used in the earliest phases of development when it comes to embryo editing (Singh et al., 2024). Because scientists may alter an embryo's genetic coding, the possibility of producing genetically altered people raises serious ethical concerns. Although there is a great deal of promise for prenatal genetic disease prevention, strong arguments have been triggered by worries about unexpected effects and the ethical limits of changing the human germline (Skapetze et al., 2023)

In addition to fueling scientific excitement, the rapid development of these technologies has spurred a demand for careful consideration of their social ramifications. The idea of "designer babies," in which certain features may be chosen or improved, raises moral questions about eugenics and the monetization of human existence. The human genome and embryo editing technologies represent a turning point in the history of biotechnology, requiring careful thought and ethical governance at the nexus of science, ethics, and social values (Qadir & Fatah, 2023).

### 2.1 Biomedical and Gene-Editing Fields: Significant Scientific Progress

A slew of significant scientific discoveries in the biomedical and gene-editing fields has led to the field's foray into new territory and its revolutionary possibilities for healthcare and beyond. The ground-breaking CRISPR-Cas9 gene-editing technique, which has emerged as a key component of the genomic toolkit, is at the vanguard of these advances.

**CRISPR-Cas9 Precision:** A naturally occurring defensive system in bacteria, CRISPR stands for Clustered Regularly Interspaced Short Palindromic Repeats. Editing certain DNA sequences with unmatched accuracy is made possible by the use of CRISPR-Cas9. The "Cas9 enzyme" is guided by the guide RNA, which is intended to match the target DNA, to precisely cut the desired regions of the DNA, allowing for the insertion, removal, or change of genetic information. The ability to precisely target medicines for a variety of illnesses and rectify genetic abnormalities has created previously unheard-of therapeutic opportunities (Skapetze et al., 2023).

**Healthcare Applications of Genome Mapping and Editing:** Thanks to developments in genome mapping technology, including high-throughput sequencing, scientists can now quickly and cheaply sequence the human genome. Personalized medicine has been made possible by the abundance of genetic data that has helped to understand the hereditary causes of many illnesses. CRISPR and other gene-editing technologies have been used to investigate possible therapies for hereditary illnesses. This involves repairing cellular abnormalities that cause illness, providing hope for ailments that were previously thought to be incurable (Doherty, 2023)

**Stem Cell Therapies:** The regenerative potential of stem cells has been greatly advanced by biomedical research. Through the exact manipulation of stem cells made possible by CRISPR technology, tailored cell treatments for a range of medical problems may one day be developed. This has the potential to transform the area of regenerative medicine by restoring damaged tissues and organs (Sharifi et al.,2 023).

**Human Germline Editing:** The prospect of editing human germlines, as shown by CRISPR, has raised both ethical questions and enthusiasm. Modifying the genetic composition of next generations has significant ethical ramifications, even if it may help avoid genetic illnesses and birth abnormalities (Singh & Kaunert, 2024). The scientific community is in constant communication to develop moral standards for the appropriate use of germline editing technology (Morrison & Buhalis, 2023).

**New Gene-Editing Technologies and CRISPR variations:** Researchers are investigating and creating novel CRISPR variations in addition to CRISPR-Cas9. Systems such as prime editing and base editing are designed to increase the accuracy and range of genetic alterations. These new technologies have the potential to alleviate some of the drawbacks and difficulties related to CRISPR-Cas9(Modarress et al.,2023).

*Figure 2. Conveys significant scientific discoveries in the biomedical and gene-editing fields*

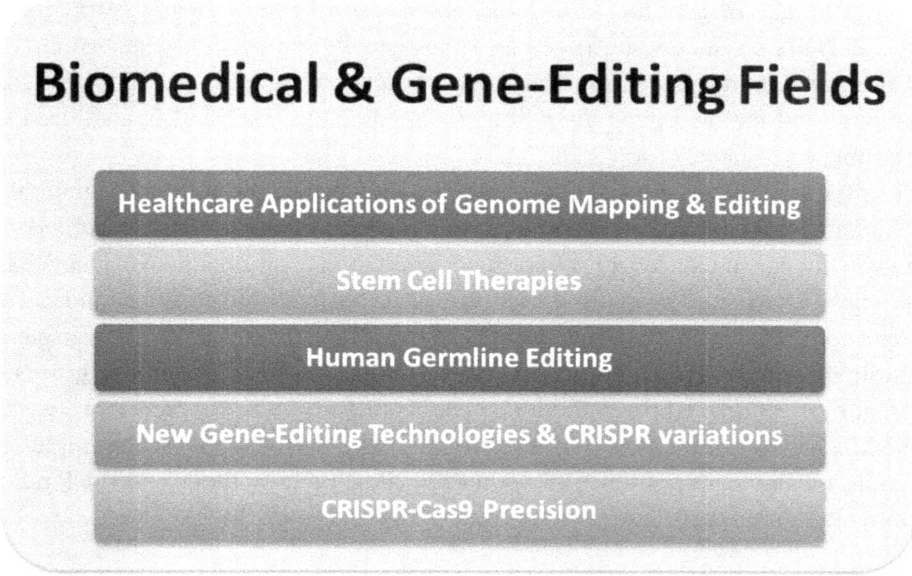


*(Source: Original)*

The rapid breakthroughs in the fields of biomedicine and gene editing highlight how revolutionary these technologies are, guaranteeing that scientific discoveries are in line with society ideals and improve health and welfare worldwide.

## 2.2 Understanding Concepts Regarding Genome Editing and Transgenic Technology

While both genome editing and transgenic technologies are effective tools in genetic engineering, their workings and applications are different. With the use of genome editing technology, an organism's DNA may be precisely altered by adding, removing, or replacing certain DNA sequences. For genome editing, tools like CRISPR-Cas9 are often used. It directly modifies the sequences of the organism's preexisting DNA. For instance, CRISPR-Cas9 targets certain DNA sequences using a guide RNA and then cuts the DNA using the Cas9 enzyme to introduce modifications via natural repair processes (Hemachandran & Rodriguez, 2023).

The process of transgenic technology entails introducing foreign genes into the genome of an organism. As a consequence, the foreign genes' encoded proteins or characteristics are expressed by the organism. It entails the introduction of alien genes into the genetic code. This is often accomplished by introducing the foreign

DNA into the cells of the host organism via vectors, such as viruses or plasmids (Kitada et al., 2023).

With the use of genome editing technology, precise modifications to certain genes or DNA sequences are possible. It has excellent precision when aiming at and altering certain areas. It is mostly used in functional genomics research, disease modeling, and targeted gene alterations for medicinal reasons. It is also used in agriculture to enhance crop yields.

Transgenic technology: Usually causes foreign genes to be randomly integrated into the host genome. When it comes to genome editing, gene insertion precision is higher. Transgenic technology is often utilized to give an organism certain characteristics. Transgenic crops in agriculture may be modified to withstand pests, tolerate herbicides, or have higher nutritional value (Singh, 2024). While transgenic technology includes inserting foreign genes into an organism's genome to give certain features, genome editing technology entails directly and very precisely altering an organism's existing DNA. While there are many uses for both technologies in research, medicine, agriculture, and other domains, their methods and the kind of genetic alterations they cause are different (Skapetze et al., 2023).

## 2.3 Editing the Human Germline and Heritable Genome

Heritable genome editing and human germline editing are two novel yet hotly debated genetic research topics. The exact alteration of genetic material in reproductive cells, such as eggs and sperm, or during the embryonic stage is known as human germline editing. The special quality of germline editing is that any modifications are inherited and will be passed on to the next generation. With the use of this technology, hereditary illnesses and disorders may be completely eradicated and their transmission stopped. However, there are significant ethical ramifications as well, including issues with "designer babies," accidentally introducing genetic effects, and the larger matter of interfering with human development (Khizar et al., 2023).

This idea is expanded upon by heritable genome editing, which highlights the goal of creating genetic alterations meant to become a permanent component of the human gene pool. Even while there are exciting scientific prospects, these techniques present more ethical challenges. The changes are inheritable and permanent, which emphasizes the need of strong moral standards and social agreement. In the conversation around new technologies, issues of permission, equality, and the possibility of unforeseen social effects are brought to the fore (Kopplin et al.,2023).

Globally, there are many different ethical and legal frameworks pertaining to heritable genome editing and human germline modification. Numerous nations have imposed stringent laws or complete prohibitions on these kinds of activities. A rising number of people are calling for international collaboration to create precise, widely-accepted rules and norms because of the global character of genetic research and the far-reaching effects of these technologies (Singh & Kaunert,2024). The ethical issues and social ramifications of human germline and heritable genome editing remain crucial to the proper development of this innovative discipline as scientists continue to push the frontiers of genetic technology (Zawish et al.,2024).

## 3. IMPLICATIONS OF HUMAN GENOME AND EMBRYO EDITING FOR WOMEN'S REPRODUCTIVE JUSTICE

The emergence of human genome editing and embryo editing has significant ramifications for reproductive justice, presenting a challenging landscape where ethical issues and technology progress collide (Periyasamy et al.,2023). On the one hand, family planning and reproductive autonomy may be improved by the prospect of eliminating genetic illnesses before birth. The moral quandaries are complex, however. Concerns about building a society where certain genetic qualities are valued arise from the potential to selectively modify genes, raising issues with equality and social expectations. Uncertainties that might disproportionately affect disadvantaged populations are introduced by the possibility of unanticipated genetic risks and unintended effects. It is also critical to address concerns of cost and fair distribution of these cutting-edge reproductive alternatives since the availability of genome editing technology has the potential to worsen already-existing imbalances. To guarantee that the application of genome editing technologies is in line with the values of reproductive justice, protecting individual choices, fostering inclusivity, and responsibly and fairly addressing societal concerns, a careful balance between scientific advancement and ethical considerations must be struck (Singh,2024).

Women's agency in reproductive decision-making is one of the ethical issues raised by modifying the human germline or editing embryos. The capacity to make knowledgeable decisions on genetic interventions raises questions regarding the possibility of excessive pressure, coercion, or restricted autonomy in women's reproductive choices, particularly in the germline or in the early stages of embryogenesis. Consent difficulties and the long-term effects of genetic changes on women's health and the health of future generations are challenges that legal systems must address. It is important to establish clear guidelines for acceptable genetic modifications and make sure that laws are consistent with moral values in order to protect women's reproductive rights (Bohan & Dumbrell, 2023).

Social conceptions of women's responsibilities in reproduction may be affected by genome and embryo editing. The idea of "designer babies" and the possibility of cultural expectations or preferences for certain genetic features might serve to further entrench stereotypes and existing gender norms (Eriksson & Regoczi,2023). This calls into doubt the viability of discrimination based on genetic traits and contradicts the goals of reproductive justice, which aim to guarantee that everyone has the freedom to make their own choices about reproduction without facing prejudice. The equitable distribution of access to these therapies is also influenced by the cost and accessibility of genome editing technology (Singh & Kaunert,2024). Maintaining the ideals of reproductive justice and avoiding the escalation of current disparities depend on making reproductive technology accessible to all women, regardless of financial background(Grassini & Ratcliffe, 2024).

A thorough and inclusive strategy is necessary to navigate the relationship between reproductive justice for women and the human genome and embryo editing. This entails taking into account a variety of viewpoints, placing an emphasis on informed consent, resolving any power disparities, and creating moral and legal frameworks that defend women's autonomy and rights when it comes to reproductive technology (Suratiningsih, 2023). In light of fast developing genetic technology, the continuing discussion around these concerns should take into account the larger implications for women's reproductive rights, health, and justice (Ishida et al., 2023).

## 4. GLOBAL GOVERNANCE FRAMEWORK: MONITORING EMBRYO EDITING AND HUMAN GENOME

The development of technology for modifying the human genome and embryos has highlighted the need for a strong global governance structure to regulate their use. Since new technologies cut beyond national boundaries, it is essential to address the ethical, legal, and social ramifications via a cogent and all-encompassing international strategy (Kumar et al., 2023). It is essential to establish protocols and benchmarks that maintain the values of openness, responsibility, and diversity in order to effectively traverse the intricate terrain of genetic engineering (Singh, 2023). International organizations like the World Health Organization (WHO) are essential in helping countries work together to create a common position on the moral use of these technologies (Tonelli & Morandi, 2023). It needs an open conversation that takes into account many cultural, ethical, and religious viewpoints to strike a balance between advancing scientific discoveries and protecting against their abuse. Establishing a global governance framework promotes international cooperation, prevents ethical transgressions, and guarantees equitable access to the advantages of these innovative technologies by guaranteeing that the responsible application of human genome and embryo editing remains at the forefront (Dobrauz-Saldapenna & Huras, 2023).

The lack of a single, worldwide regulatory framework for modifying human genomes and embryos has led to a fragmented environment. various measures have been taken by various nations, ranging from stringent laws to more lax rules (Derval,2023). This lack of consistency creates worries about the possibility of abuse and uneven access to these technologies in addition to impeding international cooperation. For the human genome and embryo editing technologies to be used responsibly and equitably, global governance guidelines must be established (Skapetze et al.,2024).

## 4.1 International Organizations and Frameworks Controlling Embryo Editing and Genome Editing

A wide range of institutions and organizations are involved in attempts to control and manage genome and embryo editing on a global basis, which reflects the intricate ethical, legal, and scientific issues these technologies entail. Leading worldwide health organization, the World Health Organization (WHO), holds talks to create guidelines for the appropriate use of genome editing on a global scale. It is essential to organizing efforts to address issues of public health and ethical concern about genetic therapies (Sharifi et al.,2024).

By offering rules and ethical standards for stem cell research, including applications requiring genome editing, the "International Society for Stem Cell Research (ISSCR)" makes a substantial contribution to the regulatory environment. These recommendations emphasize responsible behavior and ethical issues in the use of developing genetic technologies, making them an invaluable resource for researchers worldwide (Grassini & Ratcliffe, 2024).

Scientists, ethicists, and politicians get together as the Hinxton Group to discuss the moral and legal implications of genome editing technology. In order to guarantee that ethical issues continue to be at the forefront of both the research and use of genetic therapies, this worldwide consortium encourages communication and cooperation (Singh et al.,2024). The establishment of the International Commission on the Clinical Use of Human Germline Genome Editing in response to high-profile human germline editing incidents highlights the necessity for specialized organizations tasked with examining the technological, medical, and ethical ramifications of these advances. In order to address the complicated ethical situation surrounding germline editing, this committee brings together specialists from across the world (Min et al.,2024).

The United Nations Educational, Scientific, and Cultural Organization (UNESCO) participates in global dialogues on bioethics, including genetic technology-related issues. The International Bioethics Committee of UNESCO emphasizes the significance of universal ethical standards in scientific breakthroughs by offering a forum for international discussion on the ethical implications of genome and embryo editing. Even though these global frameworks and organizations provide insightful analysis and helpful suggestions, the environment is ever-changing and vulnerable to new innovations. The ongoing evolution of issues around genome and embryo editing underscores the need of international cooperation and governance systems in guiding the ethical and responsible deployment of these innovative technologies on a global scale (Matebese et al., 2024).

### 4.1.1 Treaties, Conventions and Accords Pertaining to These Technologies

#### *Human Rights and Bioethics: A Universal Declaration (UNESCO)*

Adopted in 2005, the Universal Declaration on Bioethics and Human Rights by UNESCO establishes guidelines for the moral conduct of research and medical endeavors, including genetic technology-related ones. Its tenets—human dignity, consent, and solidarity—offer a fundamental framework for ethical concerns in biomedicine even if they do not directly address genome editing (Molavi et al.,2024).

#### *Oviedo Convention is a Human Rights and Biomedical Convention*

The Oviedo Convention of the Council of Europe deals with the defense of human rights in the biomedical industry. While not specifically addressing genome editing, it does highlight the need of nondiscrimination, informed consent, and respect for human dignity—all of which are pertinent to the moral issues raised by genetic technology.

#### *CBD or Convention on Biological Diversity*

The primary goal of the United Nations-sponsored international convention known as the CBD is to conserve biological variety. Although genome editing is not formally regulated, debates in the CBD have touched on issues of the possible effects that genetically modified organisms (GMOs), particularly those produced using genetic editing technology, may have on the environment.

#### *UNESCO-published International Declaration on Human Genetic Data*

The gathering, handling, and preservation of genetic data are covered under the 2003 International Declaration on Human Genetic Data by UNESCO. It highlights permission, privacy, and genetic information protection principles, all of which are pertinent to conversations about genetic technology even if they are not specifically related to genome editing.

*World Health Organization (WHO) Frameworks for Governance*

Global governance frameworks for genome editing have been the subject of ongoing deliberations by the World Health Organization. The WHO's engagement shows a commitment to creating standards and guidelines for the appropriate use of these technologies, even if it is not a treaty. For the most current advances in the regulation of genome and embryo editing, it is important to consult the most recent information and updates from relevant international organizations and legal agencies.

*Figure 3. Shows conventions, treaties, and accords pertaining to these technologies*

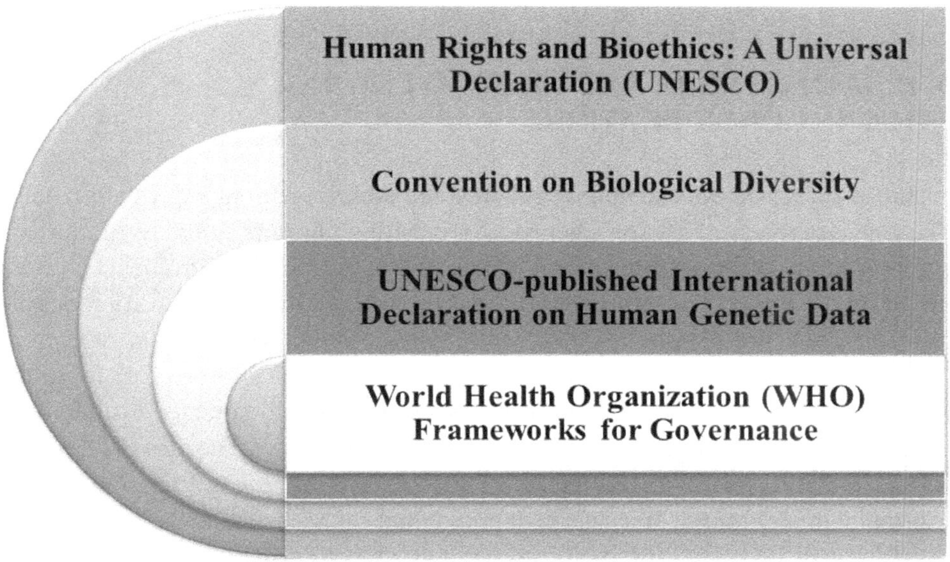


*(Source: Original)*

## 4.2 Evaluating the Current Governance Mechanisms' Effectiveness

The usefulness of the present governance frameworks for modifying the human genome and embryos is still being examined and discussed. Although several international organizations and ethical frameworks provide useful ideals, there are obstacles in the way of their actual application and enforcement. There are sometimes supervision gaps because of how quickly technology is developing at the expense of regulatory framework development. Furthermore, there is a lack of consistency in regulatory methods due to the differences in cultural, ethical, and legal settings across nations. Differences in national regulations might result in differences in ethical norms and practices since there isn't a single international convention that addresses genome editing. Furthermore, enforcing rules mostly depends on each country's desire to do so, which makes establishing a reliable and consistent global governance system difficult. In order to properly address the ethical, legal, and social aspects of human genome and embryo editing, there is a growing agreement on the necessity for more international collaboration, openness, and accountability as talks continue and scientific capabilities advance. Sustaining these governance structures calls for constant communication, cooperation, and a dedication to respecting moral principles worldwide.

## 5. HUMAN GENOME AND EMBRYO EDITING: ETHICAL CONSIDERATIONS

In the discussion of the human genome and embryo editing, ethics are crucial. The capacity to alter a person's genetic composition presents concerns of consent, autonomy, and the possibility of unforeseen outcomes. Ethical problems are also raised by the idea of "designer babies" and the potential for genetic differences to be created between people.

The essence of life, human involvement, and the possible ramifications for future generations are among the many complicated and nuanced ethical considerations raised by the human genome and embryo editing controversy. The idea of "designer babies" and the capacity to change genes selectively to improve certain features are two main ethical issues. Because of the potential for access to these technologies to create gaps between those who can purchase genetic alterations and those who cannot, this raises concerns about equality. Furthermore, since changes made today will affect countless people in the future without their express agreement, the permanence and inheritability of germline modifications generated by embryo editing create ethical challenges that span generations (Tong et al., 2024).

Another crucial ethical factor is informed permission, especially when modifying the genomes of germline cells or embryos. It is difficult to predict every possible outcome of genetic alterations, and it is yet unknown how they will affect people's health and well-being in the long run. Since those impacted by genome editing would not have the autonomy to agree or object, this calls into question established medical ethics. Editing the human germline raises questions about unknown genetic risks and unintended repercussions. Concerns about acting as "genetic gatekeepers" and possible social pressure to adhere to certain genetic standards are also raised in the ethical discussion. This raises the possibility of discrimination based on genetic traits, undercutting the values of inclusion, variety, and personal freedom. Beyond personal decisions, ethical issues have wider social ramifications, therefore careful consideration of cultural, religious, and philosophical viewpoints is required. In the rapidly developing field of genetic technologies, striking a balance between the advancement of scientific knowledge and the upholding of ethical standards in the areas of human genome and embryo editing is a constant challenge that calls for constant communication, international cooperation, and a dedication to upholding the principles of beneficence, non-maleficence, autonomy, and justice (Ahmed et al.,2024)

## 6. LEGAL ENVIRONMENT FOR WOMEN'S REPRODUCTIVE JUSTICE: EXAMINING EMBRYO EDITING AND GENOME

The legal environment pertaining to modifying human genomes and embryos is complicated and differs across nations. While some countries have passed laws governing these technologies, others still lack complete frameworks. It is difficult to guarantee the proper use of new technologies, defend individual rights, and stop any abuses when there are inconsistent legal requirements. To guarantee a unified approach to human genome and embryo editing, these gaps may be filled with the adoption of international legal rules (Singh et al.,2024).

The development of genome and embryo editing technology has created new obstacles and difficulties in the legal environment for women's reproductive justice. These cutting-edge biotechnologies bring up complex legal issues pertaining to women's autonomy, rights, and the laws that control assisted reproductive technologies. The ability of women to make knowledgeable decisions concerning genetic treatments in the context of reproduction is at the core of the issue. Legal systems have to work out what constitutes consent and make sure that women are given the knowledge they need to make choices regarding genome and embryo editing, which may have a significant impact on future generations' genetic make-up as well as their own health. The crucial element pertains to the oversight of therapeutic procedures concerning genome editing in reproductive settings. The licensing, accreditation, and supervision of reproductive clinics and genetic labs that perform these operations must be covered by legal frameworks. Legal responses to genome and embryo editing must be based on ensuring that practitioners follow ethical guidelines, provide women and couples thorough information, and get legitimate permission (Al-Dahidi et al.,2024).

Access and equality concerns must be taken into account in the legal system. These technologies' accessibility and cost may lead to inequality, preventing certain groups of women from using them. Legal frameworks should protect the ideals of reproductive justice, which stress the freedom to make reproductive choices without experiencing obstacles or inequities, by working to avoid discrimination in access to genome and embryo editing based on socioeconomic reasons. The worldwide consequences of genome editing technologies need international cooperation and the formation of generally acknowledged norms in order to navigate the legal terrain for women's reproductive rights. International treaties, conventions, and agreements may help to ensure that moral and legal principles are respected uniformly around the world and help to shape a unified global response.

However, legislative solutions must safeguard women's access to advantageous genetic therapies that help fend off inherited illnesses and promote healthier pregnancies in addition to focusing on limitations. It is a challenging issue for legal systems across the world to strike a balance between the need of monitoring and the desire to protect women's autonomy. Instead of impeding scientific advancement, the legal system should support the values of reproductive justice for women everywhere by offering a strong and moral foundation that permits responsible genome and embryo editing. The way that these legal frameworks continue to develop will probably have a significant impact on how justly and ethically genome and embryo editing technologies are used in the field of women's reproductive health (Singh & Kaunert,2024).

## 7. SOCIAL IMPLICATIONS: GENOME AND EMBRYO EDITING AND WOMEN'S REPRODUCTIVE JUSTICE

Beyond personal decisions, the societal ramifications of human genome editing and embryo editing affect society as a whole. Fairness and social justice are called into question by the possibility of generating hereditary inequities and escalating preexisting injustices. In addition, the price and accessibility of these technologies need to be taken into account in order to guarantee reproductive justice for every person, irrespective of their geographic location or socioeconomic standing. Ensuring fair access to these technologies and addressing societal problems may be facilitated by global norms for governance.

The social ramifications of genome and embryo editing technologies have a profound influence on women's reproductive justice, bringing with them a range of issues that go beyond personal preferences to have an impact on society as a whole. The most important thing to consider is how society's expectations and conventions around women's reproductive duties can change. The concept of choosing or altering certain genetic characteristics in embryos raises concerns about cultural values and preferences, as it may serve to reinforce gender stereotypes and establish new ones about the responsibilities that women should play in reproduction (Singh,2024).

The notion of "designer babies," where certain qualities may be selected or increased, is introduced by the development of genome and embryo editing. This creates questions regarding how women may be unduly pressured to adhere to desired genetic norms, perpetuating beauty standards, intellect, or other socially valued attributes. By restricting women's autonomy in choosing decisions that are consistent with their beliefs and preferences, such cultural expectations have the potential to undermine the fundamentals of reproductive justice.

The possibility of discrimination based on genetic traits is another aspect of the social ramifications. People who defy these genetic norms may be stigmatized or subjected to discrimination if certain qualities are seen to be more desirable. Reproductive justice concepts, which seek to guarantee that people may make reproductive decisions without facing discrimination, are called into question by this. Social inequality are exacerbated by genome editing technologies' price and accessibility. If wealthy people or communities are the only ones with access to these technologies, it may worsen already-existing social and economic disparities and restrict equitable access to reproductive options. This brings up important issues of justice, equality, and the ability of all women to profit from genetic technology breakthroughs, irrespective of their financial situation (Singh & Kaunert, 2024).

A comprehensive strategy that takes into account varied cultural viewpoints, encourages public discussion, and includes the voices of women from diverse backgrounds is required to address these societal ramifications. In order to enable women to make decisions that are in line with their beliefs and to increase public understanding of the societal ramifications of genome and embryo editing, educational initiatives must be developed. In the end, negotiating these technologies' social ramifications in the framework of women's reproductive justice necessitates an intelligent and inclusive public conversation to guarantee that the advantages of genetic advancements are distributed fairly and that women's autonomy and rights continue to be fundamental to the developing field of reproductive technologies (Agaton et al.,2024)

## 7.1 Social Issues' Intersectionality with Women's Reproductive Health

*Figure 4. Highlights the intersection of social issues with women's reproductive health*

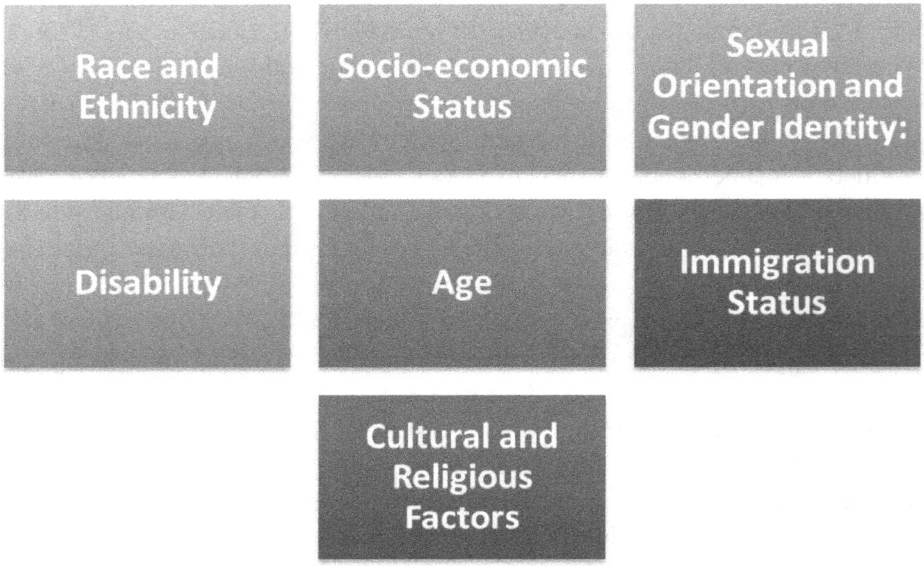


*(Source: Original)*

The intricate interaction of several social elements that shape the experiences of distinct groups of women is acknowledged by the intersectionality of social concerns in women's reproductive health (Singh,2023). This intersectionality approach recognizes that factors such as race, class, ethnicity, sexual orientation, ability, and gender influence women's reproductive health in addition to other aspects of identity. Reproductive justice requires an understanding of how these interlocking issues affect women's autonomy over reproductive decisions, access to healthcare, and general well-being (Rahimieh & Nosrati, 2024).

**Race and Ethnicity:** There are often differences in the reproductive health outcomes for women from various racial and ethnic origins. Disparities in reproductive rights, increased rates of maternal mortality, and uneven access to high-quality healthcare are all consequences of structural racism. For example, women who identify as Indigenous, Black, or Hispanic may have greater rates of maternal mortality and encounter obstacles while trying to get reproductive healthcare services.

**Socioeconomic Status:** Women's reproductive health is significantly impacted by socioeconomic variables. It may be difficult for women from lower socioeconomic backgrounds to get fertility therapies, prenatal care, and contraception. Economic inequality may affect mother and child health outcomes as well as family planning choices.

**Sexual Orientation and Gender Identity:** People who identify as LGBTQ+ may encounter particular difficulties while seeking reproductive healthcare, such as prejudice, a lack of cultural sensitivity on the part of medical professionals, and restricted access to family-building alternatives that are inclusive. Reproductive justice demands attending to the unique needs and rights of people who identify as LGBTQ+.

**Disability:** Stigmatization, inaccessibility, and insufficient support during pregnancy and delivery are some of the obstacles faced by women with disabilities while trying to receive reproductive healthcare services. Policies and services that are inclusive and take into account the various needs of women with disabilities are necessary for reproductive justice.

**Age:** Women of different ages may have different reproductive health issues. Older women may have age-related reproductive problems, while younger women may face obstacles to complete sex education and access to contraception. Support for customized reproductive healthcare is needed for both populations.

**Immigration Status:** Women who are immigrants may face particular difficulties, such as restricted access to healthcare because of linguistic or legal constraints. There are dangers to the health of mothers and children when women are deterred from obtaining essential reproductive healthcare due to fear of deportation.

**Cultural and Religious Factors:** Perceptions about abortion, family planning, and reproductive health may be influenced by religious doctrine and cultural norms. Providing reproductive healthcare treatments that are culturally competent requires an understanding of and respect for various cultural viewpoints.

Thus, tackling the interconnectedness of social concerns with women's reproductive health necessitates an all-encompassing strategy. Policies and interventions should take into account the varied needs and experiences of women, recognizing the manner in which many social variables interact to influence the course of reproduction. By aiming to eliminate structural injustices, a reproductive justice framework makes sure that all women, regardless of how their identities intersect, have the autonomy, information, and support they need to make choices about having children.

## 8. FUTURE DIRECTIONS

The rapid progress in human genome and embryo editing technology demands the creation of international guidelines for governance that tackle the moral, legal, and societal concerns related to reproductive justice. A coordinated strategy will guarantee ethical behavior, defend individual liberties, and advance fair access to these technology. We can manage the intricacies of human genome and embryo editing while respecting the values of ethics, fairness, and equality by encouraging worldwide cooperation and discourse. The landscape at the junction of social concerns and women's reproductive health is intricate and multidimensional, influenced by the interactions of age, immigrant status, gender, race, socioeconomic position, sexual orientation, disability, and cultural influences. Achieving reproductive justice—a framework that defends the rights to have children, not to have children, and to parent in secure and supportive environments—requires acknowledging and addressing these interlocking elements. The conversation around reproductive justice now emphasizes the need of accessible healthcare, inclusive legislation, and tearing down structural obstacles that disproportionately impact underprivileged communities. The creation of treatments that take into account the varied needs and experiences of women, as well as educational programs and cultural competency training for healthcare professionals, are all essential components of strategies (Singh & Kaunert,2024).

## 9. CONCLUSION AND FUTURE SCOPE

The sufficient research, activism, and policy development are crucial in addressing the dynamic state of women's reproductive health. Technology integration creates new levels of complexity and raises ethical questions, as shown by developments in genome and embryo editing. Future efforts should strive to achieve a balance between ethical protections and scientific advancement, making sure that technology advancements support reproductive justice rather than undermine it. Advocating for reproductive justice must become a worldwide movement in the future, taking into account regional differences in healthcare results and access. Fair and equitable reproductive health practices will need international cooperation and the creation of global standards. In order to ensure that policies and initiatives are informed by the stories of women from varied backgrounds and experiences, attention should also be placed on elevating the voices of these women. The core tenet of reproductive justice is empowering women to actively participate in choices about their reproductive health. The future of women's reproductive justice and health thus rests on a comprehensive, inclusive, and rights-based strategy. It entails continuing discussion, investigation, and policy formulation that take into account the complex interplay between social variables, technological developments, and the varied experiences that women have on a global scale. We can work toward a future in which every woman, regardless of her intersecting identities, has access to the full range of reproductive rights and health by promoting an all-encompassing and inclusive vision of reproductive justice.

## REFERENCES


Agaton, C. B., & Guila, P. M. C. (2024). Success Factors and Challenges: Implications of Real Options Valuation of Constructed Wetlands as Nature-Based Solutions for Wastewater Treatment. *Resources*, 13(1), 11. DOI: 10.3390/resources13010011 PMID: 38187013

Ahmed, S. F., Islam, N., Tasannum, N., Mehjabin, A., Momtahin, A., Chowdhury, A. A., Almomani, F., & Mofijur, M. (2024). Microplastic removal and management strategies for wastewater treatment plants. *Chemosphere*, 347, 140648. DOI: 10.1016/j.chemosphere.2023.140648 PMID: 37952815

Al-Dahidi, S., Alrbai, M., Al-Ghussain, L., Alahmer, A., & Hayajneh, H. S. (2024). Data-driven analysis and prediction of wastewater treatment plant performance: Insights and forecasting for sustainable operations. *Bioresource Technology*, 391, 129937. DOI: 10.1016/j.biortech.2023.129937

Alsubai, S., Dutta, A. K., Alkhayyat, A. H., Jaber, M. M., Abbas, A. H., & Kumar, A. (2023). Hybrid deep learning with improved Salp swarm optimization based multi-class grape disease classification model. *Computers & Electrical Engineering*, 108, 108733. DOI: 10.1016/j.compeleceng.2023.108733

Annoni, A., Nativi, S., Çöltekin, A., Desha, C., Eremchenko, E., Gevaert, C. M., Giuliani, G., Chen, M., Perez-Mora, L., Strobl, J., & Tumampos, S. (2023). Digital earth: Yesterday, today, and tomorrow. *International Journal of Digital Earth*, 16(1), 1022–1072. DOI: 10.1080/17538947.2023.2187467

Bohan, D., & Dumbrell, A. (Eds.). (2023). *Advances in Ecological Research: Roadmaps Part B*. Elsevier.

Chen, L., Wu, T., Wang, Z., Lin, X., & Cai, Y. (2023). A novel hybrid BPNN model based on adaptive evolutionary Artificial Bee Colony Algorithm for water quality index prediction. *Ecological Indicators*, 146, 109882. DOI: 10.1016/j.ecolind.2023.109882

De Giovanni, P. (2023). Sustainability of the Metaverse: A transition to Industry 5.0. *Sustainability (Basel)*, 15(7), 6079. DOI: 10.3390/su15076079

Derval, D. (2023). Frontiers in Product Innovation Strategy: Predicting Market Outcomes and Creating Winning Products for a People and Planet-friendly Future.

Dobrauz-Saldapenna, G., & Huras, N. (Eds.). (2023). *Circular Economy: New solutions for a better tomorrow*. Stämpfli Verlag.

Doherty, P. (2023). *Smart Cities: Reimagining the Urban Experience*. Quality Press.

Eriksson, R. O., & Regoczi, B. (2023). Diving into venture creation: An exploratory study of how external enabler combinations facilitate sustainable venture creation in the marine sector.

Esposito, M., Halkias, D., Tse, T., & Harkiolakis, T. (2023). Environmental and Climate Impacts of the Metaverse. *Available atSSRN* 4616695. DOI: 10.2139/ssrn.4616695

Grassini, S., & Ratcliffe, E. (2024). The Virtual Wild: Exploring the Intersection of Virtual Reality and Natural Environments. *Managing Protected Areas*, 327.

Grassini, S., & Ratcliffe, E. (2024). The Virtual Wild: Exploring the Intersection of Virtual Reality and Natural Environments. *Managing Protected Areas*, 327.

Hemachandran, K., & Rodriguez, R. V. (Eds.). (2023). *The Business of the Metaverse: How to Maintain the Human Element Within this New Business Reality*. CRC Press.

Ishida, S., Matsui, T., Haga, C., Hori, K., Hashimoto, S., & Saito, O. (2023). Twitter Mining for Detecting Interest Trends on Biodiversity: Messages from Seven Language Communities. *Sustainability (Basel)*, 15(17), 12893. DOI: 10.3390/su151712893

Khan, A., Pin, K., Aziz, A., Han, J. W., & Nam, Y. (2023). Optical coherence tomography image classification using hybrid deep learning and ant colony optimization. *Sensors (Basel)*, 23(15), 6706. DOI: 10.3390/s23156706 PMID: 37571490

Khizar, H. M. U., Younas, A., Kumar, S., Akbar, A., & Poulova, P. (2023). The progression of sustainable development goals in tourism: A systematic literature review of past achievements and future promises. *Journal of Innovation & Knowledge*, 8(4), 100442. DOI: 10.1016/j.jik.2023.100442

Kitada, M., Johannesen, E., Ojwala, R. A., Buckingham, S., Sun, Z., Rodríguez-Chaves, M., ... & Schofield, C. (2023). Barriers to the Collection of Gender-Disaggregated Data in Ocean Science. *Human Factors in Management and Leadership*, 71

Kopplin, C. S. (2023). Sports fashion and sustainability: A perfect match? *International Journal of Sports Marketing & Sponsorship*, 24(5), 891–912. DOI: 10.1108/IJSMS-04-2023-0078

Krishnamoorthy, G. D., Balasubramanian, K., Govindaraj, S., Ayyavu, P. G., & Geetha, D. A. D. (2023, June). Energy management system using binary particle swarm optimization technique. In *AIP Conference Proceedings* (Vol. 2766, No. 1). AIP Publishing. DOI: 10.1063/5.0139459

Kumar, R., Gupta, S. K., Wang, H. C., Kumari, C. S., & Korlam, S. S. V. P. (2023). From Efficiency to Sustainability: Exploring the Potential of 6G for a Greener Future. *Sustainability (Basel)*, 15(23), 16387. DOI: 10.3390/su152316387

Kuranga, C., Muwani, T. S., & Ranganai, N. (2023). A multi-population particle swarm optimization-based time series predictive technique. *Expert Systems with Applications*, 233, 120935. DOI: 10.1016/j.eswa.2023.120935

Matebese, F., Mosai, A. K., Tutu, H., & Tshentu, Z. R. (2024). Mining wastewater treatment technologies and resource recovery techniques: A review. *Heliyon*, 10(3), e24730. DOI: 10.1016/j.heliyon.2024.e24730 PMID: 38317979

Min, X. Z., Zhang, Z. F., Lu, X. M., Chen, J. C., Ma, W. L., Liu, L. Y., & Kallenborn, R. (2024). Occurrence and fate of pharmaceuticals and personal care products in a wastewater treatment plant with Bacillus bio-reactor treatment. *The Science of the Total Environment*, 924, 171589. DOI: 10.1016/j.scitotenv.2024.171589 PMID: 38461988

Modarress-Fathi, B., Ansari, A., & Ansari, A. (2023). Examining Sustainability Alignment of Supplier Selection Criteria during Industrial Revolutions. *Sustainability (Basel)*, 15(22), 15930. DOI: 10.3390/su152215930

Molavi, H., Mirzaei, K., Jafarpour, E., Mohammadi, A., Salimi, M. S., Rezakazemi, M., Nadagouda, M. M., & Aminabhavi, T. M. (2024). Wastewater treatment using nanodiamond and related materials. *Journal of Environmental Management*, 349, 119349. DOI: 10.1016/j.jenvman.2023.119349

Morrison, A. M., & Buhalis, D. (Eds.). (2023). *Routledge Handbook of Trends and Issues in Global Tourism Supply and Demand.* Taylor & Francis. DOI: 10.4324/9781003260790

Obiuto, N. C., Ugwuanyi, E. D., Ninduwezuor-Ehiobu, N., Ani, E. C., & Olu-lawal, K. A. (2024). Advancing wastewater treatment technologies: The role of chemical engineering simulations in environmental sustainability. *World Journal of Advanced Research and Reviews, 21*(3), 019-031.

Periyasamy, A. P., & Periyasami, S. (2023). Critical Review on Sustainability in Denim: A Step toward Sustainable Production and Consumption of Denim. *ACS Omega*, 8(5), 4472–4490. DOI: 10.1021/acsomega.2c06374 PMID: 36777581

Qadir, A. M. A., & Fatah, A. O. (2023). Platformization and the metaverse: Opportunities and challenges for urban sustainability and economic development. *EAI Endorsed Transactions on Energy Web, 10*(1).

Rahimieh, A., & Nosrati, M. (2024). A Review on Biochemistry, Microbiology and Thermodynamic Aspects of Propionate: The Key Intermediate in the Anaerobic Digestion and Wastewater Treatment. *Desalination and Water Treatment*, 317, 100191. DOI: 10.1016/j.dwt.2024.100191

Sharifi, A., Allam, Z., Bibri, S. E., & Khavarian-Garmsir, A. R. (2024). Smart cities and sustainable development goals (SDGs): A systematic literature review of co-benefits and trade-offs. *Cities (London, England)*, 146, 104659. DOI: 10.1016/j.cities.2023.104659

Sharifi, A., Allam, Z., Bibri, S. E., & Khavarian-Garmsir, A. R. (2024). Smart cities and sustainable development goals (SDGs): A systematic literature review of co-benefits and trade-offs. *Cities (London, England)*, 146, 104659. DOI: 10.1016/j.cities.2023.104659

Simões-Marques, M., Água, P., Frias, A., & Correia, A. (2023). Metaverse and Digital Twins: Contributions, Opportunities and Challenges to a Sustainable Use of the Ocean. *Human Factors and Systems Interaction, 84*(84).

Singh, B. (2023). Blockchain Technology in Renovating Healthcare: Legal and Future Perspectives. In Kaushik, K., Dahiya, S., Aggarwal, S., & Dwivedi, A. (Eds.), *Revolutionizing Healthcare Through Artificial Intelligence and Internet of Things Applications* (pp. 177–186). IGI Global., DOI: 10.4018/978-1-6684-5422-0.ch012

Singh, B. (2024). Lensing Legal Dynamics for Examining Responsibility and Deliberation of Generative AI-Tethered Technological Privacy Concerns: Infringements and Use of Personal Data by Nefarious Actors. In Ara, A., & Ara, A. (Eds.), *Exploring the Ethical Implications of Generative AI* (pp. 146–167). IGI Global., DOI: 10.4018/979-8-3693-1565-1.ch009

Singh, B. (2024). Evolutionary Global Neuroscience for Cognition and Brain Health: Strengthening Innovation in Brain Science. In Prabhakar, P. (Ed.), *Biomedical Research Developments for Improved Healthcare* (pp. 246–272). IGI Global., DOI: 10.4018/979-8-3693-1922-2.ch012

Singh, B. (2024). Social Cognition of Incarcerated Women and Children: Addressing Exposure to Infectious Diseases and Legal Outcomes. In Reddy, K. (Ed.), *Principles and Clinical Interventions in Social Cognition* (pp. 236–251). IGI Global., DOI: 10.4018/979-8-3693-1265-0.ch014

Singh, B., Dutta, P. K., & Kaunert, C. (2024). Replenish Artificial Intelligence in Renewable Energy for Sustainable Development: Lensing SDG 7 Affordable and Clean Energy and SDG 13 Climate Actions With Legal-Financial Advisory. In Derbali, A. (Ed.), *Social and Ethical Implications of AI in Finance for Sustainability* (pp. 198–227). IGI Global., DOI: 10.4018/979-8-3693-2881-1.ch009

Singh, B., Jain, V., Kaunert, C., Dutta, P. K., & Singh, G. (2024). Privacy Matters: Espousing Blockchain and Artificial Intelligence (AI) for Consumer Data Protection on E-Commerce Platforms in Ethical Marketing. In Saluja, S., Nayyar, V., Rojhe, K., & Sharma, S. (Eds.), *Ethical Marketing Through Data Governance Standards and Effective Technology* (pp. 167–184). IGI Global., DOI: 10.4018/979-8-3693-2215-4.ch015

Singh, B., & Kaunert, C. (2024). Computational Thinking for Innovative Solutions and Problem-Solving Techniques: Transforming Conventional Education to Futuristic Interdisciplinary Higher Education. In Fonkam, M., & Vajjhala, N. (Eds.), *Revolutionizing Curricula Through Computational Thinking, Logic, and Problem Solving* (pp. 60–82). IGI Global., DOI: 10.4018/979-8-3693-1974-1.ch004

Singh, B., & Kaunert, C. (2024). Augmented Reality and Virtual Reality Modules for Mindfulness: Boosting Emotional Intelligence and Mental Wellness. In Hiran, K., Doshi, R., & Patel, M. (Eds.), *Applications of Virtual and Augmented Reality for Health and Wellbeing* (pp. 111–128). IGI Global., DOI: 10.4018/979-8-3693-1123-3.ch007

Singh, B., & Kaunert, C. (2024). Harnessing Sustainable Agriculture Through Climate-Smart Technologies: Artificial Intelligence for Climate Preservation and Futuristic Trends. In Kannan, H., Rodriguez, R., Paprika, Z., & Ade-Ibijola, A. (Eds.), *Exploring Ethical Dimensions of Environmental Sustainability and Use of AI* (pp. 214–239). IGI Global., DOI: 10.4018/979-8-3693-0892-9.ch011

Singh, B., & Kaunert, C. (2024). Salvaging Responsible Consumption and Production of Food in the Hospitality Industry: Harnessing Machine Learning and Deep Learning for Zero Food Waste. In Singh, A., Tyagi, P., & Garg, A. (Eds.), *Sustainable Disposal Methods of Food Wastes in Hospitality Operations* (pp. 176–192). IGI Global., DOI: 10.4018/979-8-3693-2181-2.ch012

Singh, B., & Kaunert, C. (2024). Revealing Green Finance Mobilization: Harnessing FinTech and Blockchain Innovations to Surmount Barriers and Foster New Investment Avenues. In Jafar, S., Rodriguez, R., Kannan, H., Akhtar, S., & Plugmann, P. (Eds.), *Harnessing Blockchain-Digital Twin Fusion for Sustainable Investments* (pp. 265–286). IGI Global., DOI: 10.4018/979-8-3693-1878-2.ch011

Singh, B., & Kaunert, C. (2024). Wind and Solar Energy as Renewable Energy for Sustainable Global Future: Projecting Future Multi-Sector Sustainable Policies and Innovation. In Ara, A., & Thakore, R. (Eds.), *Promoting Multi-Sector Sustainability With Policy and Innovation* (pp. 210–245). IGI Global., DOI: 10.4018/979-8-3693-2113-3.ch009

Singh, B., & Kaunert, C. (2024). Aroma of Highly Smart Internet of Medical Things (IoMT) and Lightweight EdgeTrust Expansion Medical Care Facilities for Electronic Healthcare Systems: Fortified-Chain Architecture for Remote Patient Monitoring and Privacy Protection Beyond Imagination. In Hassan, A., Bhattacharya, P., Tikadar, S., Dutta, P., & Sagayam, M. (Eds.), *Lightweight Digital Trust Architectures in the Internet of Medical Things (IoMT)* (pp. 196–212). IGI Global., DOI: 10.4018/979-8-3693-2109-6.ch011

Singh, B., & Kaunert, C. Reinventing Artificial Intelligence and Blockchain for Preserving Medical Data. In *Ethical Artificial Intelligence in Power Electronics* (pp. 77–91). CRC Press. DOI: 10.1201/9781032648323-6

Singh, B., Vig, K., Dutta, P. K., & Kaunert, C. (2024). Unraveling Agile Transformation for Customer Satisfaction in Changing Market Conditions: Roadmap for Industry Embracing Change in Project Management. In Misra, S., Jadeja, R., & Mittal, M. (Eds.), *Practical Approaches to Agile Project Management* (pp. 305–321). IGI Global., DOI: 10.4018/979-8-3693-3318-1.ch017

Skapetze, L., Zha, C., Yin, X., von Brueck, D., & Önkü, E. (2023). Promoting Pro-Environmental Behavior based on the Psychology of Perception. *Briefe zur Interdisziplinarität*, (31).

Skapetze, L., Zhao, C., Yin, X., von Brueck, D., & Önkü, E. (2023). 6 Promoting pro-environmental behaviour based on the. *Balanced Sustainability In A Changing World, 10*, 111.

Skapetze, L., Zhao, C., Yin, X., von Brueck, D., & Önkü, E. (2024). Promoting pro-environmental behaviour based on the psychology of perception—Can the metaverse be a potential solution? In *Balanced Sustainability in a Changing World* (pp. 111-136).

Skapetze, L., Zhao, C., Yin, X., von Brueck, D., & Önkü, E. (2024). Promoting pro-environmental behaviour based on the psychology of perception—Can the metaverse be a potential solution? In *Balanced Sustainability in a Changing World* (pp. 111-136).

Suratiningsih, D. (2023). Strategy for Establishing the World Mangrove Center as a Climate Change Mitigation Effort. *Journal of Namibian Studies: History Politics Culture*, 34, 2474–2494.

Tonelli, C., & Morandi, A. (2023). The impact of 3D technology on sustainability in fashion luxury product design: evidences from an exploratory analysis.

Tong, Y., Liao, X., He, Y., Cui, X., Wishart, M., Zhao, F., & Chen, G. (2024). Mitigating greenhouse gas emissions from municipal wastewater treatment in China. *Environmental Science and Ecotechnology*, 20, 100341. DOI: 10.1016/j.ese.2023.100341 PMID: 38094258

Zawish, M., Dharejo, F. A., Khowaja, S. A., Raza, S., Davy, S., Dev, K., & Bellavista, P. (2024). AI and 6G into the metaverse: Fundamentals, challenges and future research trends. *IEEE Open Journal of the Communications Society*, 5, 730–778. DOI: 10.1109/OJCOMS.2024.3349465

Zhan, J., Xu, S., Zhu, Y., Han, Y., Li, L., Liu, J., & Guo, X. (2024). Potential pathogenic microorganisms in rural wastewater treatment process: Succession characteristics, concentration variation, source exploration, and risk assessment. *Water Research*, 254, 121359. DOI: 10.1016/j.watres.2024.121359 PMID: 38428237

# Compilation of References


Abadi, M., & Gal, S. (2018, May 2). *The rust belt, the corn belt, and every other "belt" in the USA: Business insider india*. Business Insider. https://www.businessinsider.in/the-rust-belt-the-corn-belt-and-every-other-belt-in-the-usa/articleshow/64002711.cms

Abebe, M., Tebeje, T. M., Molla, W., & Melaku, G. (2023). *Male involvement in family planning services*. IntechOpen., DOI: 10.5772/intechopen.111949

Abie, A., Belay, G., Asmare, E., Ayalew, N., Feyisa, W., & Kassie, N. (2023). Male partner involvement in postnatal care service utilization and associated factors: A community-based cross-sectional study in Motta district, Northwest Ethiopia. *PLoS One*, 18(1), e0276477. DOI: 10.1371/journal.pone.0276477

Adamczyk, A. (2022). Religion as a micro and macro property: Investigating the multilevel relationship between religion and abortion attitudes across the globe. *European Sociological Review*, 38(5), 816–831. DOI: 10.1093/esr/jcac017

Adamson, D. (2002). Regulation of assisted reproductive technologies in the United States. *Fertility and Sterility*, 78(5), 932–942. DOI: 10.1016/S0015-0282(02)04199-7 PMID: 12413975

Adamus, R. (2020). Przesłanka eugeniczna (embriopatologiczna) jako przesłanka legalnego przerywania ciąży – glosa do wyroku Trybunału Konstytucyjnego z 22.10.2020 r. (K 1/20). *Palestra*, 11, 95–105.

Agaton, C. B., & Guila, P. M. C. (2024). Success Factors and Challenges: Implications of Real Options Valuation of Constructed Wetlands as Nature-Based Solutions for Wastewater Treatment. *Resources*, 13(1), 11. DOI: 10.3390/resources13010011 PMID: 38187013

Agochukwu, N. Q., & Wittmann, D. (2019). Stress, depression, mental illness, and men's health. In Elsevier eBooks (pp. 207–221). https://doi.org/DOI: 10.1016/b978-0-12-816665-9.00010-x

Ahmed, S. F., Islam, N., Tasannum, N., Mehjabin, A., Momtahin, A., Chowdhury, A. A., Almomani, F., & Mofijur, M. (2024). Microplastic removal and management strategies for wastewater treatment plants. *Chemosphere*, 347, 140648. DOI: 10.1016/j.chemosphere.2023.140648 PMID: 37952815

AIWC. All India Women's Conference. (n.d.). https://www.aiwc.org.in/achievements.html#:~:text=In%201932%2C%20AIWEFA%20 established%20Lady,Indian%20 Council%20 for%20 Child%20 Welfare.

Al-Bar, M. A. (2021). *Abortion: Shafi'i Perspective. Abortion: Global Positions and Practices*. Religious and Legal Perspectives.

Albertyn, C. (2019). Abortion, reproductive rights and the possibilities of reproductive justice in South African courts. *University of Oxford Human Rights Hub Journal*, 2019, 87–119.

Al-Dahidi, S., Alrbai, M., Al-Ghussain, L., Alahmer, A., & Hayajneh, H. S. (2024). Data-driven analysis and prediction of wastewater treatment plant performance: Insights and forecasting for sustainable operations. *Bioresource Technology*, 391, 129937. DOI: 10.1016/j.biortech.2023.129937

Aliesio, L. D., E, V., E, A., & R, A. (2009). The Positive Effects of Father's Attendance to Labour and Delivery : A Quasi Experimental Study. International Nursing Perspectives, 9. https://www.researchgate.net/profile/Ercole-Vellone/publication/236679605_The_positive_effects_of_father's_attendance_to_labour_and_delivery_A_quasi_experimental_study/links/00463526ea2d2d7fce000000/The-positive-effects-of-fathers-attendance-to-labour-and-delivery-A-quasi-experimental-study.pdf

Ali, S., & Ahmed, Z. (2016). Islamic Perspectives on Assisted Reproductive Technology (ART) and Ethical Challenges. *Journal of Islamic Ethics*, 3(1), 45–60.

Allotey, P., Ravindran, T. S., & Sathivelu, V. (2021). Trends in abortion policies in low-and middle-income countries. *Annual Review of Public Health*, 42(1), 505–518. DOI: 10.1146/annurev-publhealth-082619-102442 PMID: 33138701

Alston, P. (1990). The Unborn Child and Abortion under the Draft Convention on the Rights of the Child. *Human Rights Quarterly*, 12(1), 156–178. DOI: 10.2307/762174 PMID: 11655994

Alsubai, S., Dutta, A. K., Alkhayyat, A. H., Jaber, M. M., Abbas, A. H., & Kumar, A. (2023). Hybrid deep learning with improved Salp swarm optimization based multi-class grape disease classification model. *Computers & Electrical Engineering*, 108, 108733. DOI: 10.1016/j.compeleceng.2023.108733

Altruistic Surrogacy and Dispute Resolution:Dyer, J. (2020). The role of arbitration in resolving disputes in altruistic surrogacy agreements. *Journal of Family Law*, 58(2), 145–162.

Anil Kumar Malhotra v. Ajay Pasricha Civ. Appeal 4704 of 2013

Annoni, A., Nativi, S., Çöltekin, A., Desha, C., Eremchenko, E., Gevaert, C. M., Giuliani, G., Chen, M., Perez-Mora, L., Strobl, J., & Tumampos, S. (2023). Digital earth: Yesterday, today, and tomorrow. *International Journal of Digital Earth*, 16(1), 1022–1072. DOI: 10.1080/17538947.2023.2187467

Ansari, M. (2020). A Comparative Study of Reproductive Law: An Analysis of Saudi Arabia, Iraq, and Malaysia. *Dalhousie Journal of Legal Studies*, 29, 11.

Anwar, S., Anwar, A. (2016). Infertility: A Review on Causes, *Treatment and Management. Women's Health & Gynaecology*, no. 2(6), pp. 1–5

Appleton, S. F. (2016). The Forgotten Family Law of Eisenstadt v Baird. *Yale Journal of Law and Feminism*, 28(1), 1–9.

Arbitration and Conciliation Act. 1996., Act, No. 26, Acts of Parliament, 2021 (India).

Arbitration in Family Law:Rivas, C. (2021). Arbitration in family law: An emerging tool for resolving disputes in surrogacy agreements. *Family Law Review*, 12(1), 88–103.

Archard, D., & Tobin, J. (2019). The Definition of a Child. In J. Tobin (Ed.). *The UN Convention on the Rights of the Child.* Oxford: Oxford University Press.

Ashford, L. (2003). *The importance of reproductive health to development: Linking fertility, poverty, and population growth.* Population Reference Bureau.

Asman, O. (2004). Abortion in Islamic countries-legal and religious aspects. *Med. & L.*, 23, 73. PMID: 15163077

Babor, D. D. M. (1999). Population growth and reproductive rights in international human rights law. *Connecticut Journal of International Law*, 14(1), 83–122.

Bacchi, C. (2012). Why Study Problematizations? Making Politics Visible. *Open Journal of Political Science*, 02(01), 1–8. DOI: 10.4236/ojps.2012.21001

Bacchi, C. L. (2009). *Analysing policy: What's the problem represented to be?* Pearson.

Bachman, S. (2023). Lessons from Ukraine: Shifting international surrogacy policy to protect women and children. Journal of Public and International Affairs. https://jpia.princeton.edu/news/lessons-ukraine-shifting-international-surrogacy-policy-protect-women-and-children

Bagheri, A. (2021). *Abortion: Shi'ite Perspective. Abortion: Global Positions and Practices*. Religious and Legal Perspectives.

Baillie, A. (2018). The effectiveness of arbitration in resolving surrogacy disputes: A comparative analysis. *International Journal of Law and the Family*, 32(4), 300–316.

Balaiah, D., Naik, D. D., Parida, R. C., Ghule, M., Hazari, K. T., & Juneja, H. S. (1999). Contraceptive knowledge, attitude and practices of men in rural Maharashtra. *Advances in Contraception*, 15(3), 217–234. DOI: 10.1023/a:1006753617161

Ball, R. (2021). *Egg Donation and the Ethics of Compensation* (Vol. 18). Reproductive Ethics Review.

Banerjee, S. (2015). Hindu Ethics and Assisted Reproductive Technologies: A Study in Reproductive Ethics. *Indian Journal of Ethics in Medicine*, 9(2), 23–34.

Baruah, M. (2022). International and national legal framework on Sustainable Development Goal (Gender equality). *Indian Journal of Law and Legal Research*, 4, 1–20.

Baylis, F. (2011). The Ethics of Commercial Surrogacy, *Journal of Medical Ethics*, vol. 37, Baylis, Françoise, 2019. Human Germline Gene Editing: The Trouble with 'Designer Babies, *Journal of Medical Ethics*, vol. 45, Bhatia, Rekha, 2021. Surrogate Rights and Legal Protection in India, *Journal of Family Law*, vol. 9, no. 3, Chang, M. C. (1959). Fertilization of Rabbit Ova in vitro. *Nature*, 184(4694), 466–467.

Beniwal, A. (2013). Gender Discrimination and Empowerment of Women in India: A View. *Indian Journal of Poultry Science*, 74(1), 27–38.

Berer, M. (2000). Reproductive Rights, Advocacy and Changing the Law. *Reproductive Health Matters*, 8(16), 6–9. DOI: 10.1016/S0968-8080(00)90182-4 PMID: 11424251

Berer, M. (2002). Making Abortion a Woman's Right Worldwide. *Reproductive Health Matters*, 10(19), 1–8. DOI: 10.1016/S0968-8080(02)00010-1 PMID: 12369311

Berer, M. (2017). Abortion law and policy around the world: In search of decriminalization. *Health and Human Rights*, 19(1), 13–27. https://www.hhrjournal.org/2017/06/abortion-law-and-policy-around-the-world-in-search-of-decriminalization/ PMID: 28630538

Berer, M. (2023). Challenging the US Supreme Court's Majority Ruling on Roe v. Wade at the International Human Rights Level. *Health and Human Rights*, 25(1), 195–206. PMID: 37397425

Berk, H. L. (2020). Savvy Surrogates and Rock Star Parents: Compensation Provisions, Contracting Practices, and the Value of Womb Work. *Law & Social Inquiry*, 45(2), 398–431. DOI: 10.1017/lsi.2019.57

Bhalotra, S., Clots-Figueras, I., & Iyer, L. (2021). Religion and abortion: The role of politician identity. *Journal of Development Economics*, 153, 102746. DOI: 10.1016/j.jdeveco.2021.102746

Bhandari, A. (2022). Navigating the Sociological and Legal Aspects of Abortion in India in the Context of the MTP Amendment Act 2021. *Jus Corpus LJ*, 3, 258.

Bharathram, S. M. M. (2023, October 19). The measure of the working woman. The Hindu. https://www.thehindu.com/opinion/op-ed/the-measure-of-the-working-woman/article67435724.ece#:~:text=India's%20first%20 national%20Time%20 Use,compared%20with%2026.1%25%20of%20men.

Bhatia, G. (2016): "The Bombay High Court's Abortion Judgment: Some UnansweredQuestions," *Live Law*, 22 September, http://www.livelaw.in/bombay-high-courts-abortion-judgmentunanswered- questions/

Biden, J. R.Jr. (2022). *Executive Order on Securing Access to Reproductive and Other Healthcare Services*. The White House.

Blagojević, A. (2020). Rethinking the Right to Abortion. *Balkan Social Science Review*, 15, 136–157. DOI: 10.46763/BSSR20150136b

Blazier, J., & Janssens, R. (2020). Regulating the international surrogacy market:the ethics of commercial surrogacy in the Netherlands and India. *Medicine, Health Care, and Philosophy*, 23(4), 621–630. DOI: 10.1007/s11019-020-09976-x PMID: 32929622

Bobyn, C. (2018, December 14). *Inside Ukraine's surrogacy industry where Australians are travelling to have a family*. ABC. Retrieved September 8, 2024, from https://www.abc.net.au/news/2018-12-15/inside-ukraines-surrogacy-industry/10614172

Bohan, D., & Dumbrell, A. (Eds.). (2023). *Advances in Ecological Research: Roadmaps Part B*. Elsevier.

Brodsky, A. (2019). Alternative dispute resolution in family law: Navigating the complexities of surrogacy agreements. *Family Law Quarterly*, 53(2), 147–170.

Bromham, D. R. (1995). Surrogacy: Ethical, legal, and social aspects. *Journal of Assisted Reproduction and Genetics*, 12(8), 509–516. DOI: 10.1007/BF02212913 PMID: 8589569

Brown, L. Louise Brown on 40 years of IVF: 'I was the world's first IVF baby; this is my story'. The Independent [Internet]. 2018 Jul 25 [cited 2024 Jul 17]. Available from: https://www.independent.co.uk/life-style/health-and-families/ivf-baby-louise-brown-story-test-tube-world-first-40th-anniversary-a8455956.html

Caamano, J. M. (2016). International, commercial, gestational surrogacy through the eyes of children born to surrogates in Thailand: A cry for legal attention. *BUL Rev.*, 96, 571.

Calkin, S., & Berny, E. (2021). Legal and non-legal barriers to abortion in Ireland and the United Kingdom. *Medicine Access @ Point of Care*, 5, 23992026211040023. Advance online publication. DOI: 10.1177/23992026211040023 PMID: 36204506

Campbell, J. (2021). Gestational Surrogacy Contract Terms Under the 2017 Uniform Parentage Act. *Barry L. Child & Fam. LJ*, 9, 1.

Carpenter, M. (2020). The OHCHR background note on Human Rights Violations Against Intersex People. *Sexual and Reproductive Health Matters*, 28(1), 1731298. Advance online publication. DOI: 10.1080/26410397.2020.1731298 PMID: 32204689

Carr-Saunders, A. M. (1922). *The population problem: A study in human evolution*. Clarendon Press.

Caruso, E. (2020). The Ambivalence of Law: Some Observations on the Denial of Access to Abortion Services in Italy. *Feminist Review*, 124(1), 183–191. DOI: 10.1177/0141778919894965

Caruso, E. (2023). The hyper-regulation of abortion care in Italy. *International Journal of Gynaecology and Obstetrics: the Official Organ of the International Federation of Gynaecology and Obstetrics*, 163(1), 1036–1042. DOI: 10.1002/ijgo.15150 PMID: 37724041

Cassen, R. H. (1978). Health and family planning. In Palgrave Macmillan UK eBooks (pp. 145–209). https://doi.org/DOI: 10.1007/978-1-349-06522-6_3

CAT. Concluding observations of the Committee against Torture: El Salvador. CAT/C/SLV/CO/2.

CAT. Concluding observations of the Committee against Torture: Nicaragua. CAT/C/NIC/CO/1.

CEDAW, *L.C. v. Peru*, CEDAW/C/50/D/22/2009, 4 November 2011.

CEDAW. Concluding comments of the Committee on the Elimination of Discrimination against Women: Brazil. CEDAW/C/BRA/CO/6.

CEDAW. Concluding comments of the Committee on the Elimination of Discrimination against Women: Chile. CEDAW/C/CHI/CO/4.

CEDAW. Concluding comments of the Committee on the Elimination of Discrimination against Women: Congo. CEDAW/C/COG/CO/6.

CEDAW. Concluding comments of the Committee on the Elimination of Discrimination against Women: Costa Rica. CEDAW/C/CRI/CO/7.

CEDAW. Concluding comments of the Committee on the Elimination of Discrimination against Women: El Salvador. CEDAW/C/SLVCO/8-9.

CEDAW. Concluding comments of the Committee on the Elimination of Discrimination against Women: Honduras. CEDAW/C/HND/CO/7-8.

CEDAW. Concluding comments of the Committee on the Elimination of Discrimination against Women: Indonesia. CEDAW/C/IND/CO/8.

CEDAW. Concluding comments of the Committee on the Elimination of Discrimination against Women: Kenya. CEDAW/C/KEN/CO/7.

CEDAW. Concluding comments of the Committee on the Elimination of Discrimination against Women: Lichtenstein. CEDAW/C/LIE/CO/5/Rev.1.

CEDAW. Concluding comments of the Committee on the Elimination of Discrimination against Women: Mauritius. CEDAW/C/MUS/CO/8.

CEDAW. Concluding comments of the Committee on the Elimination of Discrimination against Women: Nicaragua. CEDAW/C/NIC/CO/6.

CEDAW. Concluding comments of the Committee on the Elimination of Discrimination against Women: Paraguay. CEDAW/C/PRY/CO/6.

CEDAW. Concluding comments of the Committee on the Elimination of Discrimination against Women: Saint Lucia. CEDAW/C/LCA/CO/6.

CEDAW. Concluding observations on the combined initial to third periodic reports of Monaco. CEDAW/C/MCO/CO/1-3.

CEDAW. Concluding observations on the combined seventh and eight periodic reports of Hungary adopted by the Committee at its fifty fourth session. CEDAW/C/HUN/CO/7-8.

CEDAW. Concluding observations on the eight periodic report of Sri Lanka. CEDAW/C/LKA/CO/8.

CEDAW. Concluding observations on the seventh periodic report of Chile. CEDAW/C/CHLCO/7.

CEDAW. General Recommendation 21: Equality in Marriage and Family Relations. A/49/38.

CEDAW. General Recommendation 24: Article 12 of the Convention on the Elimination of All Forms of Discrimination against Women. A/54/38/Rev.1.

CEDAW. Inquiry concerning Poland conducted under article 8 of the Optional Protocol to the Convention. CEDAW/C/POL/IR/1.

CEDAW. Report of the Committee on the Elimination of Discrimination against Women, Twentieth Session (19 January – 5 February 1999). A/54/38/Rev.1.

Center for Reproductive Rights. (2024). *The world's abortion laws*. https://reproductiverights.org/maps/worlds-abortion-laws/

Center for Reproductive Rights. (n.d.). The world's abortion laws. Available from https://reproductiverights.org/maps/worlds-abortion-laws/

CENTER FOR REPRODUCTIVE RIGHTS. WHO'S NEW ABORTION GUIDELINE: HIGHLIGHTS OF ITS LAW AND POLICY RECOMMENDATIONS (2022) available at https://reproductiverights.org/wpcontent/uploads/2022/03/CRR-Fact-sheet-on-WHO-Guidelines.pdf

Chamakala, L. (2009). *Quality of Life Versus Sanctity of Life*. Dharmaram Publications.

Chang, R. C., Rao, A., Zhong, Q., Wojcieszak, M., & Lerman, K. 2023, June. # RoeOverturned: Twitter Dataset on the Abortion Rights Controversy. In *Proceedings of the International AAAI Conference on Web and Social Media* (Vol. 17, pp. 997-1005). DOI: 10.1609/icwsm.v17i1.22207

Charlesworth, H., & Chinkin, C. (2022). *The Boundaries of International Law: A Feminist Analysis*. Manchester University Press. DOI: 10.7765/9781526163592

Chaturvedi, M. (2018). Surrogacy and Assisted Reproductive Technologies: Ethical Challenges in Hinduism. *The Journal of Hindu Studies*, 12(3), 120–136.

Chaudhary, R. (2014). Ethical Dilemmas in Assisted Reproductive Technology in Hinduism. *Journal of Reproductive and Genetic Ethics*, 10(4), 89–95.

Chen, L., Wu, T., Wang, Z., Lin, X., & Cai, Y. (2023). A novel hybrid BPNN model based on adaptive evolutionary Artificial Bee Colony Algorithm for water quality index prediction. *Ecological Indicators*, 146, 109882. DOI: 10.1016/j.ecolind.2023.109882

Chen, R., Gordon, M., Chervenak, F., & Coverdale, J. (2023). Addressing Moral Distress after Dobbs v. Jackson Women's Health Organization: A Professional Virtues-Based Approach. *Academic Medicine*, 99(1), 12–15. DOI: 10.1097/ACM.0000000000005476 PMID: 37816216

Chhabra, R. K., & Kaur, V. (2022). Comparative Analysis of Abortion Laws through the lens of Human Rights Laws. *International Journal of Law Management and Humanities*, 5(3), 47–66.

Chiinhauching, S. Alam, S. N., Bhutia, S. P., Singh, S. P., & PARLIAMENT LIBRARY AND REFERENCE, RESEARCH, DOCUMENTATION AND INFORMATION SERVICE. (2022). Population control in India. In PARLIAMENT LIBRARY AND REFERENCE, RESEARCH, DOCUMENTATION AND INFORMATION SERVICE, PARLIAMENT LIBRARY AND REFERENCE, RESEARCH, DOCUMENTATION AND INFORMATION SERVICE. https://loksabhadocs.nic.in/Refinput/New_Reference_Notes/English/15072022_141200_1021205175.pdf

Chmaj, M., . . .. (2020). Ekspertyza prawna w przedmiocie oceny prawnej orzeczenia TK z 22 października 2020 r. sygn. K 1/20, sporządzona w ramach Zespołu Doradców ds. kontroli konstytucyjności prawa przy Marszałku Senatu X kadencji. Retrieved October 9, 2024 from www.senat.gov.pl, pp. 1-43.

Chodorow, N. (1978). The reproduction of mothering. In University of California Press eBooks. https://doi.org/DOI: 10.1525/9780520924086

Cline, E. H. (2015). *1177 B.C.: The year civilization collapsed*. Princeton University Press.

CNN. (2024, September 30). *Abortion access restrictions and bans in the U.S.* CNN. https://edition.cnn.com/us/abortion-access-restrictions-bans-us-dg/index.html

Cohen, D. S., Donley, G., & Rebouché, R. (2023). The new abortion battleground. *Colum. L. Rev.*, 123, 1.

Cohen, J., Trounson, A., Dawson, K., Jones, H., Hazekamp, J., Nygren, K.-G., & Hamberger, L. (2005). The early days of IVF outside the UK. *Human Reproduction Update*, 11(5), 439–460. DOI: 10.1093/humupd/dmi016 PMID: 15923202

Colker, R. (1994). Equality theory and reproductive freedom. *Texas Journal of Women and the Law*, 3(1), 99–122. PMID: 12645608

Coltrane, S. (1996). *Family Man: Fatherhood, Housework, and Gender Equity*. Oxford University Press.

Combellick-Bidney, S. (2017). Reproductive rights as human rights: Stories from advocates in Brazil, India and South Africa. *International Journal of Human Rights*, 21(7), 800–822. DOI: 10.1080/13642987.2016.1276446

Connelly, M. (2003). Population Control is History: New Perspectives on the International Campaign to Limit Population Growth. *Comparative Studies in Society and History*, 45(1), 122–147. DOI: 10.1017/S0010417503000069

Contributor, S. C. R. C. (2016, November 29). https://blog.scrcivf.com/ivf-the-history-and-evolution-of-fertility-treatments

Cook, R. J., Dickens, B. M., & Fathalla, M. F. (2011). Reproductive health and human rights: Integrating medicine, ethics, and law (Oxford, 2003; online edn, Oxford Academic). Oxford University Press. https://doi.org/DOI: 10.1093/acprof:oso/9780199241323.001.0001

Cook, R. J. (1992). International protection of women's reproductive rights. *New York University Journal of International Law & Politics. New York University. International Law Society*, 24(2), 645–728. PMID: 11656212

Cook, R. J. (2020). International Human Rights and Women's Reproductive Health. In Sherwin, S., & Parish, B. (Eds.), *Women, Medicine, Ethics and the Law* (pp. 37–50). Routledge. DOI: 10.4324/9781003073789-3

Cook, R. J., & Dickens, B. M. (2003). Human Rights Dynamics of Abortion Law Reform. *Human Rights Quarterly*, 25(1), 1–59. DOI: 10.1353/hrq.2003.0003 PMID: 15719517

Corbin, C. M. (2023). Religious liberty for all? A religious right to abortion. *Wisconsin Law Review*, •••, 475.

Costa, J.-P. (2008). *The links between democracy and human rights under the case-law of the European Court of Human Rights*. Paper presented in Helsinki on 5 June 2008. Retrieved September 12, 2024 from https://www.echr.coe.int/documents/d/echr/Speech_20080605_Costa_Helsinki_ENG, pp. 1-8.

Council on Foreign Relations. (2023, April 28). *Abortion law: Global comparisons*. Council on Foreign Relations.https://www.cfr.org/article/abortion-law-global-comparisons

CRC. Concluding comments of the Committee on the Elimination of Discrimination against Women: Malta. CRC/C/MLT/CO/3-6.

CRC. Consideration of reports submitted by States parties under article 44 of the Convention, Concluding observations: Argentina. CRC/C/Arg/CO/3-4.

CRC. General Comment no. 15 (2013) on the right of the child to the enjoyment of the highest attainable standard of health (art. 24). CRC/C/GC/15.

Crosbie, T., & Kirkman, S. (2023). From war to law? The role of the rule of law in international peacebuilding. *International Peacekeeping*, 28(4), 515–537.

CRR (Centre for Reproductive Rights). (2023). Women's Health Protection Act (WHPA). https://reproductiverights.org/the-womens-health-protection-act-federal-legislation-to-protect-the-right-to-access-abortion-care/

Czech, B. (2011). Wykładnia prawa i niezawisłość sędziowska a zdrowy rozsądek (zagadnienia wybrane). In Gudowski, J., & Weitz, K. (Eds.), *Aurea praxis. Aurea theoria. Księga pamiątkowa ku czci Profesora Tadeusza Erecińskiego. Tom II.* LexisNexis.

Dakic, D. (2015). Requirements of informed consent in the reproductive sphere under the European Convention on Human Rights. Ave Maria International Law Journal, 4, 72-105.

Dalvie, S. (2017). Right to Safe Abortion, 52 (33). *Economic and Political Weekly*, •••, 30–32.

David, H. P. (1992). Abortion in Europe, 1920-91: A public health perspective. *Studies in Family Planning*, 23(1), 1–22. DOI: 10.2307/1966824 PMID: 1557791

Davis, M. F. (2018, August 1). *Truth is Truth: U.S. Abortion Law in the Global Context*. Retrieved September 18, 2024, from https://papers.ssrn.com/sol3/papers.cfm?abstract_id=3264833

De Giovanni, P. (2023). Sustainability of the Metaverse: A transition to Industry 5.0. *Sustainability (Basel)*, 15(7), 6079. DOI: 10.3390/su15076079

Demirel, S. (2011). Abortion from an Islamic ethical point of view. *International Journal of Business and Social Science*, 2(1), 230–237.

Department of Health. New York. (2021, February 15). *The Child-Parent Security Act: Gestational Surrogacy Agreements, Acknowledgment of Parentage and Orders of Parentage*. New York State Department of Health. Retrieved September 8, 2024, from https://www.health.ny.gov/vital_records/child_parent_security_act/

Department of Health. New York. (n.d.). https://www.health.ny.gov/vital_records/child_parent_security_act/#:~:text=The%20Child%2DParent%20Security%20Act%20(CPSA)%20is%20a%20law,(ART)%20to%20have%20children

Derval, D. (2023). Frontiers in Product Innovation Strategy: Predicting Market Outcomes and Creating Winning Products for a People and Planet-friendly Future.

Detrick, S. (1999). *A Commentary on the United Nations Convention on the Rights of the Child*. Martinus Nijhoff Publishers. DOI: 10.1163/9789004638693

Devika Biswas v. Union of India (2016) 10 SCC 726.

Dobbs v. Jackson Women's Health Organization (2022) 19-1392 U.S. 597.

Dobbs v. Jackson Women's Health Organization, 597 U.S. 215 (2022)

Dobrauz-Saldapenna, G., & Huras, N. (Eds.). (2023). *Circular Economy: New solutions for a better tomorrow*. Stämpfli Verlag.

Doherty, P. (2023). *Smart Cities: Reimagining the Urban Experience*. Quality Press.

Dolzhenko, (n.d.). *Surrogacy Laws In Ukraine*. https://nccconline.org/blog/article/14#:~:text=In%20 addition%20to%20clear%20and,created%20and%20 frozen%20 FET%20 embryos (19/03/2024

Dorff, E. N. 2021. Conservative Judaism on abortion and related issues. *Abortion: Global positions and practices, religious and legal perspectives*, pp.9-22.

Dudgeon, M., & Inhorn, M. (2004). Men's Influence on Women's Reproductive Health : Medical Anthropological Perspectives. Social Science and Medicine. https://marciainhorn.com/wp-content/uploads/docs/inhorn-article-mens-influence-womens-reproductive-health.pdf

Dushina, . (2016). he Legitimation of Commercial Surrogacy in Russia. *Russian Education & Society*, (58), 12.

Dushina, A. D., Kersha, Y. D., Larkina, T. Y., & Provorova, D. D. (2017). The Legitimation of Commercial Surrogacy in Russia. *Russian Education & Society*, 58(12), 789–815. DOI: 10.1080/10609393.2017.1353835

Ebeku, K. S. A. (2004). New dawn for African women: Prospects of Africa's Protocol on women's rights. *Sri Lanka Journal of International Law*, 16, 83–138.

Edwards, A. (2010). *Violence Against Women Under International Human Rights Law*. Cambridge University Press. DOI: 10.1017/CBO9780511779671

Edwards, R. G., & Steptoe, P. C. (1980). *A Matter of Life: The Story of a Medical Breakthrough*. Hutchinson.

Ehrlich, J. S. (2006). *Who Decides? The Abortion Rights of Teens*. Praeger. DOI: 10.5040/9798216035404

Eisenstadt v. Baird (1972) 405 U.S. 438.

Ekmekci, P. E. (2017). Abortion in Islamic ethics, and how it is perceived in Turkey: A secular, Muslim country. *Journal of Religion and Health*, 56(3), 884–895. DOI: 10.1007/s10943-016-0277-9 PMID: 27364347

EngenderHealth. (n.d.). [Enhancing Male Engagement in Family Planning: Lessons Learned from EngenderHealth's Broadening Accountability of Men Campaign in Karnataka and Maharashtra]. In EngenderHealth (pp. 1–3). https://www.engenderhealth.org/wp-content/uploads/imported-files/Enhancing-Male-Engagement-in-Family-Planning-Lessons-Learned-from-EngenderHealths-Broadening-Accountability-of-Men-Campaign-in-Karnataka-and-Maharashtra.pdf

Epstein, R. A. (1995). Surrogacy: The Case for Full Contractual Enforcement,. *Va. L. Rev., 81*.

Erdman, J. N. (2017). Theorizing Time in Abortion Law and Human Rights. *Health and Human Rights*, 19(1), 29–40. PMID: 28630539

Eriksson, R. O., & Regoczi, B. (2023). Diving into venture creation: An exploratory study of how external enabler combinations facilitate sustainable venture creation in the marine sector.

Eskandar, K. (2024). Advancements in Gynecology: A Comprehensive Review of Emerging Research and Innovations. *J Med Clin Nurs Stud*, 2(1), 1–12.

Esposito, M., Halkias, D., Tse, T., & Harkiolakis, T. (2023). Environmental and Climate Impacts of the Metaverse. *Available atSSRN* 4616695. DOI: 10.2139/ssrn.4616695

European Parliament resolution of 26 November 2020 on the de facto ban on the right to abortion in Poland (2020/2876(RSP)), OJ C 425, 20.10.2021, pp. 147-154

Family Planning. (n.d.). National Health Mission. https://nhm.gov.in/index1.php?lang=1&level=2&sublinkid=821&lid=222

Fayokun, K. O. (2015). Reproductive rights and female education in Nigeria. *US-China Law Review*, 12(11), 906–921.

Fidan, A., Alagoz, R., & Karaman, N. (2021). Liberal sexual morality, religion, and attitudes toward abortion in Turkey. *Journal for the Scientific Study of Religion*, 60(4), 914–933. DOI: 10.1111/jssr.12755

Field, M. A. (2014). Compensated Surrogacy. *WASH. L. REV., 89*, 1155,1161.

Fine, J. B., Mayall, K., & Sepúlveda, L. (2017). The role of international human rights norms in the liberalization of abortion laws globally. *Health and Human Rights*, 19(1), 69–80. DOI: 10.1111/1467-9280.00006 PMID: 28630542

Fine, J. B., Mayall, K., & Sepúlveda, L. (2017). The Role of International Human Rights Norms in the Liberalization of Abortion Laws Globally. *Health and Human Rights*, 19(1), 69–80. PMID: 28630542

Finer, L. B., Frohwirth, L. F., Dauphinee, L. A., Singh, S., & Moore, A. M. (2005). Reasons U.S. women have abortions: Quantitative and qualitative perspectives. *Perspectives on Sexual and Reproductive Health*, 37(3), 110–118. DOI: 10.1363/3711005 PMID: 16150658

Fisher, A., & Tallant, J. (2016). Judith Jarvis Thomson on Abortion. In *How To Get Philosophy Students Talking: An Instructors Toolkit*. essay, Routledge.

Francome, C. (2024). *Abortion freedom: A worldwide movement*. Taylor & Francis. DOI: 10.4324/9781003478348

Freeman, M. (1999). Does surrogacy have a future after Brazier? *Medical Law Review*, 7(1), 1–20. DOI: 10.1093/medlaw/7.1.1 PMID: 11658024

Ganatra, B., Gerdts, C., Rossier, C., Johnson, B. R.Jr, Tunçalp, Ö., Assifi, A., Sedgh, G., Singh, S., Bankole, A., Popinchalk, A., Bearak, J., Kang, Z., & Alkema, L. (2017). Global, regional, and subregional classification of abortions by safety, 2010–14: Estimates from a bayesian hierarchical model. *Lancet*, 390(10110), 2372–2381. DOI: 10.1016/S0140-6736(17)31794-4 PMID: 28964589

Gaur, K. D. (1986). Abortion and the law in India. *Journal of the Indian Law Institute*, 28(3), 348–363.

Gender norms and sexual and reproductive health. (n.d.). Align Platform. https://www.alignplatform.org/gender-norms-and-sexual-and-reproductive-health#:~:text=and%20romantic%20relationships-,Women%20and%20girls%20are%20conditioned%20to%20prioritise%20purity%20and%20modesty,employ%20control%20over%20their%20partners

Georges, E. (1996). Abortion policy and practice in Greece. *Social Science & Medicine*, 42(4), 509–519. DOI: 10.1016/0277-9536(95)00174-3 PMID: 8643977

Ghosh, A., & Khaitan, N. (2017). A womb of one's own: Privacy and reproductive rights. *Economic and Political Weekly*, 52(42-43).

Gilmore, S., & Herring, J. (2017). Mediation in surrogacy: Legal and ethical considerations. *Child and Family Law Quarterly*, 29(1), 25–43.

Gomez, J. (2022). North Africa and the Middle East. Women and Sexuality: Global Lives in Focus, 93.

Gov.si. (2023, October 6). *Pravica do splava je civilizacijski dosežek*. Retrieved September 18, 2024, from https://www.gov.si/novice/2023-10-06-pravica-do-splava-je-civilizacijski-dosezek/

Government of India. (2005). National Health Mission: Framework for Implementation. https://nhm.gov.in/

Government of India. (2022). National Family and Health Survey V. https://dhsprogram.com/pubs/pdf/FR375/FR375.pdf

Government of India. (n.d.). Collaboration with and Commitments from Industry. https://main.mohfw.gov.in/sites/default/files/26953755641410949469%20%281%29.pdf

Government of India. (n.d.). Maternal Health. National Health Mission. https://nhm.gov.in/index1.php?lang=1&level=2&sublinkid=822&lid=218

Grassini, S., & Ratcliffe, E. (2024). The Virtual Wild: Exploring the Intersection of Virtual Reality and Natural Environments. *Managing Protected Areas*, 327.

Greene, M. E.. (2006). Involving men in reproductive health: Contributions to development. UN Millennium Project. Ezeh, A. C. (1993). The influence of spouses over each other's contraceptive attitudes in Ghana. *Studies in Family Planning*, 24(3), 163–174.

Greene, M. E., & Biddlecom, A. E. (2000). Absent and problematic men: Demographic accounts of male reproductive roles. *Population and Development Review*, 26(1), 81–115.

Griffiths, S., & Martin, L. (2006). Assisted Reproduction and Colorado Law: Unanswered Questions and Future Challenges. *Colorado Lawyer*, 35(11), 39.

Griswold v. Connecticut (1965) 381 U.S. 479.

Gupta, Kavita, 2022. *Legal Parentage under Indian Surrogacy Law,* Indian Journal of Legal Studies Handyside, A. H. et al. (1990). Pregnancies from Biopsied Human Preimplantation Embryos Sexed by Y-Specific DNA Amplification. *Nature,* 344(6268), 768-770.

Gutowski, M., & Kardas, P. (2020). Trybunał Konstytucyjny nie mógł rozstrzygnąć gorzej, czyli o dewastacji systemu jednym rozstrzygnięciem. *Palestra*, 10, 5–12.

Guttmacher Institut. (2022). *Unintended Pregnancy and Abortion Worldwide*. Retrieved September 18, 2024, from https://www.guttmacher.org/fact-sheet/induced-abortion-worldwide

Guzman Alejandro, P. A. (2020). Reproductive rights. *Revista Juridica de la Universidad de Puerto Rico*, 89(1), 249–298.

Gwatkin, D. R. (1979). Political will and family planning: The implications of India's emergency experience. *Population and Development Review*, 5(1), 29. DOI: 10.2307/1972317

Hallidya, E. R., de Proost, L., & Verweij, E. (2023). The (mis)use of fetal viability as the determinant of non-criminal abortion in the Netherlands and England and Wales. *Medical Law Review*, 31(4), 538–563. DOI: 10.1093/medlaw/fwad015 PMID: 37253391

Han, L. K. (2023, March 7). *The commercial surrogacy industry is booming as demand for babies rises*. CNBC. Retrieved September 8, 2024, from https://www.cnbc.com/2023/03/07/womb-for-rent-more-women-are-working-in-commercial-surrogacy-industry.html

Han, L., Rodriguez, M. I., & Caughey, A. B. (2018). Blurred lines: Disentangling the concept of fetal viability from abortion law. *Women's Health Issues*, 28(4), 287–288.

Harris, S. (2020). Women's Rights as Human Rights: A Study of Muslim Women's Reproductive Justice in Contemporary Saudi Arabia and Egypt.

Hatun, D., & Yılmaz, M. (2020). Religiosity and public attitudes toward abortion among Turkish adults: From an Islamic perspective. *Sakarya Üniversitesi İlahiyat Fakültesi Dergisi*, 22(42), 433–456.

Hatzis, A. N. (2009). From soft to hard Paternalism and back: The Regulation of Surrogate Motherhood in Greece [PORT. EcON. J.]. *Portuguese Economic Journal*, 8(3), 8. DOI: 10.1007/s10258-009-0049-5

Hellman, L. M., & Pritchard, J. A. (1971). *Williams obstetrics* (14th ed.).

Hemachandran, K., & Rodriguez, R. V. (Eds.). (2023). *The Business of the Metaverse: How to Maintain the Human Element Within this New Business Reality*. CRC Press.

Heri, C. (2024). Deference, Dignity and 'Theoretical Crisis': Justifying ECtHR Rights Between Prudence and Protection. *Human Rights Law Review*, 24, 1–19.

Hervey, T., & Banerjee, T. (2023). Abortion rights in EU law: Recent developments. BioLaw Journal – Rivista di BioDiritto, 1, 331-341.

Hevia, M., & Vacaflor, C. H. (2013). The legal status of in vitro fertilization in Latin America and the American Convention on Human Rights. *Suffolk Transnational Law Review*, 36(1), 51–88.

Hibina, Y. (2023). The advantages and disadvantages of altruistic and commercial surrogacy in India. *Philosophy, Ethics, and Humanities in Medicine; PEHM*, 18(8), 8. DOI: 10.1186/s13010-023-00130-y PMID: 37420245

High Court on Its Own Motion v The State of Maharashtra, Suo Motu Public Interest Litigation (2016): No 1 of 2016, Judgment dated 20 September 2016.

Hippocrates. (1931). *Hippocratic Writings.* (Translated by J. Chadwick and W. N. Mann). Penguin Classics. Originally written in 400 B.C.E.

*History of IVF: Origin and Developments of the 20th Century | PFCLA.* (2022, July 25). Pacific Fertility Center Los Angeles. Retrieved October 19, 2024, from https://www.pfcla.com/blog/history-of-ivf

Hogan, L. (2021). Women's reproductive rights and the legacy of religion in Ireland: The Eighth Amendment and its repeal. *Religion & Human Rights*, 16(2-3), 143–172. DOI: 10.1163/18710328-bja10021

Horn, A. (2019, August 19). *Damaged babies and broken hearts: Ukraine's commercial surrogacy industry leaves a trail of disasters.* ABC. Retrieved September 8, 2024, from https://www.abc.net.au/news/2019-08-20/ukraines-commercial-surrogacy-industry-leaves-disaster/11417388

Human Rights Committee (2018). General comment No. 36 (2018) on article 6 of the International Covenant on Civil and Political Rights, on the right to life, 30 October 2018. CCPR/C/GC/36,.

Human Rights Committee. (2005). K. L. v. Peru. 24 October 2005. CCPR/C/85/D/1153/2003.

Human Rights Committee. (2016). Mellet v. Ireland. 31 March 2016. CCPR/C/116/D/2324/2013.

*Human rights crisis: Abortion in the United States after Dobbs.* Human Rights Watch. (2023, April 18). https://www.hrw.org/news/2023/04/18/human-rights-crisis-abortion-united-states-after-dobbs

Hunter, J. (1786). Observations on the Inflammation of the Internal Coats of Veins. *Transactions of a Society for the Improvement of Medical and Chirurgical Knowledge.*

Huss, B., & Kaiser, F. (2022). Induced abortion and life satisfaction in Germany: The role of selection processes and short-term effects. *Zeitschrift für Soziologie*, 51(4), 404–419. DOI: 10.1515/zfsoz-2022-0022

Huzaimah, A., Abdillah, M., Laila, N. Q., Tamudin, M., & Astuti, T. M. P. (2023). Disregarding the Reproductive Rights of Women in Child Marriage in Indonesia. *Samarah: Jurnal Hukum Keluarga Dan Hukum Islam*, 7(2), 1097–1120. DOI: 10.22373/sjhk.v7i2.17392

Iemelianenko, V., Gornostay, A., & Ivantsova, A. (2019). Reproductive rights violations: Forced sterilization and restriction of voluntary sterilization. *Wiadomosci Lekarskie (Warsaw, Poland: 1960), 72*, 2536-2540.

Igareda González, N. (2020). I. (2020). Legal and ethical issues in cross-border gestational surrogacy. *Fertility and Sterility*, 113(5), 916–919. DOI: 10.1016/j.fertnstert.2020.03.003 PMID: 32327242

Ikeatu, E. G. (2020). Violations of women's reproductive rights in Nigeria. *Nnamdi Azikiwe University Journal of International Law and Jurisprudence*, 11(2), 157–174.

Indian Council of Medical Research. (2005). *National Guidelines for Accreditation, Supervision and Regulation of ART Clinics in India.* Retrieved from https://www.icmr.nic.in

Indian Penal Code, No.45 of 1860.

*Information series: Sexual and Reproductive Health and Rights*. UN Human Rights Office. (2020). https://www.ohchr.org/en/women/information-series-sexual-and-reproductive-health-and-rights

Inhorn, M. C. (2020). Two 'quiet'reproductive revolutions: Islam, gender, and (in) fertility. In *The Routledge Handbook of Islam and Gender* (pp. 343–357). Routledge. DOI: 10.4324/9781351256568-23

Initiatives for pregnant women. (n.d.). https://pib.gov.in/PressReleaseIframePage.aspx?PRID=1843841

Intihar, A. (2023). *Možnost za varno prekinitev nosečnosti rešuje življenja. Delo.si*. Retrieved September 18, 2024, from https://www.delo.si/novice/slovenija/moznost-za-varno-prekinitev-nosecnosti-resuje-zivljenja/

IPPF. (2014). Stories of Gender Justice and Sexual and Reproductive Health and Rights. International Planned Parenthood Federation. https://www.ippf.org/sites/default/files/web_ippf_menboyscollection.pdf

Ishida, S., Matsui, T., Haga, C., Hori, K., Hashimoto, S., & Saito, O. (2023). Twitter Mining for Detecting Interest Trends on Biodiversity: Messages from Seven Language Communities. *Sustainability (Basel)*, 15(17), 12893. DOI: 10.3390/su151712893

Ishola, F., Ukah, U. V., & Nandi, A. (2021). Impact of abortion law reforms on women's health services and outcomes: A systematic review protocol. *Systematic Reviews*, 10(1), 192. DOI: 10.1186/s13643-021-01739-w PMID: 34183064

Jacquart, D., & Thomasset, C. (1988). *Sexuality and Medicine in the Middle Ages*. Polity Press.

Jaffe, S. (2020). US Supreme Court upholds abortion rights, for now. *Lancet*, 396(10244), 85–86. DOI: 10.1016/S0140-6736(20)31518-X PMID: 32653060

Jain, D. (2023). Supreme Court of India judgement on abortion as a fundamental right: Breaking new ground. *Sexual and Reproductive Health Matters*, 31(1), 2225264. Advance online publication. DOI: 10.1080/26410397.2023.2225264 PMID: 37395544

Jain, D., & Shah, P. K. (2020). Reimagining reproductive rights jurisprudence in India: Reflections on the recent decisions on privacy and gender equality from the supreme court of India. *Colum. J. Gender & L.*, 39, 1.

Jalnawalla, S. F. (1974). Medical Termination of Pregnancy Act: A Preliminary Report of the First Twenty Months of Implementation. *Journal of Obstetrics and Gynecology of India*, •••, 588–592. PMID: 1228023

Jargilo, I. (2016). Regulating the Trade of Commercial Surrogacy in India. *Journal of International Business and Law*, 15(2), 12.

Jaswal, P. S., & Kaur, J. (2021). SURROGATE MOTHERHOOD IN INDIA: An Analysis of Surrogacy (Regulation) Act, 2021. *Shimla Law Review*, IV, 257.

Jatlaoui, T. C., Shah, J., Mandel, M. G., Krashin, J. W., Suchdev, D. B., Jamieson, D. J., & Pazol, K. (2017). Abortion surveillance d United States, 2014. *MMWR. Surveillance Summaries*, 66(24), 1–48. DOI: 10.15585/mmwr.ss6624a1 PMID: 29166366

Jejeebhoy, S. J., & Sathar, Z. A. (2001). Women's autonomy in India and Pakistan: The influence of religion and region. *Population and Development Review*, 27(4), 687–712. DOI: 10.1111/j.1728-4457.2001.00687.x

Jerebič, T. (2018, May 28). *Pravica do splava. HomoCumolat.com*. Retrieved September 18, 2024, from https://homocumolat.com/2018/05/28/pravica-do-splava/

Jerman, J., Jones, R. K., & Onda, T. (2023, August 11). *Characteristics of U.S. Abortion Patients in 2014 and Changes Since 2008*. Guttmacher Institute. https://www.guttmacher.org/report/characteristics-us-abortion-patients-2014

Jha, A., & Rituraj, A. Assistant Professor of Law, School of Legal Studies, The Neotia University, West Bengal, & Visiting Faculty, School of Legal Studies, The Neotia University, West Bengal. (2023). X v. Principal Secretary, Health and Family Welfare Dept, Govt. of NCT of Delhi & Anr. In CMR UNIVERSITY JOURNAL FOR CONTEMPORARY LEGAL AFFAIRS (Vol. 5, Issue 1, pp. 315–320).

Joachim, J. M. (2007). *Agenda Setting, The UN, and NGOs*. Georgetown University Press.

Johari, V., & Jadhav, U. (2017): "Abortion Rights Judgment: A Ray of Hope!" *Indian Journal of Medical Ethics*, 28 February 2017, http://ijme. in/wp-content/uploads/2017/02/20170228_ abortion_rights_judgment.pd

John Paul, I. I. (1987). *Donum Vitae: Instruction on Respect for Human Life in its Origin and on the Dignity of Procreation*. Congregation for the Doctrine of the Faith.

Johnson v. Calvert, 5 Cal. 4th 84, 19 Cal. Rptr. 2d 494, 851 P.2d 776 (1993).

Johnson, P. (2012). Sexism. In Elsevier eBooks (pp. 84–90). https://doi.org/DOI: 10.1016/b978-0-12-373932-2.00296-9

Johnson, D. (2021). Surrogacy Laws in California: A Model for the Nation, *Journal of Family Law*, vol. *29,* Jones, H. W., & Jones, G. S. (1981). Elizabeth Carr: The First American IVF Baby. *Fertility and Sterility*, 35(1), 1–2.

Joseph, S., Schultz, J., & Castan, M. (2024). *The International Covenant on Civil and Political Rights. Cases, Materials, and Commentary*. Oxford University Press.

Jubert, A., Bayen, M., Serman, F., Robin, G., Catteau-Jonard, S., Ollivon, J., Tilly, A., Messaadi, N., & Bayen, S. (2023). Medical tourism for late abortion: Women's profile and circumstances. A quantitative study among women who travelled within Europe for late abortion. *Sexual & Reproductive Healthcare : Official Journal of the Swedish Association of Midwives*, 36, 100824. DOI: 10.1016/j.srhc.2023.100824 PMID: 36893521

Justice K S Puttaswamy v. Union of India (2017) 10 SCC 1.

Kamiński, I. C., & Wróbel, A. (2020). *Karta Praw Podstawowych Unii Europejskiej. Komentarz* (Wróbel, A., Ed.). C.H. Beck.

Kandiyoti, D. (1988). Bargaining with patriarchy. *Gender & Society*, 2(3), 274–290.

Kapoor, S. (2023, May 10). Abortion: Comparative Study between Indian Laws and US Laws. Retrieved August 18, 2024,.

Kapoor, P. (2023). Exploring Abortion Laws. *Economic and Political Weekly*, 58(29), 59–63.

Kapoor, P., & Laws, E. A. (2023). A Case Study of Bangladesh, India, Russia, and the United States, 53 (29). *Economic and Political Weekly*, •••, 59–63.

Kaufman, R., Brown, R., Martínez Coral, C., Jacob, J., Onyango, M., & Thomasen, K. (2022). Global impacts of Dobbs v. Jackson Women's Health Organization and Abortion Regression in the United States. *Sexual and Reproductive Health Matters*, 30(1), 2135574. Advance online publication. DOI: 10.1080/26410397.2022.2135574 PMID: 36383177

Kaur, J. (2012). The Role of Litigation in Ensuring Women's Reproductive Rights: An Analysis of the Shanti Devi Judgment in India. *Reproductive Health Matters*, 20(39), 21–30. DOI: 10.1016/S0968-8080(12)39604-3 PMID: 22789079

Kaur, J., & Bhardwaj, C. (2023). Right to Abortion in India: A Critical Appraisal of Legislative and Judicial Initiatives., No. 1 Int'l JL Mgmt. &. *Human.*, 6, 2223.

Kelsen, H. (2007). *General Theory of Law and State* (transl. by A. Wedberg). Clark: The Lawbook Exchange Ltd.

Kelsen, H. (2015). Wesen und Entwicklung der Staatsgerichtsbarkeit. In L. Vinx, *The Guardian of the Constitution : Hans Kelsen and Carl Schmitt on the Limits of Constitutional Law*. Cambridge: Cambridge University Press.

Keown, J. (1988). Anti-abortion legislation 1803–1861 and medical influence thereon. In *Abortion, doctors and the law: Some aspects of the legal regulation of abortion in England from 1803 to 1982* (pp. 26–48). Cambridge University Press. DOI: 10.1017/CBO9780511563683.004

Kerian, C. L. (1997). Surrogacy: A Last Resort Alternative for Infertile Women or a Commodification of Women's Bodies and Children. *WIS. WOMEN's L.J., 12*.

Keynes, E., & Miller, R. K. (1989). *The Court v. Congress*. Duke University Press.

Khan, A., Pin, K., Aziz, A., Han, J. W., & Nam, Y. (2023). Optical coherence tomography image classification using hybrid deep learning and ant colony optimization. *Sensors (Basel)*, 23(15), 6706. DOI: 10.3390/s23156706 PMID: 37571490

Khan, S. I., Hudson-Rodd, N., Saggers, S., Bhuiyan, M. I., Bhuiya, A., Karim, S. A., & Rauyajin, O. (2008). Phallus, performance and power: Crisis of masculinity. *Sexual and Relationship Therapy*, 23(1), 37–49. DOI: 10.1080/14681990701790635

Khizar, H. M. U., Younas, A., Kumar, S., Akbar, A., & Poulova, P. (2023). The progression of sustainable development goals in tourism: A systematic literature review of past achievements and future promises. *Journal of Innovation & Knowledge*, 8(4), 100442. DOI: 10.1016/j.jik.2023.100442

Khurtsidze, I. (2016). *Legal regulation of surrogacy in Georgia* (Special Edition). European Scientific Journal.

Ki-moon, B., Osotimehin, B., & United Nations. (1994). Programme of action. In International Conference on Population and Development (20th Anniversary Edition). United Nations Population Fund. https://www.unfpa.org/sites/default/files/pub-pdf/programme_of_action_Web%20ENGLISH.pdf

Kitada, M., Johannesen, E., Ojwala, R. A., Buckingham, S., Sun, Z., Rodríguez-Chaves, M., ... & Schofield, C. (2023). Barriers to the Collection of Gender-Disaggregated Data in Ocean Science. *Human Factors in Management and Leadership*, 71

Kitson, M. (2018, October 1). *Surrogacy in Spain: The dark side of Ukraine's surrogacy boom | Spain*. EL PAÍS English. Retrieved September 8, 2024, from https://elpais.com/elpais/2018/09/27/inenglish/1538051520_476218.html

Kluchin, R. M. (2011). *Fit to be Tied: Sterilization and Reproductive Rights in America, 1950-1980*. Rutgers University Press.

Kochhar, R. (2023, March 1). *The Enduring Grip of the Gender Pay Gap*. Pew Research Center. https://www.pewresearch.org/social-trends/2023/03/01/the-enduring-grip-of-the-gender-pay-gap/

Komanovics, A. (2009). Effective enforcement of human rights: The Tysiac v. Poland case. Studia Iuridica Auctoritate Universitatis Pecs Publicata, 143, 186-225.

Kopplin, C. S. (2023). Sports fashion and sustainability: A perfect match? *International Journal of Sports Marketing & Sponsorship*, 24(5), 891–912. DOI: 10.1108/IJSMS-04-2023-0078

Kozub-Ciembroniewicz, K., & Szumiło-Kulczycka, D. (2022). Czy aborcja naprawdę jest sprawą Konstytucji? *Palestra*, 10, 33–49.

Kranz, R. (2002). *Reproductive Rights and Technology*. Facts on File.

Krawiec, K., & Rampell, A. (2020). Power dynamics in surrogacy arbitration: Legal representation and fairness. *Harvard Journal of Law & Gender*, 43(2), 95–118.

Krishnamoorthy, G. D., Balasubramanian, K., Govindaraj, S., Ayyavu, P. G., & Geetha, D. A. D. (2023, June). Energy management system using binary particle swarm optimization technique. In *AIP Conference Proceedings* (Vol. 2766, No. 1). AIP Publishing. DOI: 10.1063/5.0139459

Kumar, A. P. (2016). 'Right to Choose'as a Fundamental Right. *Economic and Political Weekly*, •••, 10–11.

Kumar, R., & Das, P. (2011). Ethical and legal issues in assisted reproductive technologies. *The Journal of Reproductive Medicine*, 56(2), 79–85. DOI: 10.1037/jrm0001

Kumar, R., Gupta, S. K., Wang, H. C., Kumari, C. S., & Korlam, S. S. V. P. (2023). From Efficiency to Sustainability: Exploring the Potential of 6G for a Greener Future. *Sustainability (Basel)*, 15(23), 16387. DOI: 10.3390/su152316387

Kunchit. (2023). Women's Health and Reproductive Rights. Issue 4 Int'l JL Mgmt. & Human., 6, 1008.

Kuranga, C., Muwani, T. S., & Ranganai, N. (2023). A multi-population particle swarm optimization-based time series predictive technique. *Expert Systems with Applications*, 233, 120935. DOI: 10.1016/j.eswa.2023.120935

Kurland, A. S. (2006). Access to contraception. *The Georgetown Journal of Gender and the Law*, 7(3), 1129–1142.

Law Commission of India. (2009). Need for Legislation to Regulate Assisted Reproductive Technologies *(Report No. 228). Retrieved from*https://lawcommissionofindia.nic.in

Laxmi Mandal v. Deen Dayal Harinagar Hospital 2010 (172) DLT 9.

Le Bouthillier, Y. (2011). Article 32 Supplementary means of interpretation. In Corten, O., & Klein, P. (Eds.), *The Vienna Convention on the Law of Treaties: A Commentary*. Oxford University Press.

Ledbetter, R. (1984). Thirty years of family planning in India. *Asian Survey*, 24(7), 736–758. DOI: 10.2307/2644186

Leeuwenhoek, A. (1677). *Observationes D. Anthonii Leeuwenhoek, de Natis e semine genitali Animalculis*. Philosophical Transactions of the Royal Society.

Lennerhed, L. (2019). No backlash for Swedish women? The right to abortion on demand, 1975–2000. *Journal of Modern European History*, 17(3), 326–336. https://www.jstor.org/stable/26832829. DOI: 10.1177/1611894419854681

Lewis, J. (Ed.). (2024). *Women's welfare, women's rights*. Taylor & Francis. DOI: 10.4324/9781003469865

Lieber, K. B. (1992). Selling the Womb: Can the Feminist Critique of Surrogacy Be Answered?,. *68 IND. L.J.*, 205.

Lindgren, Y. (2022). Dobbs v. Jackson Women's Health and the Post-Roe Landscape. J. Am. Acad. Matrimonial Law., 35, 235.

Loksabha debates, 17th March, 2020 available at https://eparlib.nic.in/bitstream/123456789/794800/1/lsd_17_03_17-03-2020.pdf

Lorimer, K., McMillan, L., McDaid, L., Milne, D., Russell, S., & Hunt, K. (n.d.). Exploring masculinities, sexual health and wellbeing across areas of high deprivation in Scotland: The depth of the challenge to improve understandings and practices. *Health & Place*, 50, 27–41. DOI: 10.1016/j.healthplace.2017.12.002

Loving v. Virginia (1967) 388 U.S. 1.

Luckey, C. (2011). Commercial Surrogacy: Is Regulation necessary to manage Industry. *Commercial Surrogacy: Is Regulation necWISCONSIN JOURNAL OF LAW. Gender & Society*, 26(2).

Luckey, C. (2011). Commercial Surrogacy: Is Regulation Necessary to Manage the Industry. *Wisconsin Journal of Law. Gender & Society*, •••, 26.

Luna, Z. (2020). *Reproductive Rights as Human Rights: Women of Color and the fight for Reproductive Justice*. New York University Press. DOI: 10.18574/nyu/9781479894369.001.0001

MacDonnell, V., & Hughes, J. (2013). The German abortion decisions and the protective function in German and Canadian constitutional law. *Osgoode Hall Law Journal*, 50(4), 999–1050. DOI: 10.60082/2817-5069.1008

Machaj, Ł. (2023). Dobbs v. Jackson Women's Health Organization: The epitaph for Roe v. Wade. Bialostockie Studia Prawnicze, 28(3), 259-278.

Machalow, D. (2021). Religious Diversity and a Women's Right to Choose: The Religious Right's Mistakenly Assumed Monopoly on Belief and Religious Support for Abortion. *Rutgers JL & Religion*, 22, 476.

Machinton,, N. (1987). urrogate Motherhood: Boon or Baby-Selling - The Unresolved Questions,. *71 Marq. L. Rev., 115*.

MacKinnon, C. A. (1994). Toward Feminist Jurisprudence. In A. M. Jaggar (Ed.), *Living with Contradicitons* (1st ed.). essay, Routledge.

Macpherson, C. B. (1962). *The political theory of possessive individualism: Hobbes to Locke*. Clarendon Press.

Maffi, I., & Tønnessen, L. (2023). Abortion, law, and health in the Arab world. In *Research Handbook on International Abortion Law* (pp. 303–320). Edward Elgar Publishing. DOI: 10.4337/9781839108150.00027

Magill, S. (2020). The Right to Privacy and Access to Abortion in a Post Puttaswamy World. *University of Oxford Human Rights Hub Journal*, 3(2), 160–194.

Maharatna, A. (2002). India's Family Planning Programme: An Unpleasant Essay. *Economic and Political Weekly*, 37(10), 971–981. http://www.jstor.org/stable/4411847

Mankowski, E., & Smith, R. (2016). Men's Mental Health and Masculinities. In Elsevier eBooks (pp. 66–74). https://doi.org/DOI: 10.1016/b978-0-12-397045-9.00182-8

Margolin, T. A. (2007). Abortion as a Human Right. *Women's Rights Law Reporter*, 29(77), 77–98.

Marinelli, S., Del Rio, A., Straccamore, M., Negro, F., & Basile, G. (2022). The armed conflict in Ukraine and the risks of inter-country surrogacy: The unsolved dilemma. European Review for Medical and Pharmacological Sciences, 26(5646 Malavika R. A Critical Analysis of the Surrogacy Regulation Bill 2016 [Internet]. Feminism in India. 2016 Aug 31 [cited 2024 Jul 17]. Available from: https://feminisminindia.com/2016/08/31/critical-analysis-surrogacy-regulation-bill-2016/

Marty, R., & Pieklo, J. M. (2019). *The End of Roe V. Wade: Inside the Right's Plan to Destroy Legal Abortion*. IG Publishing.

Masculinities. (2022, December 2). Gender Matters. https://www.coe.int/en/web/gender-matters/masculinities

Mason, C. (2016). Challenges in arbitration of surrogacy agreements: Addressing power imbalances and fairness. *International Journal of Law, Policy and the Family*, 30(4), 369–387.

Matebese, F., Mosai, A. K., Tutu, H., & Tshentu, Z. R. (2024). Mining wastewater treatment technologies and resource recovery techniques: A review. *Heliyon*, 10(3), e24730. DOI: 10.1016/j.heliyon.2024.e24730 PMID: 38317979

Maternal health. (n.d.). UNICEF. https://www.unicef.org/india/what-we-do/maternal-health

McBride, D. E., & Mazur, A. G. (2008). *Women's Movements, Feminism, and Feminist Movements*. Cambridge University Press.

McDermott, R. C., Pietrantonio, K. R., Browning, B. R., McKelvey, D. K., Jones, Z. K., Booth, N. R., & Sevig, T. D. (2019b). In search of positive masculine role norms: Testing the positive psychology positive masculinity paradigm. *Psychology of Men & Masculinity*, 20(1), 12–22. DOI: 10.1037/men0000160

McDougall, S. (2021). Pardoning infanticide in late medieval France. *Law and History Review*, 39(2), 229–253. DOI: 10.1017/S0738248020000267

McNamara, K., Poverman, M., Nádas, M., Mallow, M., & Gerber, S. (2023). Privileging Midwives for Abortion Care. *Journal of Midwifery & Women's Health*, 68(6), 769–773. DOI: 10.1111/jmwh.13577 PMID: 37850529

Medical Termination of Pregnancy Act, Act No. 34 of 1971

Mehlman, M. J. (2015). Reproductive information and reproductive decision-making. *The Journal of Law, Medicine & Ethics*, 43(2), 241–244. PMID: 26242944

Meinke, S. A. (1990). Surrogate motherhood: ethical and legal issues.

Merali, I. (2000). Advancing women's reproductive and sexual health rights: Using the international human rights system. *Development in Practice*, 10(5), 609–624. https://www.jstor.org/stable/4029536. DOI: 10.1080/09614520020008797

Meyer v. Nebraska (1923) 262 U.S. 390.

Miasi, A. (2022, November 28). *Abortion is a right: Pursuing international remedies for U.S. human rights law violations*. Platform for Peace and Humanity. https://peacehumanity.org/2022/11/28/abortion-is-a-right-pursuing-international-remedies-for-u-s-human-rights-law-violations/

Millbank, J. (2018). Transparency and accountability in ADR processes for surrogacy disputes. *Journal of Legal Ethics*, 41(3), 271–288.

Millett, K. (1970). *Sexual Politics*. University of Illinois Press.

Ministry of Health and Family Welfare. (2020). *Assisted Reproductive Technologies (Regulation) Bill, 2020*. Government of India. Retrieved from http://mohfw.gov.in

Ministry of Health and Family Welfare. https://main.mohfw.gov.in/?q=acts-rules-and-standards-health-sector/acts/mtp-act-amendment-2002

Ministry of Health. (n.d.). *Surrogacy in Israel*.

Minkoff, H., Vullikanti, R. U., & Marshall, M. F. (2024). The two front war on reproductive rights—When the right to abortion is banned, can the right to refuse obstetrical interventions be far behind? *The American Journal of Bioethics*, 24(2), 11–20. DOI: 10.1080/15265161.2023.2262960 PMID: 37830758

Min, X. Z., Zhang, Z. F., Lu, X. M., Chen, J. C., Ma, W. L., Liu, L. Y., & Kallenborn, R. (2024). Occurrence and fate of pharmaceuticals and personal care products in a wastewater treatment plant with Bacillus bio-reactor treatment. *The Science of the Total Environment*, 924, 171589. DOI: 10.1016/j.scitotenv.2024.171589 PMID: 38461988

Mishtal, J. (2014). Reproductive Governance in the New Europe: Competing Visions of Morality, Sovereignty and Supranational Policy. *Anthropological Journal on European Cultures*, 23(1), 59–76. DOI: 10.3167/ajec.2014.230104

Mitra, A. (2017). "We're always going to argue about abortion" – International law's changing attitudes towards abortion. *New Zealand Women's Law Journal*, 1, 142–181.

Modarress-Fathi, B., Ansari, A., & Ansari, A. (2023). Examining Sustainability Alignment of Supplier Selection Criteria during Industrial Revolutions. *Sustainability (Basel)*, 15(22), 15930. DOI: 10.3390/su152215930

Moen, E. (1981). Women's Rights and Reproductive Freedom. *Human Rights Quarterly*, 3(2), 53–60. DOI: 10.2307/761857

Molavi, H., Mirzaei, K., Jafarpour, E., Mohammadi, A., Salimi, M. S., Rezakazemi, M., Nadagouda, M. M., & Aminabhavi, T. M. (2024). Wastewater treatment using nanodiamond and related materials. *Journal of Environmental Management*, 349, 119349. DOI: 10.1016/j.jenvman.2023.119349

Mondal, V.. (2012). Genetic and Gestational Surrogacy: An Overview. *Walailak Journal of Science and Technology*, 9(3), 189–193.

Morgan, L. M. (2021). Costa Rica's oversized role in Latin American sexual and reproductive rights lawfare. *Revista Direito GV*, 17(3), 1–31. DOI: 10.1590/2317-6172202137

Morrison, A. M., & Buhalis, D. (Eds.). (2023). *Routledge Handbook of Trends and Issues in Global Tourism Supply and Demand*. Taylor & Francis. DOI: 10.4324/9781003260790

Morrissey, J. F. (2015). Surrogacy: The Process, the Law, and the Contracts,. *WILLAMETTE L. REV., 51.*

Mouliarova, E. (2019). The Legal Regulation of Surrogacy in Russia. *11 ITALIAN J. PUB. L.*

Mullany, B. C. (2006). Barriers to and attitudes towards promoting husbands' involvement in maternal health in Katmandu, Nepal. *Social Science & Medicine*, 62(11), 2798–2809.

Murray, M. (2021). Race-ing Roe: Reproductive Justice, Racial Justice, and the Battle for Roe v.vs. Wade. *Harvard Law Review*, 134(6), 2025–2102. Retrieved September 18, 2024, from https://harvardlawreview.org/print/vol-134/race-ing-roe/

Myers, R. S. (2014). Re-reading Roe v. Wade. *Washington and Lee Law Review*, 71(2), 1025–1046.

N. M. N., & Kuruvilla, M. (2022). The Sexual Politics of the Manusmriti: A Critical Analysis with Sexual and Reproductive Health Rights Perspectives. In Journal of International Women's Studies (Vol. 23, Issue 6, pp. 21-). https://vc.bridgew.edu/jiws/vol23/iss6/3

N1info.si. (2023). V *Ljubljani so se zbrali podporniki in nasprotniki pravice do splava*. Retrieved September 18, 2024, from https://n1info.si/novice/slovenija/v-ljubljani-so-se-zbrali-podporniki-in-nasprotniki-pravice-do-splava-video/

N1info.si. (2024). *Institut 8. marec z vseevropsko kampanjo: Borili se bodo za pravico do splava*. Retrieved September 18, 2024, from https://n1info.si/novice/slovenija/institut-8-marec-z-vseevropsko-kampanjo-borili-se-bodo-za-pravico-do-splava/

National Legal Services v. Union of India, (2014) 5 SCC 438.

Neel, M. M. (2019). Carrying capacity: Should Georgia enact surrogacy regulation? *Georgia Law Review (Athens, Ga.)*, 54(1), 333–360.

NFHS-5. (2021). Men's participation in family planning & reproductive health in India. https://india.unfpa.org/sites/default/files/pub-pdf/brief3_-_mens_participation_in_fp_and_rh.pdf

Ngo, N. V., Pemunta, N. V., Basil, N., Fokunang, E. T., Mbong, S. E., Ezra, K., Che, H. N., & Umbugadu, E. S. (2024). Reproductive health policy Saga: Restrictive abortion laws in low-and middle-income countries (LMICs), unnecessary cause of maternal mortality. *Health Care for Women International*, 45(1), 5–23. DOI: 10.1080/07399332.2021.1994971 PMID: 34726567

Ngwena, C. G. (2013). *Reforming African abortion laws to achieve transparency : arguments from equality*. Retrieved September 18, 2024, from https://repository.up.ac.za/handle/2263/41812?show=full

Ngwena, C. G. (2013). A Commentary on LC v Peru: The CEDAW Committee's First Decision on Abortion. *Journal of African Law*, 57(2), 310–324. DOI: 10.1017/S0021855313000107

*NIH Study Suggests Women with Disabilities have Higher Risk of Birth Complications and Death.* National Institutes of Health. (2021, December 15). https://www.nih.gov/news-events/news-releases/nih-study-suggests-women-disabilities-have-higher-risk-birth-complications-death

Ninatti, S., & Arcari, M. (2015). Patterns of Democracy In The Case Law of The EU Court of Justice And The European Court of Human Rights. *Polish Yearbook of International Law*, XXXV, 171–192.

Noursi, S., Clayton, J. A., Bianchi, D. W., & Fink, D. (2021). Maternal morbidity and mortality. *Journal of Women's Health*, 30(2), 145–146. DOI: 10.1089/jwh.2020.8851

Obiuto, N. C., Ugwuanyi, E. D., Ninduwezuor-Ehiobu, N., Ani, E. C., & Olu-lawal, K. A. (2024). Advancing wastewater treatment technologies: The role of chemical engineering simulations in environmental sustainability. *World Journal of Advanced Research and Reviews, 21*(3), 019-031.

Office of Population and Reproductive Health. Bureau for Global Health, Sanicki, A., Betron, M., Brown, J., Greene, M., Hardee, K., Kapungu, C., Martinez, L., Shattuck, D., Skinner, J., Underwood, C., & Van Lith, L. (2018). Essential considerations for engaging men and boys for improved family planning outcomes [Report]. https://www.usaid.gov/sites/default/files/2022-05/Engaging-men-boys-family-planning-508.pdf

Osman, A. (2022). Abortion laws in Muslim countries: Modern reconfiguration of pre-modern logic. *Muslim World Journal of Human Rights*, 19(1), 19–52. DOI: 10.1515/mwjhr-2021-0007

Ostergren, R., & Bossé, K. (Eds.). (2004). *The Europeans: A history* (pp. 79–80). Guilford Press.

Outka, G. (2021). *Islamic ethics of life: abortion, war, and euthanasia*. Univ of South Carolina Press.

Pacelle, R. L. (2003). *Between Law and Politics*. A & M University Press.

Pagden, A. (Ed.). (2000). *The Oxford illustrated history of prehistory*. Oxford University Press.

Pagoto, S. L., Palmer, L., & Horwitz-Willis, N. (2023). The next infodemic: Abortion misinformation. *Journal of Medical Internet Research*, 25, e42582. DOI: 10.2196/42582 PMID: 37140975

Palepu, J. (2020, September) *Will the Medical Termination of Pregnancy Amendment Bill reduce abortion cases before Indian High Courts?* THE LEAFLET, https://www.theleaflet.in/will-the-medical-termination-ofpregnancy- amendment-bill-reduce-abortion-cases-before-indian-high-courts/#

Pandey, B. G. (2022, June 27). NFHS-5: Why birth control remains a woman's burden in India. https://www.bbc.com/news/world-asia-india-61906015

Pandey, M. K., & Rao, T. S. (2023). Sexuality education in India yet remains a Taboo—An attempt to Dust-Off. *Journal of Psychosexual Health*, 5(1), 11–12. DOI: 10.1177/26318318231155993

Parliament. (1971). THE MEDICAL TERMINATION OF PREGNANCY ACT, 1971 [Legal]. In THE MEDICAL TERMINATION OF PREGNANCY ACT, 1971. https://www.indiacode.nic.in/bitstream/123456789/1593/1/A1971-34.pdf

Patel, N. H., Jadeja, Y. D., Bhadarka, H. K., Patel, M. N., Patel, N. H., & Sodagar, N. R. (2018). Insight into Different Aspects of Surrogacy Practices. *Journal of Human Reproductive Sciences*, 11(3), 212–218. DOI: 10.4103/jhrs.JHRS_138_17 PMID: 30568349

Pathak, A. (2021). LGBTQ+ Access to ART: The Indian Legal Context, *Journal of Reproductive Rights*, R.H. Blank & J.C. Merrick, (1995) Human Reproduction Emerging Technolog*ies, CQ Press, Washington, 1995,* Rahman, A. (2018). Islamic Bioethics: The Shia Perspective on Surrogacy and Assisted Reproductive Technologies. *Middle East Journal of Reproductive Ethics*, 15(4), 200–214.

Pathfinder International. (n.d.). PRACHAR: Advancing young people's sexual and reproductive health and rights in India. In Pathfinder International. https://www.youthpower.org/sites/default/files/YouthPower/files/resources/Prachar%20report.pdf

Patton, M. (2021). Hybrid approaches to resolving surrogacy disputes: Combining mediation and arbitration with litigation safeguards. *Journal of Dispute Resolution*, 2021(2), 200–215.

Perdue, M., & Jenkinson, L. (2018). Surrogacy and mediation: A study of outcomes and satisfaction among parties involved in surrogacy disputes. *Journal of Mediation & Arbitration*, 10(1), 55–74.

Periyasamy, A. P., & Periyasami, S. (2023). Critical Review on Sustainability in Denim: A Step toward Sustainable Production and Consumption of Denim. *ACS Omega*, 8(5), 4472–4490. DOI: 10.1021/acsomega.2c06374 PMID: 36777581

Petchesky, R. P. (1980). Reproductive Freedom: Beyond “a Woman’s Right to Choose.”. *Signs (Chicago, Ill.)*, 5(4), 661–685. DOI: 10.1086/493757

Petchesky, R. P. (2024). *Abortion and woman’s choice: the state, sexuality and reproductive freedom*. Verso Books.

Pheterson, G., & Azize, Y. (2005). Abortion practice in the northeast Caribbean: “Just write down stomach pain.”. *Reproductive Health Matters*, 13(26), 44–53. DOI: 10.1016/S0968-8080(05)26201-8 PMID: 16291485

Pillai, G. (2024). *India’s Push-and-Pull on Reproductive Rights*. Verfassungsblog., DOI: 10.59704/41b437064b3e88d3

Pillay, V., & Wang, G. (1999). Social Structural Model of Women’s Reproductive Rights: A Cross-National Study of Developing Countries. *Canadian Journal of Sociology*, 24(2), 255–281. DOI: 10.2307/3341731

Pizzarossa, L. B., & Skuster, P. (2021). Toward Human Rights and Evidence-Based Legal Frameworks for (Self-Managed) Abortion: A Review of the Last Decade of Legal Reform. *Health and Human Rights*, 23(1), 199–212. PMID: 34194213

Planned Parenthood v. Casey (1992) 505 U.S. 833.

Population Fund of India. (n.d.). Men’s Participation in Family Planning & Reproductive Health Learnings and opportunities for India. https://india.unfpa.org/sites/default/files/pub-pdf/brief3_-_mens_participation_in_fp_and_rh.pdf

Prakash, S., & Asthana, N. (2019). Reproductive rights of women: Constitutional and global perspective. *Supremo Amicus*, 10, 294–303.

Prasad, V., & Confusions, C. (2015). 50 (10). *Economic and Political Weekly*.

Presser, H. B., Gordon, L., Rich, A., & Norton, W. W. (1978). Review: Birth Control and the Control of Motherhood. *Family Planning Perspectives*, 10(6), 374–376. DOI: 10.2307/2134425

Price, K. (2010). What is Reproductive Justice? How Women of Color Activists are Redefining the Pro-Choice Paradigm? *Meridians (Middletown, Conn.)*, 10(2), 42–65. DOI: 10.2979/meridians.2010.10.2.42

Prokopijević, M. (1994). In Defense of Abortion. *Archives for Philosophy of Law and Social Philosophy*, 80(3), 363–382.

Promoting Men’s Involvement in Maternal and Child Health. (2016). https://men-care.org

Pust, S. (2023). *Zato se toliko splavov pri nas opravi samoplačniško. Žurnal24.* Retrieved September 18, 2024, from https://www.zurnal24.si/zdravje/zato-se-toliko-splavov-pri-nas-opravi-samoplacnisko-403232

Qadir, A. M. A., & Fatah, A. O. (2023). Platformization and the metaverse: Opportunities and challenges for urban sustainability and economic development. *EAI Endorsed Transactions on Energy Web, 10*(1).

Rahajeng, A. N. (2020). *Abortion in Islamic Law and Its Intersection with Human Rights. Journal of Islamic Law Studies* (Vol. 3). JILS.

Rahimieh, A., & Nosrati, M. (2024). A Review on Biochemistry, Microbiology and Thermodynamic Aspects of Propionate: The Key Intermediate in the Anaerobic Digestion and Wastewater Treatment. *Desalination and Water Treatment*, 317, 100191. DOI: 10.1016/j.dwt.2024.100191

Raj, O. (2022). Constitutional and criminal perspectives of women's reproductive rights. *Indian Journal of Integrated Research in Law*, 2(5), 1–10.

Ramalingam, M., Durgadevi, P., Durgadevi, P., & Mahmood, T. (2016). In vitro fertilization. *Obstetrics, Gynaecology & Reproductive Medicine, 26*(7), 200-209. //.DOI: 10.1016/j.ogrm.2016.05.006

Ramanathan, M. R. (2002). Women's Health and Reproductive Health Services in India: Balancing Rights, Responsibilities, and Needs. *Studies in Family Planning*.

Ramsey, J. (2006). Paying for reproduction—The case against paid surrogacy. *The Juridical Review*, 4, 325–349.

Ramskold, L. A. H., & Posner, M. P. (2013). Commercial surrogacy: How provisions of monetary remuneration and powers of international law can prevent exploitation of gestational surrogates. *Journal of Medical Ethics*, 39(6), 397–402. DOI: 10.1136/medethics-2012-100527 PMID: 23443211

Rebouché, R. (2016). Abortion rights as human rights. *Social &amp. Social & Legal Studies*, 25(6), 765–782. DOI: 10.1177/0964663916668391

Reichenbach, L., & Roseman, M. J. (2009). *Reproductive Health and Human Rights: The Way Forward*. University of Pennsylvania Press. DOI: 10.9783/9780812206104

Reuters. (2023, April 5). Which countries allow commercial surrogacy? https://www.reuters.com/world/which-countries-allow-commercial-surrogacy-2023-04-05/

Richard A. Posner,. (1989). The Ethics and Economics of Enforcing Contracts of Surrogate Motherhood,. *H.LTH L. & POL'Y.*

Rimm, J. (2009). Booming Baby Business: Regulating Commercial Surrogacy in India, *U. PA.J. INT'L L*, 30, 1443–1444.

Rishi, G. Government of India, Kashyap, I., National Technical Support Unit - Family Planning (NTSU-FP), & Ministry of Health and Family Welfare (MoHFW). (2016). Men Matter: Engaging men in India's reproductive health goals. https://nhm.gov.in/images/pdf/programmes/family-planing/Campaing/Coffee_Table_Book.pdf

Rizvi, H. (2015). Assisted Reproductive Technologies in Islam: Legal and Ethical Perspectives. *Journal of Islamic Law and Society*, 22(2), 76–92.

Roache, M., & Everingham, S. (2018, September 13). *Ukraine's 'baby factories': The human cost of surrogacy | Women's Rights*. Al Jazeera. Retrieved September 8, 2024, from https://www.aljazeera.com/indepth/features/ukraine-baby-factories-human-cost-surrogacy-180912201251153.html

Roe v. Wade (1973) 410 U.S. 113.

Roe v. Wade, U.S. 113 (1973).

Ross, L. (2021). Understanding Reproductive Justice. In McCann, C., Kim, S.-k., & Ergun, E. (Eds.), *Feminist Theory Reader: Global and Local Perspectives* (pp. 77–82). Routledge.

Rysavy, M. A., Li, L., Bell, E. F., Das, A., Hintz, S. R., Stoll, B. J., & Higgins, R. D. (2015). Between-hospital variation in treatment and outcomes in extremely preterm infants. *The New England Journal of Medicine*, 372(19), 1801–1811. DOI: 10.1056/NEJMoa1410689 PMID: 25946279

Sabha, R. (2021). *Parliamentary Debates on The ART (Regulation) Bill, 2021*. Government of India.

Sadurski, W. (2019). *Poland's Constitutional Breakdown*. Oxford University Press. DOI: 10.1093/oso/9780198840503.001.0001

Saha, M. (2022). Social Impacts of ART Regulation in India, *Asian Bioethics Review*, vol. 13, Sanyal, P. (2013). Assisted Reproductive Technologies in the Context of Hindu Family Life and Ethics. *Hindu Ethics Journal*, 5(1), 98–108.

Saheli. (2000). Reproductive Rights in the Indian Context. Saheli Women's Resource Centre. https://sites.google.com/site/saheliorgsite/health/reproductive-rights-in-the-indian-context

SAMA Resource Group for Women and Health & Partners for Law in Development. (2018). Country assessment undertaken for National Human Rights Commission by: SAMA Resource Group for Women and Health, Partners for Law in Development: Status of human rights in the context of Sexual Health and Reproductive Health Rights in India. https://nhrc.nic.in/sites/default/files/sexual_health_reproductive_health_rights_SAMA_PLD_2018_01012019_1.pdf

Samuel, T. J. (1966). The development of India's policy of population control. *The Milbank Memorial Fund Quarterly*, 44(1), 49. DOI: 10.2307/3349038

Sandesh Bansal v. Union of India (PIL) W. P. No. 9061/2008.

Satz, D. (2013). Feminist perspectives on reproduction and the family. Plato Stanford. https://plato.stanford.edu/entries/feminism-family/#3

Sauer, M. V. (2001). Reproductive Donation: An Overview of Egg and Sperm Donation and Surrogacy. *Human Reproduction Update*, 7(1), 1–5.

Saxena, P. (2022). Impact of ART Regulation on Accessibility and Affordability in India. *The Journal of Reproductive Medicine*, 25(2), 104–116.

Scharp Brilly, N. (2021). The Right to Abortion: A qualitative analysis of NGOs viewpoint on what hinders women's access to abortion in Tunisia.

Schwartzman, M., & Schragger, R. (2022). Religious Freedom and Abortion. *Iowa Law Review*, 108, 2299.

Scott, E. (2020). Mediation in surrogacy disputes: Balancing the interests of the surrogate and intended parents. *Journal of Family Law*, 45(3), 321–345.

Scott, J. (1998). Generational Changes in Attitudes to Abortion: A Cross-National Comparison. *European Sociological Review*, 14(2), 177–190. https://www.jstor.org/stable/522633. DOI: 10.1093/oxfordjournals.esr.a018233

Sedgh, G., Singh, S., & Hussain, R. (2016). Intended and unintended pregnancies worldwide in 2012 and recent trends. *Studies in Family Planning*, 45(3), 301–314. DOI: 10.1111/j.1728-4465.2014.00393.x PMID: 25207494

Seth, K., Nanda, S., Sahay, A., Verma, R., & Achyut, P. (2020). "IT'S ON HIM TOO" PATHWAYS TO ENGAGE MEN IN FAMILY PLANNING. International Centre for Research on Women. https://www.icrw.org/wp-content/uploads/2020/06/Couple-Engage-Evidence-Review.pdf

Sexual & reproductive health. (n.d.). United Nations Population Fund. https://www.unfpa.org/sexual-reproductive-health

Shah, K. T., Bhende, A. A., & Kanitkar, T. Lucknow university, Pillai, A. P., Mahalanobis, P. C., Mukerjee, R., Sapru, P. N., Bhose, S. J., Yeatts, W. M., Datta, R., & Chandrasekhar, S. (n.d.). HISTORY OF FAMILY PLANNING IN INDIA. http://ir.unishivaji.ac.in:8080/jspui/bitstream/123456789/3652/9/09_Chapter%203.pdf

Shah, P. K., & Jacob, J. (2023). Beyond abortion decriminalization: human rights perspectives on the role of law in creating enabling environments for abortion access. In Ziegler, M. (Ed.), *The Research Handbook on International Abortion Law* (pp. 343–373). Edward Elgar Publishing Limited. DOI: 10.4337/9781839108150.00030

Shah, S. L., Mathai, A., & Wadis, A. P.. (1967). *Report of the Committee to Study the Question of Legalization of Abortion*. Ministry of Health and Family Planning.

Shalev, C. (2000). Rights to Sexual and Reproductive Health: The ICPD and the Convention on the Elimination of all Forms of Discrimination against Women. *Health and Human Rights*, 4(2), 38–66. DOI: 10.2307/4065196 PMID: 10796970

Shanley, M. L. "Surrogate Mothering" and Women's Freedom: A Critique of Contracts for Human Reproduction. *Signs (Chicago, Ill.)*, 18(3), 618–639. DOI: 10.1086/494822 PMID: 11659996

Shantilal Shah Committee. (1966). Report of the Committee to study the question of legalisation of abortion. Government of India. https://dn790000.ca.archive.org/0/items/dli.ministry.20283/1266.pdf

Shapiro, G. K. (2014). Abortion law in Muslim-majority countries: An overview of the Islamic discourse with policy implications. *Health Policy and Planning*, 29(4), 483–494. DOI: 10.1093/heapol/czt040 PMID: 23749735

Sharifi, A., Allam, Z., Bibri, S. E., & Khavarian-Garmsir, A. R. (2024). Smart cities and sustainable development goals (SDGs): A systematic literature review of co-benefits and trade-offs. *Cities (London, England)*, 146, 104659. DOI: 10.1016/j.cities.2023.104659

Sharma, D. (2021). Regulating Assisted Reproductive Technology in India: A Critical Overview, *Indian Journal of Medical Ethics*, vol. 7, no. 2, Sharma, S. (2013). Legal and ethical considerations in ART regulation. *Indian Journal of Medical Ethics*, 10(4), 234–238. DOI: 10.20529/IJME.2013.061

Sherman, C., Witherspoon, A., Glenza, J., & Noor, P. (2024, July 29). Tracking abortion laws across the united states. *The Guardian*. Retrieved from https://www.theguardian.com/us-news/ng-interactive/2024/jul/29/abortion-laws-bans-by-state

Shozi, B. (2020). Something old, something new: Applying reproductive rights to new reproductive technologies in South Africa. *South African Journal on Human Rights*, 36(1), 1–24. DOI: 10.1080/02587203.2020.1776632

Siddiqui, N. (2017). Surrogacy in Islamic Jurisprudence: A Review of Sunni and Shia Perspectives. *Journal of Muslim Family Law*, 29(3), 80–94.

Sifris, R. (2016). Commercial surrogacy and the human right to autonomy. *Journal of Law and Medicine*, 23(2). PMID: 26939504

Sifris, R., & Belton, S. (2017). Australia: Abortion and Human Rights. *Health and Human Rights Journal*, 19, 209–220. PMID: 28630553

Simões-Marques, M., Água, P., Frias, A., & Correia, A. (2023). Metaverse and Digital Twins: Contributions, Opportunities and Challenges to a Sustainable Use of the Ocean. *Human Factors and Systems Interaction, 84*(84).

Singh, B. (2023). Blockchain Technology in Renovating Healthcare: Legal and Future Perspectives. In Kaushik, K., Dahiya, S., Aggarwal, S., & Dwivedi, A. (Eds.), *Revolutionizing Healthcare Through Artificial Intelligence and Internet of Things Applications* (pp. 177–186). IGI Global., DOI: 10.4018/978-1-6684-5422-0.ch012

Singh, B. (2024). Evolutionary Global Neuroscience for Cognition and Brain Health: Strengthening Innovation in Brain Science. In Prabhakar, P. (Ed.), *Biomedical Research Developments for Improved Healthcare* (pp. 246–272). IGI Global., DOI: 10.4018/979-8-3693-1922-2.ch012

Singh, B. (2024). Lensing Legal Dynamics for Examining Responsibility and Deliberation of Generative AI-Tethered Technological Privacy Concerns: Infringements and Use of Personal Data by Nefarious Actors. In Ara, A., & Ara, A. (Eds.), *Exploring the Ethical Implications of Generative AI* (pp. 146–167). IGI Global., DOI: 10.4018/979-8-3693-1565-1.ch009

Singh, B. (2024). Social Cognition of Incarcerated Women and Children: Addressing Exposure to Infectious Diseases and Legal Outcomes. In Reddy, K. (Ed.), *Principles and Clinical Interventions in Social Cognition* (pp. 236–251). IGI Global., DOI: 10.4018/979-8-3693-1265-0.ch014

Singh, B., Dutta, P. K., & Kaunert, C. (2024). Replenish Artificial Intelligence in Renewable Energy for Sustainable Development: Lensing SDG 7 Affordable and Clean Energy and SDG 13 Climate Actions With Legal-Financial Advisory. In Derbali, A. (Ed.), *Social and Ethical Implications of AI in Finance for Sustainability* (pp. 198–227). IGI Global., DOI: 10.4018/979-8-3693-2881-1.ch009

Singh, B., Jain, V., Kaunert, C., Dutta, P. K., & Singh, G. (2024). Privacy Matters: Espousing Blockchain and Artificial Intelligence (AI) for Consumer Data Protection on E-Commerce Platforms in Ethical Marketing. In Saluja, S., Nayyar, V., Rojhe, K., & Sharma, S. (Eds.), *Ethical Marketing Through Data Governance Standards and Effective Technology* (pp. 167–184). IGI Global., DOI: 10.4018/979-8-3693-2215-4.ch015

Singh, B., & Kaunert, C. (2024). Aroma of Highly Smart Internet of Medical Things (IoMT) and Lightweight EdgeTrust Expansion Medical Care Facilities for Electronic Healthcare Systems: Fortified-Chain Architecture for Remote Patient Monitoring and Privacy Protection Beyond Imagination. In Hassan, A., Bhattacharya, P., Tikadar, S., Dutta, P., & Sagayam, M. (Eds.), *Lightweight Digital Trust Architectures in the Internet of Medical Things (IoMT)* (pp. 196–212). IGI Global., DOI: 10.4018/979-8-3693-2109-6.ch011

Singh, B., & Kaunert, C. (2024). Augmented Reality and Virtual Reality Modules for Mindfulness: Boosting Emotional Intelligence and Mental Wellness. In Hiran, K., Doshi, R., & Patel, M. (Eds.), *Applications of Virtual and Augmented Reality for Health and Wellbeing* (pp. 111–128). IGI Global., DOI: 10.4018/979-8-3693-1123-3.ch007

Singh, B., & Kaunert, C. (2024). Computational Thinking for Innovative Solutions and Problem-Solving Techniques: Transforming Conventional Education to Futuristic Interdisciplinary Higher Education. In Fonkam, M., & Vajjhala, N. (Eds.), *Revolutionizing Curricula Through Computational Thinking, Logic, and Problem Solving* (pp. 60–82). IGI Global., DOI: 10.4018/979-8-3693-1974-1.ch004

Singh, B., & Kaunert, C. (2024). Harnessing Sustainable Agriculture Through Climate-Smart Technologies: Artificial Intelligence for Climate Preservation and Futuristic Trends. In Kannan, H., Rodriguez, R., Paprika, Z., & Ade-Ibijola, A. (Eds.), *Exploring Ethical Dimensions of Environmental Sustainability and Use of AI* (pp. 214–239). IGI Global., DOI: 10.4018/979-8-3693-0892-9.ch011

Singh, B., & Kaunert, C. (2024). Revealing Green Finance Mobilization: Harnessing FinTech and Blockchain Innovations to Surmount Barriers and Foster New Investment Avenues. In Jafar, S., Rodriguez, R., Kannan, H., Akhtar, S., & Plugmann, P. (Eds.), *Harnessing Blockchain-Digital Twin Fusion for Sustainable Investments* (pp. 265–286). IGI Global., DOI: 10.4018/979-8-3693-1878-2.ch011

Singh, B., & Kaunert, C. (2024). Salvaging Responsible Consumption and Production of Food in the Hospitality Industry: Harnessing Machine Learning and Deep Learning for Zero Food Waste. In Singh, A., Tyagi, P., & Garg, A. (Eds.), *Sustainable Disposal Methods of Food Wastes in Hospitality Operations* (pp. 176–192). IGI Global., DOI: 10.4018/979-8-3693-2181-2.ch012

Singh, B., & Kaunert, C. (2024). Wind and Solar Energy as Renewable Energy for Sustainable Global Future: Projecting Future Multi-Sector Sustainable Policies and Innovation. In Ara, A., & Thakore, R. (Eds.), *Promoting Multi-Sector Sustainability With Policy and Innovation* (pp. 210–245). IGI Global., DOI: 10.4018/979-8-3693-2113-3.ch009

Singh, B., & Kaunert, C. Reinventing Artificial Intelligence and Blockchain for Preserving Medical Data. In *Ethical Artificial Intelligence in Power Electronics* (pp. 77–91). CRC Press. DOI: 10.1201/9781032648323-6

Singh, B., Vig, K., Dutta, P. K., & Kaunert, C. (2024). Unraveling Agile Transformation for Customer Satisfaction in Changing Market Conditions: Roadmap for Industry Embracing Change in Project Management. In Misra, S., Jadeja, R., & Mittal, M. (Eds.), *Practical Approaches to Agile Project Management* (pp. 305–321). IGI Global., DOI: 10.4018/979-8-3693-3318-1.ch017

Skalts, V., & Nørgaard, M. (1965). Abortion legislation in Denmark. *Case Western Reserve Law Review*, 17(2), 498–556. https://scholarlycommons.law.case.edu/caselrev/vol17/iss2/10

Skapetze, L., Zha, C., Yin, X., von Brueck, D., & Önkü, E. (2023). Promoting Pro-Environmental Behavior based on the Psychology of Perception. *Briefe zur Interdisziplinarität*, (31).

Skapetze, L., Zhao, C., Yin, X., von Brueck, D., & Önkü, E. (2023). 6 Promoting pro-environmental behaviour based on the. *Balanced Sustainability In A Changing World, 10*, 111.

Skapetze, L., Zhao, C., Yin, X., von Brueck, D., & Önkü, E. (2024). Promoting pro-environmental behaviour based on the psychology of perception—Can the metaverse be a potential solution? In *Balanced Sustainability in a Changing World* (pp. 111-136).

Skinner v. Oklahoma (1942) 361 U.S. 535.

Smith, E. S. (2014). Reproductive justice begins with contraceptive access in the Philippines. *Pacific Rim Law & Policy Journal*, 23(1), 203–250.

Smith, R., & Robertson, J. (2019). ADR versus litigation in surrogacy disputes: A comparative analysis. *Family Court Review*, 57(4), 587–605.

Smolak, M. (2016). *Wykładnia Konstytucji. Aktualne problemy i tendencje*. Wolter Kluwer.

South California Reproductive Centre. (2016, November 29). *The Evolution of Fertility Treatments and Development of IVF*. Blog. Retrieved October 18, 2024, from https://blog.scrcivf.com/ivf-the-history-and-evolution-of-fertility-treatments

Spar, D. L. (2019). *The Baby Business: How Money, Science, and Politics Drive the Commerce of Conception*. Harvard Business Press.

Srinivas, A. (2021). The Legal and Ethical Complexities of Surrogacy in India, *Indian Law Journal*, Steinbock, Bonnie. 2020. Surrogacy: Exploitation or Empowerment? *Bioethics*, 34, •••.

Stanford's Children Health. (n.d.). *Complications of Multiple Pregnancy*. Stanford Medicine Children's Health. Retrieved September 8, 2024, from https://www.stanfordchildrens.org/en/topic/default?id=complications-of-multiple-pregnancy-85-P08021&sid=

Starbird, E., Norton, M., & Marcus, R. (2016). Investing in family planning: Key to achieving the sustainable development goals. *Global Health, Science and Practice*, 4(2), 191–210. DOI: 10.9745/ghsp-d-15-00374

Stark, B. (2011). The women's convention, reproductive rights, and the reproduction of gender. *Duke Journal of Gender Law & Policy*, 18(2), 261–304.

Starrs, A. M., Ezeh, A. C., Barker, G., Basu, A., Bertrand, J. T., Blum, R., Coll-Seck, A. M., Grover, A., Laski, L., Roa, M., Sathar, Z. A., Say, L., Serour, G. I., Singh, S., Stenberg, K., Temmerman, M., Biddlecom, A., Popinchalk, A., Summers, C., & Ashford, L. S. (2018). Accelerate progress—sexual and reproductive health and rights for all: Report of the guttmacher– lancet commission. *Lancet*, 391(10140), 2642–2692. DOI: 10.1016/S0140-6736(18)30293-9 PMID: 29753597

*State Bans on Abortion Throughout Pregnancy*. Guttmacher Institute. (2024, July 25). https://www.guttmacher.org/state-policy/explore/state-policies-abortion-bans

*Statistics at a Glance: Earnings of Women Aged 20–59, by Age Group and Race/Ethnicity*. Social Security Administration. (2023). https://www.ssa.gov/policy/docs/factsheets/at-a-glance/earnings-women-age-race-ethnicity.html

Staunton, C. (2011). As easy as A, B and C: Will A, B and C v. Ireland be Ireland's wake-up call for abortion rights? *European Journal of Health Law*, 18(2), 205–220. DOI: 10.1163/157180911X564589 PMID: 21644438

Storming the Citadels of Poverty. Family Planning under the Emergency in India, 1975-1977 on JSTOR. (n.d.). www.jstor.org. https://www.jstor.org/stable/43553297

Suchita Srivastava v. Chandigarh Administration (2009) 9 SCC 1

Suchita Srivastava v. Chandigarh Administration (2009) 9 SCC 1.

Sugarman, J., Wenner, D. M., Rid, A., Henry, L. M., Luna, F., Klitzman, R., MacQueen, K. M., Rennie, S., Singh, J. A., & Gostin, L. O. (2023). Ethical research when abortion access is legally restricted. *Science*, 380(6651), 1224–1226. DOI: 10.1126/science.adh3104 PMID: 37347876

Supreme Court of India. (2023). *Order in MA 2157 of 2023 in WP(C) 1137 of 2023*. Retrieved from https://www.livelaw.in/pdf_upload/ma-2157-of-2023-in-wpc-1137-of-2023-1-1-498107.pdf

Suratiningsih, D. (2023). Strategy for Establishing the World Mangrove Center as a Climate Change Mitigation Effort. *Journal of Namibian Studies: History Politics Culture*, 34, 2474–2494.

Surrogacy (Regulation) Act. (2021). Government of India. The Bible (King James Version), Genesis 16:1-2, 21:1-7. *Samuel*, 1, 1–20.

*Surrogacy in Ukraine: Cost*. (n.d.). IVMed. Retrieved September 8, 2024, from https://ivmed.agency/surrogacy-in-ukraine

Sutton, B., & Borland, E. (2019). Abortion and Human Rights for Women in Argentina. *Frontiers*, 40(2), 27–61. DOI: 10.1353/fro.2019.a730152

Svitnev, K. (2010). Legal regulation of assisted reproduction treatment in Russia. *Reproductive Biomedicine Online*, 20(7), 892–894. DOI: 10.1016/j.rbmo.2010.03.023 PMID: 20435519

Tanderup, M., Reddy, S., Patel, T., & Nielsen, B. B. (2015). Informed consent in medical decision-making in commercial gestational surrogacy: A mixed methods study in New Delhi, India. *Acta Obstetricia et Gynecologica Scandinavica*, 94(5), 465–472. DOI: 10.1111/aogs.12576 PMID: 25581093

Taylor, S. (2024). Abortion was a crime: Three medievalists respond to English cases dating back to the 13th century. Law and History Review. https://lawandhistoryreview.org/article/abortion-was-a-crime-three-medievalists-respond-to-english-cases-dating-all-the-way-back-to-the-13th-century-corroborate-the-treatises-statements-that-abortio/

Tella, K. K. (2024). *Abortion Rights, Reproductive Justice and the State: International Perspectives*. Routledge India.

Teman, E. (2016). *Surrogacy in Israel: state-controlled surrogacy as a mechanism of symbolic control*. Cambridge University Press. DOI: 10.1017/CBO9781316282618.023

Th Medical Termination of Pregnancy Act, 1971, No. 34, Acts of Parliament, 1971 (India).

The American College of Obstetricians and Gynecologists. (2019). *Women's Health Care Physicians. Multiple Pregnancy*https://www.acog.org/Patients/FAQs/Multiple-Pregnancy?IsMobileSet=false#risk

The Medical Termination of Pregnancy (Amendment) Rules, 2021, Rule 3B.

The Missing Piece. Valuing women's unrecognized contribution to the economy. (n.d.). UNDP. https://www.undp.org/latin-america/blog/missing-piece-valuing-womens-unrecognized-contribution-economy#:~:text=At%20the%20global%20level%2C%20women,1%20house%20and%2023%20 minutes.

The People's Archive of Rural India. (n.d.). National Family Health Survey (NFHS-5), 2019-21: India. People's Archive of Rural India. https://ruralindiaonline.org/en/library/resource/national-family-health-survey-nfhs-5-2019-21-india/

*The world's abortion laws*. Center for Reproductive Rights. (2023). https://reproductiverights.org/maps/worlds-abortion-laws/

Thomas, A. (2015). Christian Ethics and Modern Medicine: A Protestant Perspective on Assisted Reproductive Technologies. *Theological Studies*, 68(2), 145–161.

Thompson, S. (2017). Ethical implications of mediation in surrogacy disputes: Ensuring fairness and avoiding coercion. *Bioethics*, 31(6), 420–429.

Tobin, J. (2019). *The UN Convention on the Rights of the Child: A Commentary*. Oxford: Oxford University Press.

Todd-Gher, J., & Shah, P. K. (2020). Abortion in the Context of COVID-19: A Human Rights Imperative. *Sexual and Reproductive Health Matters*, 28(1), 1758394. DOI: 10.1080/26410397.2020.1758394 PMID: 32308156

Tonelli, C., & Morandi, A. (2023). The impact of 3D technology on sustainability in fashion luxury product design: evidences from an exploratory analysis.

Tong, Y., Liao, X., He, Y., Cui, X., Wishart, M., Zhao, F., & Chen, G. (2024). Mitigating greenhouse gas emissions from municipal wastewater treatment in China. *Environmental Science and Ecotechnology*, 20, 100341. DOI: 10.1016/j.ese.2023.100341 PMID: 38094258

Tsai, R. L., & Ziegler, M. (2023). Abortion Politics and the Rise of Movement Jurists. *U.C. Davis Law Review*, 57, 2149.

Tuininga, K. (2008). The Ethics of Surrogacy Contracts and Nebraska's Surrogacy Law. *CREIGHTON L. REV.*, 41, 185.

UN Committee on Economic, Cultural and Social Rights. General Comment No. 22 (2016) on the right to sexual and reproductive health (article 12 of the International Covenant on Economic, Social and Cultural Rights). E/C.12/GC/22.

UN Economic and Social Council. Concluding observations on the fifth periodic report of Costa Rica. E/C.12/CRI/CO/5.

UN Economic and Social Council. Consideration of reports submitted by State parties under articles 16 and 17 of the Covenant, Peru. E/C.12/PER/CO/2-4.

UN HRC. Concluding observations on the fifth periodic report of Senegal. CCPR/C/SEN/CO/5.

UN HRC. Concluding observations on the seventh periodic report of Colombia. 17.11.2016. CCPR/C/COL/CO/7.

UN HRC. Concluding observations on the seventh periodic report of El Salvador. CCPR/C/SLV/CO/7.

UN HRC. General Comment No. 28, Article 3 (The equality of rights between men and women). CCPR/C/21/Rev.1/Add.10.

UN HRC. General Comment No. 36, Article 6: right to life. CCPR/C/GC/36.

UN Human Rights Council. Resolution on Elimination of all forms of discrimination against women and girls. UN Doc. A/HRC/38/L.1/Rev.1.

United Nations General Assembly (1955). *Draft International Covenants on Human Rights. Annotation prepared by the Secretary-General*, document of 1 July 1955, A/2929.

United Nations Population Fund. (1994). Programme of action of the International Conference on Population and Development. https://www.unfpa.org/sites/default/files/event-pdf/PoA_en.pdf#

United Nations. (n.d.). Education as the Pathway towards Gender Equality | United Nations. https://www.un.org/en/chronicle/article/education-pathway-towards-gender-equality

URS. (1991). *Constitution of the Republic of Slovenia*. Retrieved March 11, 2024, from https://pisrs.si/Pis.web/pregledPredpisa?id=USTA1

Vasilieva, V.A., Stefanyshyn, N.B., Skhab-Buchynska, T.Ya. (2019). Surrogate Motherhood: Analysis of the Basis of the Legislation of Ukraine and Foreign Countries. *Journal of Advanced Research in Law and Economics*, no. 9(6), pp. 2176–2189. DOI: (in English).DOI: 10.14505//jarle.v9.6(36).33

Verma, R. K., Schensul, S. L., & Schensul, J. J. (2001). Risk, perception, and condom use among married men in Mumbai, India. *International Family Planning Perspectives*, 27(3), 138–145.

Viktoriya Omelchenko, V. (n.d.). *Assisted reproduction technologies in Russian Federation*. https://medlawlab.web.auth.gr/wp-content/uploads/2022/03/Assisted-reproduction-in-Russian-Federation-by-Viktoria-Omelchenko.pdf

Visaria, L., & Ramachandran, V. (2007). *Abortion in India: Ground Realities*. Routledge.

von Baer, K. E. (1827). *De Ovi Mammalium et Hominis Genesi*.

von Hagel, A., & Mansbach, D. (2016). *Reproductive Rights in the Age of Human Rights*. Macmillan. DOI: 10.1057/978-1-137-53952-6

Waldron, J. (2023). *The Rule of Law and the Importance of Procedure* (in) *Thoughtfulness and the Rule of Law*, Cambridge-London: Harvard University Press.

Wegner, M. N., Landry, E., Wilkinson, D., & Tzanis, J. (2022, August 25). Men as partners in Reproductive Health: From Issues to action. Guttmacher Institute. https://www.guttmacher.org/journals/ipsrh/1998/03/men-partners-reproductive-health-issues-action

Wen, C. (2003). Informed choice in rural Anhui. *Human Rights (Chicago, Ill.)*, 2(4), 22–23.

Wentzell, E. A., & Inhorn, M. C. (2014). Reconceiving masculinity and 'men as partners' for ICPD Beyond 2014: Insights from a Mexican HPV study. *Global Public Health: An International Journal for Research, Policy and Practice*, 9(6), 691–705. DOI: 10.1080/17441692.2014.917690

What are the international surrogacy laws by country? Surrogate.com. Available from: https://surrogate.com/intended-parents/surrogacy-laws-and-legal-information/what-are-the-international-surrogacy-laws-by-country/

Wilder, N. J. (1986). Society's Response to the New Reproductive Technologies: The Feminist Perspectives, *S.California Law Review*, •••, 59.

Williams, A. (2018). State regulatory efforts in protecting surrogate's bodily autonomy. *Seton Hall Law Review*, 49(1), 205–232. PMID: 30557923

Williams, R. (2019). The Ethical Dimensions of Assisted Reproductive Technology in Christianity. *Christian Bioethics Journal*, 15(3), 125–138.

Women, U. N. (1979). Convention on the elimination of all forms of discrimination against women. diakses melalui: http://www. un. org/womenwatch/daw/cedaw/text/econvention. htm, pada, 12.

World Health Organization. (2015). Postnatal care guidelines. In Postnatal Care for Mothers and Newborns: Vol. April 2015 (p. 2) [Report]. https://www.who.int/docs/default-source/mca-documents/nbh/brief-postnatal-care-for-mothers-and-newborns-highlights-from-the-who-2013-guidelines.pdf

World Health Organization. (2015a) *Safe abortion: Technical & policy guidance for health systems*. Retrieved September 18, 2024, from https://apps.who.int/iris/bitstream/handle/10665/173586/WHO_RHR_15.04_eng.pdf

World Health Organization. (2015b) *Sexual health, human rights and the law*. Retrieved September 18, 2024, from https://apps.who.int/iris/bitstream/10665/175556/1/9789241564984_eng.pdf

World Health Organization. (2021) *Model list of essential medicines*, 22nd List.

World Health Organization. (2024a). *Maternal Mortality.* Retrieved October 6, 2024, from: https://www.who.int/news-room/fact-sheets/detail/maternal-mortality

World Health Organization. (2024b). *Abortion.* Retrieved October 9, 2024, from: https://www.who.int/news-room/fact-sheets/detail/abortion

World Health Organization. 'Abortion Care Guideline' https://www.who.int/publications/i/item/9789240039483 28.

World Health Organization. WHO. (2019, September 23). Maternal health. https://www.who.int/health-topics/maternal-health#tab=tab_1

World Health Organization. WHO. (2024, April 10). Sexual and reproductive health and rights. https://www.who.int/health-topics/sexual-and-reproductive-health-and-rights#tab=tab_2

Worldwide Surrogacy Specialists. (2021, November 1). *3 Commercial Surrogacy v. Altruistic Surrogacy*. https://www.worldwidesurrogacy.org/blog/commercial-surrogacy-vs-altruistic-surrogacy

WWW. REPRODUCTIVE RIGHTS.ORG. (2021). Reproductive rights in India: the current situation. In Reproductive Rights in India: The Current Situation [Report]. https://reproductiverights.org/sites/default/files/documents/Reproductive-Rights-In-Indian-Courts.pdf

www.wisdomlib.org. (2018, February 16). Manusmriti Verse 9.81. https://www.wisdomlib.org/hinduism/book/manusmriti-with-the-commentary-of-medhatithi/d/doc201444.html

X v. Union of India &Anr., INSC 919, 2023 [1] Indian Penal Code, No.45 of 1860, §312 - Whoever voluntarily causes a woman with child to miscarry, shall, if such miscarriage be not caused in good faith for the purpose of saving the life of the woman, be punished with imprisonment of either description for a term which may extend to three years, or with fine, or with both; and, if the woman be quick with child, shall be punished with imprisonment of either description for a term which may extend to seven years, and shall also be liable to fine.

Xing, E., Owda, R., Loder, C., & Collins, K. (2023). Abortion rights are Health Care Rights. *JCI Insight*, 8(11), e171798. Advance online publication. DOI: 10.1172/jci.insight.171798 PMID: 37288659

Yadav, G. (2022). Abortion (Hinduism). In *Hinduism and Tribal Religions* (pp. 9–12). Springer Netherlands. DOI: 10.1007/978-94-024-1188-1_484

Yamin, A. E. (2023). Five Lessons for Advancing Maternal Health Rights in an Age of Neoliberal Globalization and Conservative Backlash. *Health and Human Rights*, 25(1), 185–194. PMID: 37397427

Yarmohammadi, H., Zargaran, A., Vatanpour, A., Abedini, E., & Adhami, S. (2013). An investigation into the ancient abortion laws: Comparing ancient Persia with ancient Greece and Rome. *Acta Medico-Historica Adriatica : AMHA*, 11(2), 291–298. PMID: 24304111

Zampas, C., & Gher, J. M. (2008). Abortion as a human right: International and regional standards. *Human Rights Law Review*, 8(2), 249–294. DOI: 10.1093/hrlr/ngn008

Zawish, M., Dharejo, F. A., Khowaja, S. A., Raza, S., Davy, S., Dev, K., & Bellavista, P. (2024). AI and 6G into the metaverse: Fundamentals, challenges and future research trends. *IEEE Open Journal of the Communications Society*, 5, 730–778. DOI: 10.1109/OJCOMS.2024.3349465

Zhan, J., Xu, S., Zhu, Y., Han, Y., Li, L., Liu, J., & Guo, X. (2024). Potential pathogenic microorganisms in rural wastewater treatment process: Succession characteristics, concentration variation, source exploration, and risk assessment. *Water Research*, 254, 121359. DOI: 10.1016/j.watres.2024.121359 PMID: 38428237

Ziegler, M. (2020). *Abortion and the Law in America: Roe v. Wade to the present.* Cambridge University Press.

Ziegler, M. (2018). *Beyond Abortion: Roe V. Wade and the Battle for Privacy.* Harvard University Press.

Zois, A. (n.d.). In Ukraine and Russia, surrogacy is seen as work. Available: https://www.zois-berlin.de/en/publications/meet-the-author/in-ukraine-and-russia-surrogacy-is-seen-as-work

Zureick, A. (2015, January 16). *(En)Gendering Suffering: Denial of Abortion as a Form of Cruel, Inhuman or Degrading Treatment.* Retrieved September 18, 2024, from https://papers.ssrn.com/sol3/papers.cfm?abstract_id=2579416

ZZNPOB. (1977). *Health Measures in Exercising Freedom of Choice in Childbearing Act.* Retrieved March 9, 2024, from https://pisrs.si/Pis.web/pregledPredpisa?id=USTA1

# About the Contributors

**Maja Pucelj** (1982) graduated from the Faculty of Public Administration in Ljubljana and the Faculty of Management in Koper and received her master's degree from the New University Faculty of government and European Studies and the European Faculty of Law. She completed her first doctorate at Alma Mater Europaea - ISH in the field of humanities and finished her second doctorate by New University Faculty of government and European Studies in the field of international studies with an emphasis on human rights. She started her career as a policewoman, where she also participated in a special police unit, she continued her career as a risk manager, head of legal services in the field of leasing and banking, as a director of marketing and auditor in an audit company. Before joining EMUNI University and Faculty of Organisation Studies (FOŠ), where she works as Assistant professor, she worked as an advisor to the Minister of Education, Science and Sport in the fields of pre-school education, primary education, secondary and higher education, adult education, and the quality of education and as an undersecretary in the Cohesion Policy department at the Ministry of Education, Science and Sports. She is an author of numerous works in the field of human rights.

**Magdalena Matusiak-Frącczak** is an Assistant Professor at University of Łódź, Faculty of Law and Administration in Poland. She is a PhD and an attorney (adwokat), lecturer at the University of Łódź (Poland), Faculty of Law and Administration and a Visiting Professor at the Chandigarh University (India).

* * *

**Sana Ahmed** has over fifteen years of HR industry and university teaching / industry consultancy experience. She earned her MSc in Employment Relations and Organisational Behaviour from the London School of Economics and Political Science (UK) in 2010. Her prior education includes a Professional Diploma of Human

Resource Management, Human Resource Development and Human Resources Information Systems from the National University of Sciences and Technology (Pakistan) in 2009 and a Masters in Public Administration from the Quaid-e-Azam University (Pakistan) in 2007. She is currently pursuing PhD from Henley Business School, University of Reading, U.K. Her research work has frequently appeared at Academy of Management and British Academy of Management conferences among others. She also regularly delivers PDWs from the platforms of AOM and BAM. She has also published research articles and book chapters in international journals of repute. She is also a Fellow of the UK HEA

**Akash Bag** is currently serving as an Assistant Professor at Adamas University in India and is also working towards a Ph.D. in Digital Forensics and Cyber Security at Amity University. He has contributed to publications in IEEE, Springer, IGI Global, and AIP, actively participating in collaborative projects on an international scale.

**Sanjum Bedi** is an Associate professor of Law at Amity University, Madhya Pradesh India and has more than 14 years of teaching experience. She secured her Law Degree and pursued LL.M from Kurukshetra University. She was always passionate about opting for Teaching as her career. However, at the same time, she wanted to explore the Court Room Experience. This made Dr. Bedi to practice for around one and a half years in the Court where she dealt mostly in Criminal Cases. It was surely a great experience but she also understood that a legal person cannot sustain without Research. Her interest in Research led her to join the Women's Studies Research Centre at Kurukshetra University. She thoroughly enjoyed working there as a Research Officer and finally delved into Teaching. While working as a Research Officer, she did extensive research on the U.G.C. Projects assigned to her on "Working Women in the Organised and Unorganised Sectors". She also worked on "Female Foeticide" and "Vrindavan WidowsShe has completed her Doctoral Research in the emerging field of Law & Artificial Reproductive Technologies (precisely Medical Jurisprudence & Bioethics) from Punjab. She has 19 publications to her credit. Her research findings have been presented on National & International platforms.

**Sushmita Das** is currently pursuing Ph.D. in Law and has done post-graduate LL.M (Corporate and Securities Laws) from Tamil Nadu National Law University, Tiruchirappalli, Tamil Nadu, India (2018-19). She pursued graduation in Law (B.A.LL.B(Hons.) from Department of Legal Studies and Research, Barkatullah University Bhopal, Madhya Pradesh, India She has also pursued PG Diploma in Environmental Laws from National Law School of India University, Bengaluru,

Karnataka, India. She has also qualified competitive level examinations in India for the Assistant Professor and began her career in academia in 2019 and has since served as an Assistant Professor of Law and guest lecturer at a number of different Universities and Law colleges in India. She has been a part of numerous workshops, and has won awards for the best research papers she has presented at both national and international conferences and seminars. Her work has been published in peer-reviewed journals, book chapters, and the UGC Care Listed Journals to her credits. She was an active intern at the National Stock Exchange in Mumbai, Maharashtra, as well as the Supreme Court, High Court, District Court, Tribunals, and a number of Commissions during her time as a student as an undergraduate and post-graduate studies. Her primary areas of interest and expertise in Legal Profession are Jurisprudence, Environmental Law, Human Rights, and Corporate and Securities Law.

**Anwesha Ghosh** is currently an Assistant Professor in the Department of Law, at Amity Law School, Amity University. Before joining Amity University, she was working with National Law University, Patiala. Prior to which she was a UGC-sponsored Senior Research Fellow (SRF) at the Central University of Punjab, India. Her topic of research is "Legislative Governance Towards Gender Diversity in Indian Corporate Boards: Review of Institutional Factors and Best Practices". She has completed the pre-submission of her Ph.D. thesis to the Department of Law, Central University of Punjab, and is now heading towards the final submission of her Ph.D. thesis. Her current Ph.D. research majorly focuses on the pivotal role of women directors in Indian companies, advocating for gender diversity and inclusive corporate governance. Ms. Ghosh achieved a University Gold Medal during her LL.B. degree at Haldia Law College affiliated with Vidyasagar University, West Bengal, India. Her academic excellence continued with a University Gold Medal for her outstanding performance in LL.M. and an Endowment Medal for securing the highest marks in Corporate and Commercial Laws from the National University of Study and Research in Law, Ranchi, India. Ms. Ghosh had previously worked.

**Shubhang Gomasta** is currently pursuing Ph.D in Law and has done post-graduate LL.M specialisation in (Corporate and Commercial Law). He has pursued five years integrated under graduation (2014-19) from Tamil Nadu National Law University, Tiruchirappalli, Tamil Nadu. He has pursued PG Diploma in Environmental Laws & Human Rights from National Law School of India University, Bengaluru, Karnataka. He has also qualified competitive level examinations in India for the Assistant Professor. He began his career in academia in 2021 and has since served as an assistant professor of law at different Universities in India. He has been a part of numerous workshops, and has won awards for the best research papers he has presented at both national and international conferences and seminars. His work has been published in peer-reviewed journals, book chapters, the UGC Care Listed Journals and more than twenty-five research papers to his credits. His primary areas of interest and expertise in Legal Profession are Arbitration Laws and Corporate and Commercial Laws.

**Laeeq Razzak Janjua** is a finance professional working in a, compliance, and academia, whose journey is characterized by dedication, expertise, and a commitment to excellence. Mr. Janjua's academic prowess is reflected in his extensive body of work, which includes the publication of a book on corporate social responsibility as co-author and over 40 academic research papers. These contributions have solidified his reputation as a thought leader and a respected authority in his field, earning him recognition and acclaim from peers and scholars alike. Currently serving as a Compliance Officer at TMF Group, Mr. Janjua brings a wealth of experience and expertise to his role, where he navigates the complex landscape of regulatory requirements with precision and proficiency. In addition to his role at TMF Group, Mr. Janjua also serves as a lecturer at WSB University in Poland, where he imparts his knowledge and insights to the next generation of professionals. Prior to his current roles, Mr. Janjua amassed over 10 years of invaluable experience in the financial industry, having worked with esteemed institutions such as Citi Bank, MoneyGram Payment International, and BNP Paribas. Driven by a passion for excellence and a dedication to making a positive impact, Mr. Janjua continues to be a guiding force in the fields of compliance and academia. His unwavering commitment to integrity, coupled with his extensive knowledge and experience, positions him as a leader and a trailblazer in his field, shaping the future of compliance and corporate social responsibility.

**Jipson Joseph** has a PhD in Ethics from DVK Bangalore. Currently, he is a Research Scholar in the School of Law at Christ University, Bangalore. His research interests are in the fields of ethics, gender studies, constitutional law, human rights, human security, environmental justice, developmental policies and global poverty.

**Ananya Pandey** is a Research Scholar in School of Law at Christ University, Bangalore. She has her research interests in the field of Constitutional Law, Human Rights, Women Rights, Intellectual Property Law and Jurisprudence.

**Bhupinder Singh** working as Professor at Sharda University, India. Also, Honorary Professor in University of South Wales UK and Santo Tomas University Tunja, Colombia. His areas of publications as Smart Healthcare, Medicines, fuzzy logics, artificial intelligence, robotics, machine learning, deep learning, federated learning, IoT, PV Glasses, metaverse and many more. He has 3 books, 139 paper publications, 163 paper presentations in international/national conferences and seminars, participated in more than 40 workshops/FDP's/QIP's, 25 courses from international universities of repute, organized more than 59 events with international and national academicians and industry people's, editor-in-chief and co-editor in journals, developed new courses. He has given talks at international universities, resource person in international conferences such as in Nanyang Technological University Singapore, Tashkent State University of Law Uzbekistan; KIMEP University Kazakhstan, All'ah meh Tabatabi University Iran, the Iranian Association of International Criminal law, Iran and Hague Center for International Law and Investment, The Netherlands, Northumbria University Newcastle UK,

**Hemendra Singh** is a Lecturer of Law at Jindal Global Law School, situated within O.P. Jindal Global University, Sonipat. He pursued his LL.M. in Intellectual Property Rights from National Law University, Jodhpur, following his graduation with a B.A. LL.B. (Hons.) from Rajiv Gandhi National University of Law, Punjab. With a focus on corporate law, intellectual property law, criminal law, and constitutional law, he has authored numerous research articles published in both national and international journals.

**Ravisha Sodha** is a distinguished legal professional who completed her B.A. LL.B. from Rajiv Gandhi National University of Law, Patiala. She is currently serving as a Legal Researcher at the Rajasthan High Court, where she contributes her expertise to legal research and analysis. Her academic background and professional experience equip her with a strong foundation in legal principles and a keen understanding of judicial processes.

**Tejaswini Tripathy**, a three-year litigation expert with a master's degree in Constitutional and Administrative Law, has published on topics such as transgender health and understanding federalism in India's reservation policies and has worked in the Delhi High Court and Supreme Court. She is currently enrolled at National Law University, Odisha, India as a Ph.D. scholar.

# Index

## A



## B



## C

## E



## F



## G

# P



# R

# S



# T



# U



# W

www.ingramcontent.com/pod-product-compliance
Lightning Source LLC
LaVergne TN
LVHW080346011026
849161LV00009B/2209
* 9 7 9 8 3 6 9 3 7 8 3 7 3 *